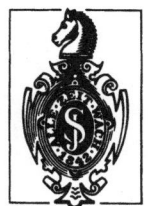

M.A. Lemp R. Marquardt (Eds.)

The Dry Eye

A Comprehensive Guide

With 89 Figures, Mostly in Color

Springer-Verlag Berlin Heidelberg GmbH

Professor Dr. Michael A. Lemp
Georgetown University Medical Center, Center for Sight
3800 Reservoir Road, NW, Washington, DC 20007, USA

Professor Dr. Rolf Marquardt
Baldingerweg 8, W-7900 Ulm, FRG

ISBN 978-3-642-63479-6   ISBN 978-3-642-58130-4 (eBook)
DOI 10.1007/978-3-642-58130-4

Library of Congress Cataloging-in-Publication Data. The Dry eye: a comprehensive guide/
M.A. Lemp, R. Marquardt (eds.). p.   cm. Includes bibliographical references and index.
ISBN 3-540-53308-7.—ISBN 0-387-53308-7 1. Dry eye syndromes. I. Lemp, Michael A.
II. Marquardt, R. (Rolf) [DNLM: 1. Dry Eye Syndromes. WW 208 D798] RE216.D78D78
1992 617.7'64—dc20 DNLM/DLC for Library of Congress

© Springer-Verlag Berlin Heidelberg 1992
Originally published by Springer-Verlag Berlin Heidelberg New York in 1992
Softcover reprint of the hardcover 1st edition 1992

Typesetting: Best-set Typesetter Ltd., Hong Kong
25/3130-5 4 3 2 1 0 – Printed on acid-free paper

Preface

There has been considerable increase in the knowledge concerning tear secretion, the ocular surface, and pathophysiologic conditions leading to the dry eye. Much of this new knowledge is not widely appreciated. Although there have been proceedings of symposia published, there is no currently available book of sufficient scope, yet reasonable length, which ties together aspects of this newly acquired knowledge. This textbook is designed to give the ophthalmic practitioner a comprehensive, yet concise, guideline concerning the diagnosis and treatment of the dry eye. We have been able to bring together leading researchers to accomplish the same. We wish to express our special thanks to the company Dr. Mann Pharma of Berlin without whose generous sponsorship we could not have completed our task. The sponsorship, in bringing together the authors in planning, preparation, and realization of this text, is gratefully acknowledged.

Washington/Ulm, March 1992

M.A. Lemp
R. Marquardt

Contents

List of Contributors

Dartt, Darlene A., Professor Dr., Eye Research Institute
of Retina Foundation, 20 Stanford Street, Boston,
MA 02114, USA

Lemp, Michael A., Professor Dr., Georgetown University
Medical Center, Center for Sight, Department
of Ophthalmology, 3800 Reservoir Road, NW, Washington,
DC 20007, USA

Lütjen-Drecoll, Elke, Professor Dr., University of Erlangen,
Department of Anatomy, Krankenhausstr. 8,
W-8520 Erlangen, FRG

Marquardt, Rolf, Professor Dr., Baldingerweg 8, W-7900 Ulm,
FRG

Murube, Juan, Professor Dr., Hospital Ramón y
Cajal, Department of Ophthalmology, Apatado 37,
28034 Madrid, Spain

Norn, Mogens, Professor Dr., Klovervej 15, 3600 Frederikssund,
Denmark

Rohen, Johannes W., Professor Dr. Dr. h.c., University
of Erlangen, Department of Anatomy, Krankenhausstr. 8,
W-8520 Erlangen, FRG

Roth, Hans Walter, Dr. med., Pfullendorfer Str. 5,
W-7900 Ulm-Wiblingen, FRG

Introduction

The sufficient and regular moistening of the human eye is essential for vision without complaints. Prerequisites for this are the presence of a sufficient quantity of lacrimal fluid, normal composition of the lacrimal fluid, normal eyelid closure, and regular blinking, which repeatedly builds up and cleans a new precorneal tear film and prevents the eye from drying. The composition and volume of the lacrimal fluid is of special importance as a "windshield washer" of the eye.

The precorneal lacrimal fluid is by no means a stable system but an instable one which easily may lose its equilibrium due to numerous disturbing factors. Between the inner mucous layer of the tear film and its outer lipid layer is situated the aqueous layer, making up the greatest part of the lacrimal fluid.

There are many reasons for disturbances, for example, constitutional or acquired diseases such as insufficient lid closure. There are also disturbances by chemicals, drugs, allergic reactions, chronic inflammations, systemic diseases, and environmental factors. The increasing use of chemical agents in our environment and the numerous pollutants discharged into it frequently cause pathological reactions of the eye. Due to its hypervascular conjunctiva the eye has a very close contact to the environment.

The consequences are irritations of the conjunctiva accompanied by a sensation of dryness, burning, rubbing, and the sensation of sand grains in the eyes. These disturbances change the quantity and composition of the lacrimal fluid and cause structural changes on the conjunctiva and cornea when they influence the eye for a longer period – this is the clinical picture of the dry eye. The increase in the number of patients suffering from dry eye has been challenging scientists and ophthalmologists for centuries, not least because the disease (which itself is annoying for the patient) may lead to severe impairment of vision in serious cases.

Especially in the past 20 years the number of dry eye patients has increased in all developed countries – approximately every fifth patient who sees an ophthalmologist is suffering from this disease.

If possible, treatment of the basic disease constitutes the most appropriate therapy. Otherwise, the disturbing factors of irritating substances, insufficient air humidity, errors of refraction, or impairment in binocular vision must be eliminated. Drug therapy includes pharmaceutical preparations that enhance the secretion of tears. This measure is called for only if enough lacrimal tissue is still present. In other cases, the pathological or insufficient tear film is augmented. For this purpose, viscous tear film substitutes or ophthalmic gels are available. The temporary or permanent blockage of the efferent lacrimal ducts represents a further type of measure. In severe cases the eye may be protected by a wet chamber.

Unfortunately, this disease is often misinterpreted as infectious, allergic, or irritative conjunctivities. The consequence of this false diagnosis is often incorrect treatment with eye drops against conjunctivitis. These drops contain vasoconstrictors, which aggravate the clinical picture, or antibiotics or corticoids, which are virtually ineffective in these cases.

To close a gap in our knowledge, this book was compiled by ophthalmologists and scientists who have been investigating the physiology, pathophysiology, diagnosis, and therapy of this clinical picture, and who have built up international reputations. This book is intended for the ophthalmologist who is confronted with this problem in his medical practice.

Chapter 1

History of the Dry Eye

J. Murube

1 Introduction

Three hundred and sixty million years ago, the crosopterygian fishes, either as a result of the ecological pressure of other animals or because of drastic climatic changes in their environment, evolved into amphibians. Amongst the many changes undergone by these animals was the formation of the lacrimal apparatus, the function of which was to maintain a moist eye and to avoid a dry eye. This apparatus developed in different ways in the various terrestial species. Throughout human evolution, the structure of the lacrimal system has changed very little; the most important change occurred in prehistoric times with the appearance of affective lacrimation, which can be viewed as an unconscious attempt to solicit help when in a state of fear, solitude, or desperation. Darwin [1] hypothesized that weeping was brought about by the mechanical compression of the lacrimal glands when crying. Montagu [2] believed that tearing was originally a reflex to keep the nasopharynx moist when sobbing. García de la Torre [3] saw it as being a characteristic result of nervous tension. Frey et al. [4] regarded it as a means of eliminating some biological products which enter the blood system when emotions are aroused. At a later date, another type of outwardly directed emotional tearing appeared, accompanying more sublime emotions (love, beauty, feelings, mysticism). I have hypothesized [5] that there has been a transformation of a preexistent mannerism, and that nowadays tearing can express the opposite of what was originally intended. The showing of teeth as an expression of either attacking or laughing, is an example of such transformation.

The first awareness of tears developed during prehistory. In Indoeuropean languages the various words for tears, appear to spring from a common origin: *dakru*.

M.A. Lemp/R. Marquardt (Eds.) The Dry Eye
© Springer-Verlag Berlin Heidelberg 1992

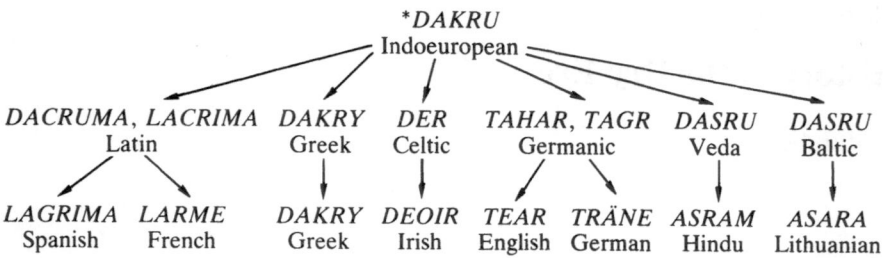

*DAKRU
Indoeuropean

DACRUMA, LACRIMA   DAKRY   DER   TAHAR, TAGR   DASRU   DASRU
Latin   Greek   Celtic   Germanic   Veda   Baltic

LAGRIMA   LARME   DAKRY   DEOIR   TEAR   TRÄNE   ASRAM   ASARA
Spanish   French   Greek   Irish   English German   Hindu   Lithuanian

According to Bopp [6], the word *dakru* was formed by joining the stem *dans* (to bite) and the suffix *-ru*. Pokorny [7] proposed the prefix *d-* and *akru* (acrid, saline). I propose [5,8] a third hypothesis: that *dakru* is a combination of *udar* (flowing water) and *oku* (eye). This hypothesis is somewhat borne out by comparison with the corresponding words in other languages: Mandarin, *yen-lei* (eye water); Korean, *nun-mul* (eye water); Indonesian, *air-mata* (water eye); Madagascan, *ranu-masu* (water eye); Ibo (Nigeria), *anya-miri* (eye water); Nahuatl (Mexico), *ixayotl* (face water).

The concept of tears was always related to the idea of drops falling out of the eye, and it therefore received a plural name "tears", as if they were numerous small units. When generic reference is made to the lacrimal liquid, I believe it is better to give it a singular name "tear", as with saliva or urine.

About the time of 1500 B.C., (Eber's papyrus) [9] the Egyptians believed that tears came from the heart. Hippocrates (fifth, fourth centuries B.C.) [10] believed that they originated from the brain, while Plato (fourth century B.C.) [11] thought them to be a mixture of the eye's natural moisture with "visual fire." Galen (second century A.D.) [12] noticed the lacrimal puncta and showed them to have a double function: the elimination of tears to the nose and the pouring of tears into the eyes by means of two glands, one superior, the other inferior. With the influence of Arabic culture in the following centuries, the concept of the lacrimal glands was lost, as the Arabs regarded tears as coming from the veins of the forehead and temples or from the brain [13,14]. Debate continued into the modern era as to whether tears are produced in the brain and transported to the lacrimal basin through the lamina cribrosa [15], or along the nerves [16], or even produced directly in the conjunctiva [17]. However, after Stensen [18] described the dacryodoches and the main lacrimal gland, it was accepted that tears originated there. The nineteenth century saw the discovery of the accessory lacrimal glands [19–26]. The existence of tear components from other sources came with the discovery of the meibomian glands [15,27], Zeis glands [28], Moll's glands [20,29], and mucin-secretory cells [30,31,32].

Although reflex and affective tearing have been known since the beginning of human history, basic lacrimation remained unknown until very recent times. In the past it was thought that the external surface of the eye was spontaneously wet and fatty (Aristotle, fourth century B.C.) [33].

The idea that secretion could come from the conjunctiva arose in the seventeenth and eighteenth centuries [17,34,35], and the possibility of a basal secretion in the main and accesory lacrimal glands developed during the nineteenth [36,32].

2 The Concept of the Dry Eye

Primitive man suffered frequently from various diseases, particularly from neurosis, wounds, fractures, dermatosis, intestinal parasitosis, bronchitis, gynecological infections, and inflammation of the eyes, the latter of which was known to the Greeks as ophthalmia. When associated with an evident dryness, this was known as xerophthalmia, dry in Hippocratic Greek being *aûos* and *xërós*, where the latter had the connotation of hardness. Hippocrates divided the ophthalmic disorders into humid and dry, and the latter was seen as being due to the personal constitution of the patient and the air. The combination of a southerly wind in winter bringing with it mild, rainy weather, and a northerly wind in spring, bringing dry, cold weather, was believed to cause xerophthalmia, mainly in those with a bilious constitution. Xerophthalmia is more severe than the humid condition, and quickly evolves into ulcerations, and ultimately to perforation of the eye if the wind persists into summer [37–39]. It appears that in ancient Greece mild xerophthalmic conditions were not detected as dry eyes, and that many such conditions may have been named under other concepts such as myopia, trachoma, or sycosis (roughness of the conjunctiva). Myopia (*myo*, contract; *óps*, eye, face) expresses the contraction of the lids and was applied not only to myopia but to astigmatism, photophobia, conjunctivitis, etc. Trachoma (*trachys*, rough, scabrous) and sykosis (*sykon*, fig, and, by extension, roughness of the fig's leaf) probably sometimes included the concept of the dry eye as well.

The Romans defined xerophthalmia, or *arida lippitudo*, as an ocular disease in which there was neither swelling nor tearing; the eyes are red, heavy, and itching, and during the night the eyelids, which are not hard, stick together as with gum or mucus [40]. Other types of conjunctivitis, such as *aspritudo* (asperity, roughness) and *scabrities* (scabrousness, asperity), could also cover some types of dry eye as well. Special stamps (*sigilla*) for collyrium presciptions for dry eye (*ad siccam lipp*) have been [41] found.

In Graecoroman medicine, Galen (second century A.D.) [42] defined xerophthalmia as a condition of asperity and pruritus of the eye, canthal ulcer, palpebral redness, and saline lacrimation, and scleropthalmia as the redness of the eye, with a hardness and difficulty in moving the lids. In ancient Greek, *sklërós* meant hard (as opposed to *hygrós*, wet); both terms may be considered today as corresponding to types of dry eyes. Among xerophthalmia, sclerophthalmia, and other diseases of the eye, Aëtius of Amida [43] included psorophthalmia, as red eyes and lids, canthal ulcers, and salty and corrosive tears. In the writings of the ancients, the term xerophthalmia is also seen in other works [44–47]. The term *knipótes*, used by Erotianus [44] as synonymous with xerophthalmia, was also cited by Hippocrates [48], Galen [49], and Aëtius [43].

During the middle ages and at the beginning of the modern era, few advances were made with respect to knowledge concerning the dry eye. Two broad but poorly differentiated diagnostic categories were recognized: those with and those without night blindness. These were thought to arise from the personality, or humor, of the patient, as well as the type of climate, diet, and even supernatural forces.

In the nineteenth century the description of a different clinical picture began. Mackenzie [50] distinguished the dry eyes arising from a lack of tears from those due to a lack of mucus. Hubbenet [51] described conjunctival xerotic spots in patients with hemeralopia, and Leber [52], filamentary keratitis. At the same time, knowledge of the previous etiological causes (humoral, vitamin deficiency, etc.) was augmented with that of the extirpation of the lacrimal glands and of the microbiological infections. The latter was seen as the cause of almost all types of dry eye. Even at the beginning of the present century, Parsons [53] still divided dry eye conditions into two types. The first, in its milder form, was characterized by Bitot's spots and in its more severe form by keratomalacia. The second type was seen as resulting from cicatricial degeneration following trachoma, burns, pemphigus, diphtheria, etc., or exposure due to ectropion or lagophthalmos.

When Wolff [57] expressed the concept of a layered structure of the tear film, the concept had its antecedents in Terson [54], Schirmer [55] and Magnani [56]. But Wolff [57,58] went further by describing a lipid, an aqueous, and a mucin layer. Subsequent studies examined mucin dispersed in the aqueous layer [59], mucin secreted by the epithelium [60], and the surface forces of the tear and cornea [61–68]. With the evolution of new concepts and ideas about the make-up of the tear film, qualitative aqueous-, mucin-, or lipid-deficient dry eye states, association with systemic diseases, immunological responses, and new perspectives as to the causes of the dry eye syndrome began to emerge. In the following section we consider how these ideas developed.

3   The History of the Causes of the Dry Eye

3.1   The Infectious Dry Eye

Throughout history, the most frequently occurring condition known under the term of xerophthalmia is most probably trachoma. This form of conjunctivitis was not properly identified clinically and etiologically until the end of the last century and the beginning of this. Until the microbiological era it was not possible scientifically to classify the different types of dry eye produced by infections. The discovery of *Bacillus xerosis* gave rise to a debate as to whether this was the cause or the consequence of dryness, Bitot's spots, or keratomalacia. Nowadays other types of infectious conjunctivitis have been identified, such as viral keratoconjunctivitis [69], which can provoke a mucin deficiency, corneal hypesthesia, and an aqueous deficiency. Infectious dacryoadenitis, an illness more frequent in the past than today, was not a common cause of dry eye. Nowadays, lacrimal gland infections are less frequent, though still cited as a cause of dry eye, by direct [70] or indirect [71] effect. More recently some viral infections – infectious mononucleosis, cytomegalovirus, and AIDS – have been considered causes of dry eye due to a immune response or to direct involvement of the lacrimal glands [72–75]. Alterations in the meibomian glands, both seborrheic and nonseborrheic, may provoke a shortened break-up time, keratoconjunctivitis, and dryness [76–79].

3.2 Dry Eye Due to Nutritional Deficiency

It is accepted that hypovitaminosis is another cause of dry eye. The Schola Hippocratica [39] described "people who have hyperlacrimation or become nyctalop [night blind]," but this does not mean that we can assume that they suspected a syndromelike relationship between eye irritation and night blindness. Despite having very specific symptoms, this association was not clearly defined until much later. Hubbenet [51] and Bitot [80] described the conjunctival spot-shaped degeneration; and Leber [52] identified hemeralopia and keratomalacia as the same picture when they are associated with the dry eye, but he attributed its cause to an infectious encephalitis. Vitamins were discovered in 1909, and experiences during the First World War began to show that foods lacking in fat produced eye dryness and night blindness [81,82]. However, it was Venco [83] who produced specific evidence showing that it was the deficiency of vitamin A which caused the disease. Numerous other studies, performed about the same time or since have thrown more light on the subject [84–90]. Avitaminosis A, which is frequently and erroneously classified under the generic term of xerophthalmia, is nowadays in underdeveloped countries, a frequent cause of dry eye and blindness, its principal cause being malnutrition. Less significant causes of dry eye include other nutritional conditions such as hyponutrition [91,92], alcoholism [89], and dehydratation [93,94].

3.3 Dry Eye Due to Glandular Destruction

The destruction of the lipid-producing and mucin-producing glands in the lids, caruncle, or conjunctiva, by ablation, burns, or cauterization was an old accidental or therapeutic experience, which sometimes produced dry eye, but more frequently epiphora by destruction of the normal anatomical architecture of the lacrimal basin. Galen [42] saw the caruncle as the gate-keeper of the lacrimal puncta, because, when it was destroyed, the normal flux of the tear was altered. Throughout history many such cases have been reported, even at the present time [95].

Although today seen to have little significance, the ablation of the lacrimal glands played an early and important role in the development of new concepts of the dry eye. In the first half of the nineteenth century, it was observed that extirpation of the main lacrimal gland [96,97,35], due to tumors or hypertrophies, did not produce a dry eye. This led Bernard [208] and Textor [98] to remove the gland in cases of chronic epiphora. In the second half of the nineteenth century, hundreds of operations involving the removal of a part or all of the gland were performed [99–103,54,55]. The frequency of these operations fell when dacryocystitic epiphora began to be resolved with Toti's dacryocystorhinostomy. In the postoperative phase there occasionally appeared a clinical dry eye [70,104–108]. Sub-stantial information was gained through these operations, for example, on the absence of a response to the innervational stimuli of the accessory lacrimal glands [109], and the fall of the albumin and muramidasic com-ponent of tears with the removal of the main lacrimal gland [110]. Some of these concepts are now under revision.

3.4 The Neurological Dry Eye

The first causes of neurogenic dry eye were seen as being due to neurosecre-tory deprivation. In 1868 Herzenstein [111] wrote that the section of the first trigeminal branch suppressed reflex and affective weeping, and in 1876 Goldzieher [112] and Hutchinson [113] reported various cases of unilateral dry eye with homolateral facial paralysis. At that time the secretory inner-vation of the lacrimal glands was not as yet well known, and it was not established until the beginning of the twentieth century that the lesion in the facial nerve, between its nucleus and the geniculate ganglion, was a cause of dry eye. Later in this century studies were published showing a connection between dry eye and lesions in the greater superficial petrosal nerve [114], the vidian nerve [115], and the sphenopalatine ganglion [116,117]. During the present century many cases of hypolacrimation have been reported in patients with alterations in the central nervous system [55,118–121]. The neurosensorial deprivation of the lacrimal basin caused by an interruption of the trigeminal nerve and its subsidiary corneal damage due to dryness, scarce or incomplete blinking, traumatic aggression, or a lack of neuro-trophic stimuli was reported in the rabbit by Decker [122], and later in the human by Feuer [123], Gaule [124], and Ollendorff [125].

3.5 Dry Eye Associated with Systemic Skin Disorders

Cases of dry eye associated with systemic diseases of the skin and mucosae have doubtless been known to man since antiquity. It was only in the present century, however, that entities such as eczema [126], pemphigoid [127–130], dysplasia ectodermica anhydrotica [131], dysplasia ectodermica hydrotica [132], Fiessinger-Rendu-Stevens-Johnson's syndrome [133–135], Curtius' syndrome [136], Zinsser-Engman-Cole syndrome [137,138], Lyell's syndrome [139], and primary epitheliopathy [140] were better identified and separated, and their relation with the dry eye better understood.

3.6 Dry Eye Associated with Endocrinopathies

In Graves-Basedow's disease there is generally hyperlacrimation; nevertheless, von Graefe [141] reported in 1857 its association with hypolacrimation, an observation which has also been made occasionally by other authors [142,143]. In the present century, hypolacrimation has been also observed in relation with diabetes mellitus [144,145], pheochromocytoma [146], ovariectomy [147,148], premature ovarian failure and hypothyroidism [149], and various physiological endocrinological conditions involving, for example, the menstrual cycle [150], menopause [151,152], and involutio senilis, which has an endocrinological component [153].

3.7 Dry Eye Associated with Exocrinopathies

The existence of simultaneous affections of tear and salival glands has been known since the last century [154,155]. Fuchs [156] reported simultaneous painless hypertrophy of lacrimal glands and parotids with lymphomatous infiltration, and Mikulicz [157] added a similar case in which the salivary glands were infiltrated with small round cells. Fraser [158] published a case of dryness of eyes, mouth, and nose; Haeckel [159] symmetrical disturbances of lacrimal and salival glands; and Gougerot [160] cases of dryness of eyes, mouth and vulva. Sjögren published at least 17 papers on the subject, between 1930 [161] and 1940 [162], and by the end of the decade this association was called Sjögren's syndrome.

3.8 Dry Eye Associated with Autoimmune Connective Tissue Disease

The Schola Hippocratica [36,39] held that patients with xerophthalmia are prone to arthritis, lumbago, dysentery, and other diseases, that the dry eye is less severe if the patient develops fever or lumbago, that women with chronic flux should be asked whether they also have amblyopia, odontopathies, or lumbalgia, and that people with severe dry eye improve if lumbalgia appears. As concerns the association of dry eye with rheumatism, it should be pointed out that *rheuma* had a meaning different from that today [163,164], and referred to a discharge or flux in any part of the body. Inflammation or pain in the joints was termed arthritis. The association of arthritis deformans chronica with keratopathia filamentosa was first published by Fisher [165] and was later supported by other authors [126,166, 167]. Rheumatoid arthritis thus came to be added to the list of disabilities under Sjögren's syndrome. In the 1950s and 1960s researchers noted the frequent association of the syndrome with malignant lymphoblastoma [168, 169]. At approximately the same time it was also discovered that other connective tissue diseases such as lupus erythematosus, scleroderma, and polymyositis may also belong to a syndrome that involves the dry eye.

A frequent association was later detected between Sjögren's syndrome and certain alloantigens [170,171] and to particular autoantibodies [172–174]. As the findings differed according to whether or not the patients had connective tissue disease, Frost Larsen et al. [175] proposed classifying Sjögren's syndrome as primary or secondary, depending upon whether there was not or was an association with connective tissue disease, respectively. More recently, dry eye after chronic graft-versus-host disease has been reported in cases of bone marrow transplantation [176,177]. As Sjögren's syndrome is not well defined, different diagnostic criteria have been proposed such as Copenhagen's [178], La Joya's [179], Greece's [180], and Pisa's [181] criteria.

3.9 Dry Eye Associated with Congenital Malformations

Hypolacrimation with or without clinical manifestations has been reported recently in: Riley-Day syndrome [120], first branchial arch syndromes [182, 183], absence of goblet cells associated with dysgenesia irides [184,185], absence of lacrimal gland and lacrimal caruncle in Bonnevie-Ullrich syndrome [186], absence of meibomian glands [187], and absence of the lacrimal puncta [188,189].

3.10 Pharmacological and Toxic Dry Eye

Homer [190] knew that some drugs stop lacrimal secretion, and it has been known since the last century that atropine momentarily diminishes the exocrine secretions [191,142]. This can either produce a clinical dry eye [192] or increase the levels of lysozyme in deficiency cases [193]. Other drugs reported as being influential in the reduction of lacrimal secretion are contraceptives [94,194,195], tranquilizers [195,196], the antipyretic acetylsalicylic acid [196], the antineoplastic busulfan [197], the antiangina pectoris perhexiline [198] di hydroergotamine [199], alpha-adrenergic stimulants [200,201], and beta-adrenergic blockers [202].

Some toxic chemicals may desiccate the eyes, for example, denaturalized colza oil [203], botulinum toxin [204], or typhoid fever [71].

3.11   The Mechanical Dry Eye

Dry eye caused by incomplete closure of the eyelids, ectropion, lid deformities, exophthalmos, or lagophthalmos has been noted since antiquity. More recently, it has been observed that certain surface abnormalities impede a good spreading of the tear and provoke dry eyes [205], i.e., pterygium [206] or extrusion of keratoprosthesis [206]. Limbic corneal ulcers or Dellen may stimulate the pterygium [207]. Inadequate, weak blinking (facial palsy, senile weakness, enophthalmos) or less blinking than usual (neurosensorial deprivation, neurological disease) is an uncommon cause of dry eye.

3.12   Dry Eye Due to Excessive Evaporation

The importance of the evaporation of the lacrimal sea was hypothesized in the past century [208,209,123] and has been confirmed in the present one [55,59,210–214]. The evaporation is more intense in hot climates [215], when the lipid layer of the tear film is deficient [57], in aircraft [93], or in drafts while motoring [216].

3.13   The Hysteric Dry Eye

Hysteria has been identified by Borel [217] and Garcia Mansilla [218] as a cause of dry eye.

4   The History of the Diagnosis of the Dry Eye

In ancient times the dry eye was diagnosed by the direct observation of very advanced objective signs and subjective symptoms: a lack of brightness, ulcers or scars on the surface of the eyeball, a lack of reflex or emotional tears, and dryness during sleep due to lagophthalmos. As a result, only severely dry eyes were diagnosed. A condition of only medium severity was frequently confused with other entities, especially when occurring with other collateral symptoms such as redness, reflex tearing, or lid hardness. The mildly dry eye, as such, always passed unnoticed. A more sophisticated diagnostic examination of the dry eye began in recent centuries and became more sophisticated in the present one. This diagnosis can be divided into four types; these are considered individually below.

4.1 Visual Examination

The first type of diagnosis is based on the simple visual examination of the eye. Formerly, such direct examination showed only gross lesions: ectropion, symblepharon, lagophthalmos, corneal ulcers, vascularization, opacifications, etc. In the past century, examination was carried out with oblique illumination, but nowadays this is performed with a slit lamp, which allows a more detailed study. One can see the shrinkage of caruncular and conjunctival folds or the leukoplakia [219] in the mucosa, the height of or the debris in the tear meniscus [76], corneal gloss or other characteristics [220–222] in the tear film, incipient edema in the cornea [223], and the state of the meibomian glands in the lid margins, etc.

Incipient damage to the corneal and conjunctival epithelium was initially observed in the past century with vital dyes: Fluorescein was synthesized in 1871 and was used to dye the cornea of rabbits by Pflüger [224] in 1882, and of humans by Straub [225] in 1888. Its derivative, rose bengal, was synthesized in 1882 and later used as external eye vital dye by Schirmer [226] and many others [108,140,227–230]. Rose bengal staining in cases of dry eye has been graded by van Bijsterveld [231]. Other dyes used in this way include eosin, blue water, nigrosin plus indulin [232], methylene blue, scarlet red plus mercurochrome [108], bromothymol blue [233], red tetrazolium [130], formazan plus trypan blue [130], and lissamine green [234].

Filaments, composed of epithelial cells and mucin and formed on the cornea as a result of epithelial damage, were first described by Leber [52] and others [235,236,165] in the nineteenth century, and have been studied by many others in the present century [69,126,161,237]. These occur frequently not only in the dry eye but also in herpes simplex, herpes zoster, vernal conjunctivitis, and other conditions. Mucous threads and mucous plaques of the lacrimal lake are usually better observed if they are stained with alcian blue and tetrazolium [130] or with periodic acid–Schiff stain [238].

The formation on the ocular surface of dry spots was initially observed in cases of keratitis neuroparalytica. Decker [122] (1876) observed them in a rabbit after sectioning the trigeminal nerve. Later they were described in humans [123,124,207,239]. Different manifestations of the dry spots of the cornea were described as Gaule's pits and [124] as Fuchs' Dellen [207]. Dry spots of the cornea were not well studied until Marx [240] and Go Ing Hoen et al. [241], observing the dry spots without a slit lamp and without dyeing the tear film, determined the normal breakup time to be 60–67 s, but with substantial variability. The topic nevertheless received little attention [205] until recent times [64–66,242–246]. The dry spots are better observed with fluorescein and ultraviolet light, but a grid pattern keratoscope [247] avoids the need for such.

The interference color patterns of the lipid layer of the tear film were first described by Marx [240], but he believed them to be formed in the whole lacrimal film, or at least did not realize that they were in the lipid layer. The first to identify this was Klein in 1949 [248]. In the past decades, Hamano [220] has studied them in Sjögren's syndrome. Very recently, Kilp [221] and Olsen [125] introduced a catoptric photometric method for measuring the lipid layer.

4.2 Quantification of the Lacrimal Secretion

The second set of tests to be developed represented an attempt to quantify the lacrimal secretion. The first measurements were done in the eighteenth and nineteenth centuries by direct collecting of tears and deducing the normal production: 60 g/day [34], 3.18 g/day [191], one drop each half hour [249]. Absorbent papers were also used in the past century in experimental animal studies by Demtschenko [250] and Tepliachine [251]. In humans the method was pioneered in 1900 by Köster [252], who put pieces of filter paper 10 × 10–20 mm in the conjunctival sac, stimulating the nasal mucosa with a brush. In 1903 Schirmer [55] used filter paper in strips of 5 × 35 mm, placing one end of them inside the inferolateral conjunctival cul-de-sac for 5 min, elaborating upon method I, with only the stimulation of blinking. Method II involved ocular cocaine anesthesia and the rubbing of nasal mucosa with a brush. Method III involved a local anesthesia and looking at the sun. Schirmer's test found very little use in the following decades [153,253], until in 1941, de Rötth [147] proposed a standardized test using Whatman 41 filter paper. The test soon developed a number of variants: tests with closed eyes [254], after topical ocular anesthesia [255], putting the paper beside the lacrimal punctum [256], diminishing [147] or increasing [257] the time, with litmus paper [258,259], with strips dyed with fluorescein in the aerial portion [260], with lipid-extracted paper in an envelope [261], with cotton threads instead of filter papers [262], etc. Method I of Schirmer's test served to estimate the absolute quantity of tear secretion [263,264], but its more frequent use was in the clinical diagnosis of relative tear secretion by the length of moistening, especially in Sjögren's syndrome. Sjögren [108], however, wrote: "The lacrimal test of Schirmer is an inexact method, even if it is performed strictly according to the rules."

The dilution of a tracer instilled in the lacrimal basin has also been used in the past six decades to estimate the quantity of lacrimal secretion. The first of these tracers were colorants: starch evidenced with lugol [265], argyrol [266], fluorescein [267–270], or fluorescein plus rose bengal [271]. The dilution of desquamated epithelial cells [272,213] and scintillographic techniques [273–275] were also used to quantify lacrimal secretion and lacrimal flux.

The above methods are used to determine the total tear secretion, composed mainly of the aqueous component. Some methods, on the other hand, were developed with the aim of measuring only the mucin or the lipid component. Mucin can be measured by dyeing the chondroitin and mucoitin sulfate of its conglomerates with alcian blue [130], but more precise quantification has been achieved by determining some of its compounds and deducing the total mucin; such compounds have been sialic acid [276], hexosamine [238], and oligosaccharides [95].

The lipid secretion has been, from a historical point of view, the most recent to be quantified. This is achieved by staining with Sudan IV [277] or Sudan III [234,278], interferential colorimetry [220], or photometry [125]. A general idea of the lipid layer may be obtained by tear evaporimetry [279].

4.3 Quality of the Tear

The normal composition of tear was determined first by Fourcroy et al. in 1791 [280], and thereafter by many others in the past [35,281,191,91] and present [282–286] centuries. Crystallization of the residue of spontaneous dessication of the tear was observed by Fourcroy et al. [280]. Solé [287] observed 160 years later that these crystals conformed to specific patterns which he called stagograms, and which Tabbara [288] later called "fernlike" figures. Alterations in the various components of the tear in different types of dry eye have been studied by many authors in this century [65,238, 289–291]. Some components have special interest and have been used in diagnostic tests because they decrease in the dry eye; these include muramidase [292,86,61,231] and lactoferrin [295]. The tonicity of the tear was examined empirically at the end of the nineteenth century by Massart [293]. In the first decade of the present century, it was more accurately determined by hemolysis [294], by using the histologic response of the corneal epithelium [296], and by freezing point [296]. Mastman et al. [297] found tear osmolarity to be equivalent to a NaCl water solution of $9.53\,pM$ in normal persons and $9.70\,pM$ in patients with keratoconjunctivitis sicca. Increasing attention has since been given to the hypertonicity of the tear as a test of dry eye [298]. The pH of the tear decreases early after death (Lecha Marzo's test of death, 1916), but it is not clear whether this is related to the dryness of the conca lacrimalis or to the postmortem tissue changes [298]. The surface tension of the tear was determined for the first time by Cerrano [299]. In the dry eye this may be increased [64,66], but its evaluation has not been used as a diagnostic test because inflammatory products in the lacrimal sea may significativatly modify its value [238,290].

4.4 Examination of the Glands

The simple examination in situ by observation or palpation of swollen lacrimal glands, altered palpebral rims, or inflamed or atrophic conjunctiva was the first step to be developed. The following step came in the past century with the biopsy of the lacrimal gland [155–157], and more recently, to establish the criteria of diagnosis, the biopsy of the major [157] or minor [300–302] salivary glands. Recently developed is the scintillographic study of the lacrimal glands [303].

The goblet cells and epithelium of the conjunctiva may be studied by biopsy [89,304] or by impression cytology [305–307]. In many dry eyes there is an innervational problem that affects not only the secretion but decreases the sensation of the lacrimal basin as well [308].

5 The History of the Treatment of the Dry Eye

5.1 Stimulants of Tear Secretion

Irritants which act through a hyperlacrimatory trigeminal reflex have been used for millenia. Eber's papyrus [9] advises that in blear eyes (which includes trachoma and similar clinical entities) one should apply onion and verdigris in equal parts to the eyes. Later, various other irritants were used: cold air, smoke, pricking vapors, mustard, etc. [309]. Their current use is reduced to provoking hyperlacrimation to collect samples of the tear: onion [208,310], lemon juice [193], petroleum [311], jointed charlock and mustard oil [109], sodium chloride [91], absolute alcohol [193], ammoniac vapor [310,109], tear gases [312,282], atmospheric pollutants [313], tobacco smoke [314], formol vapors [283], and nasal mechanical stimulation [280,252,55].

Among the direct stimulant drugs, pilocarpine is the oldest [91,200], but its lacrimatory effect in patients with dry eye has proven very poor [315,150,140] and frequently decreases the level of lysozyme in the tear [316]. Other lacrimal stimulants introduced more recently include physalemin [317], eledoisin [318–320], vasoactive intestinal polypeptide [321], and certain beta-adrenergics [322].

Some drugs specifically stimulate and liquify the mucin component of the tear such as bromhexine [324,175] and vitamin A.

5.2 Vitamins

Hippocrates knew that night blindness was cured with ox liver, and Dioscorides [325] knew that it was cured with goat's liver by inhaling the fumes when smoked, as eye drops when used as an extract, or eaten when baked. At that time, however the occasional association between night blindness and xerophthalmia had not yet been noticed; this was identified only in following centuries. The cure for nyctalopic xerophthalmia, through the ingestion of mammal and fish liver, especially cod liver oil, was known in the past century [326]. It was not until the second decade of the present century that it was noticed that the fatty extract of foods has an antixerophthalmic subfraction (vitamin A) and an antirachitic one (vitamin D). The effectiveness of the vitamin A in counteracting this specifc type of vitamin deficiency dry eye was well documented in the 1920s and 1930s. Viusa [327] used lemon to improve the condition. Kreiker [84] showed that the first lesion of the avitaminotic A dry eye was the degeneration of goblet cells. The ingestion of vitamin A has been shown to increase the conjunctival mucus secretion [328,89], and the local application of retinoic acid to improve the ocular symptoms of avitaminosis A, in rats [329] and humans [90]. It has recently been suggested that vitamins C [330] and B1 [331] also have a hyperlacrimatory effect.

5.3 Hormones

During the present century various experiments on animals have shown the hyperlacrimatory effect of tiroxin [332], parotin [260], testosterone [333, 86,148], and estrogens [334]. The castration of male and female guinea pigs reduces their lacrimal secretion [335]. Contraceptives are believed to decrease lacrimal secretion (although certain studies indicate the opposite [336]) or to liquify the fatty component [195].

5.4 Anti-inflammatories, Antipaludian Agents, Immunosuppressors

Corticosteroids [337], hydroxychloroquine [338], azathioprine and cyclosporin A [339] have all been used, since being introduced into clinics, for the treatment of certain types of dry eye.

5.5 Substitutes

Running water was the first tear substitute in the dry eye of primitive humans. Saline solutions isosmolar to natural tear were used by Berger in 1894 [142,71]. Cantonnet [296] in 1908 made an isosmolar collyrium, which was first given the name of *larmes artificielles*. Recent decades have seen hypo-osmolar collyria aimed at reestablishing the normal osmolarity of the lacrimal sea of patients with dry eye. Hyperosmolar collyria and ointments have also been used, not only as tear substitutes, but also to attract water from the tissues. Lipids such as olive, almond, colocynth, linseed, or castor oil were used in antiquity to treat the dry eye [9,43,340]. Many of these products, for example, almond oil, have been used in modern times [192], but have gradually been substituted by mineral oil, paraffin (petrolatum, vaseline), or lanolin. Frequently these lipids serve as an excipient of another active product, providing a double effect, such as the collyrium of vitamin D in an oily solution [341].

Gums also had an ancient use. At that time there was no precise concept of the mildly dry eye; however, empirical knowledge had accumulated of the benefits of gum's collyria in some ophthalmic conditions, many of wich were probably xerophthalmic. From the 188 recipes of Alcoatí of Toledo [340] 73 contained glues (e.g., sarcocolla, gum arabic, tragacanth gum). In recent times the most frequently used have been arabic (acacia) gum and tragacanth [129,342].

Mucilages or related substances such as cellulose, starch, and semola, had a similar use. Eber's papyrus [9] advises the use of a mixture of water, boiled papyrus, acacia gum, incense, and antimony for irritated and watery eyes. Alcoati [340] used starch and semola. The collyria of ethers of cellulose have recently been introduced in dacryology [343,344] because of their surfactant and viscous properties, and these now have a widespread use.

Synthetic polymers are of more recent use as tear substitutes; Krishner et al. [345] introduced the polyvinyl polymers and Marquardt [346] the polyacrylics. Organic animal products such as gelatins extracted from collagen were the main component of some ancient collyria, and more recently these have formed part of some artificial tears [347]. In recent decades collyria of mucin [85] has also been used, as well as autologous blood serum [348,349], colostrum [350], chondroitin sulfate [351], sodium hyaluronate [352], and whole saliva. The application of saliva to the eyes of the blind goes back to Biblical times (Mark 8:23; John 9:6). In the past years it has been used in patients with dry eye by direct application [142], by means of derivations [353], and, recently, in glandular transplants [354]. Saliva restores to the tear film many of its physiological components such as epidermal growth factor, which has been reported as a normal component of the lacrimal fluid [323,286].

5.6 Liquefying Agents

In the attempt to maintain natural tear, but make it more liquid, fibrolysin [355], N-acetyl-L-cysteine [356], and bromhexine [324,175] have been used.

5.7 Hyperosmolar Agents

The idea that there is a physiological flux from the walls of the lacrimal basin to the lacrimal sea [17,34,35,357,358,210] suggested to some authors in this century that its flow using hyperosmolar collyria or ointments of sodium chloride [91,359] or sugar [360] could be increased in patients with dry eye.

In cases of chronic bullous keratopathy, the superficial petrosal nerve has been denervated producing a more dense basal tear and diminishing the discomfort [361].

5.8 Physical Treatment

Massaging of the dacryoglands has recently been advised for the meibomian glands in cases of lipodeficient dry eye; due to its expressory effect in mucin-deficient and serodeficient dry eye as well, it was probably also known empirically in ancient times. In the present century, radiotherapy [362] on the lacrimal glands has been used in cases of Mikulicz' disease, and the soft laser [363] in cases of keratoconjunctivitis sicca.

5.9 Mechanical Devices

In the past centuries cups and cannulas for ocular baths and irrigations were frequently used. Recent decades have seen the appearance of deposits for artificial tears, which are fixed to the spectacles, clothes, or body and deliver their liquid into the lacrimal basin [364–368]. To avoid evaporation from the lacrimal sea and to protect the cornea, various protective measures have been used: wet ambients, ocular pads, etc. Among those of particular interest are modified goggles [369–371] and hydrophilic contact lenses [372,94].

5.10 Surgical Treatment

Apart from general ophthalmological interventions to correct some of the causes of dry eye (e.g., ectropion, coloboma, lagophthalmos) specific surgery for the dry eye has also appeared. Tarsorrhaphy has been prac-tised since the past century [373,56]. Canalicular occlusion, impeding tear drainage by burning the lacrimal puncta with galvanic current, was first conducted experimentally in animals by Römer [374] in 1899. Later, various other procedures of electrocoagulation were carried out in patients with dry eye [355,253,375,348]. Occlusion has also been attempted with laser photo-coagulation [376] sutures [368], or plugs of gelatin [377], silicone, [378–380] and N-butyl-cyanoacrylate [381]. One means of affecting the drainage sys-tem without destroying it has been to transfer the lacrimal punctum to dry dock in the anterior part of the lid rim [382]. Nevertheless, the most widely used procedure remains electrocoagulation [383].

The transposition of Stensen's duct, to pour saliva into the lacrimal basin, was first introduced by Filatov and Chevaljev in the 1950s [353]. And found widespread use in the 1960s, however, its use has subsequently declined [369]. The most recent method of using saliva is transplantation of the autologous sublingual gland and the auto- and homotransplant of the submandibular gland [354,384,385]. Transplanting the lacrimal glands has never been attempted, but remains a possibility, as experiments in rabbits have shown that autoimplants can survive [332], and those in rats that the culture of lacrimal cells is possible [386,387].

6 The Social Response to the Dry Eye

Apart from the individual contributions of the above mentioned scientists and of many others, the World Health Organization, the International Agency for the Prevention of Blindness, and various governmental and non-governmental organizations have developed specific programs aimed at combating the different diseases which cause dry eye, principally trachoma and avitaminosis A. The foundation of the Internationalis Societas Dakryologiae, (Madrid, 1983) and the Europaea Societas Dacryologiae (Milan, 1988) has led to a greater interest in the topic.

Four congresses of the International Society of Dakryology have taken place (Lubbock, 1984; Budapest, 1987; Amsterdam, 1990; Madrid, 1993) as well as seven international symposia on dacryology (México, 1970; Budapest, 1973; Kyoto, 1978; Milan-Pavia, 1986; Lisbon, 1988; Singapore, 1990; Brussels, 1992), and three symposia on Sjögren's syndrome (Holth, Denmark, 1986; San Antonio, USA, 1989; Ionnina, Greece, 1992). Discovery of the high frequency of dry eye – 20%–25% of patients who come to an eye clinic [388,389] –, with its commercial implications has attracted the interest of the health industries. In the United States in 1985, Harris [390] founded the first self-help society for patients with dry eye, Sjögren's Syndrome Foundation, and within a short time such organizations have also been founded in Holland, Israel, Spain, and other countries.

The dry eye still presents us with more questions than answers. Efforts to resolve these continue, and are proving increasingly successful as our knowledge grows. However, the most interesting aspect of this topic lies in the future, and will be written by our descendants.

References

1. Darwin C (1872) The expression of the emotions in man and animals. Murray, London
2. Montagu A (1960) Natural selection and the origin and evolution of weeping in man. JAMA 174:392–397
3. García de la Torre JM (1980) Las lágrimas y el llanto. Arch Soc Canar Oftalmol 5:102–110

4. Frey WH, Hoffman-Ahern C, Johnson RA, Lykken DT, Tuason VB (1983) Crying behavior in the human adult. Integr Psychiat 1:94–100
5. Murube del Castillo J (1981) Dacriología básica. Royper, Las Palmas, pp 400, 768, 778–780, 785
6. Bopp F (1874) Grammaire comparé des langues indo-européennes, vol 1. Impr Nationale, Paris, pp 51, 105, 106, 179
7. Pokorny J (1959) Indogermanisches etymologisches Wörterbuch, vol 1. Francke, Bern, pp 23, 64, 66, 243, 249, 261, 326–338, 775, 776
8. Murube del Castillo J (1986) History of dakryology. In: Holly FJ (ed) The preocular tear film. Dry Eye Inst, Lubbock, pp 3–30
9. Ebers GM (1985) Das hermetische Buch über die Arzneimittel der alten Aegypter in hieratischer Schrift, 2 vols. Engelmann, Leipzig
10. Hippocraticum Corpus (5th–4th centuries B.C.) Perì adénön (On the glands), sect 3, no 65
11. Plato (427–347 B.C.) Quoted by Wood [391]
12. Galen (2nd century A.D.) De comp medicam sec, loc, lib 5, chap 2
13. Hunain Ibn Ishak (245 A.Hg., 860 A.D.) Ashr maqalat fil ain (Ten treatises of the structure of the eye)
14. Al-Rhazes (10th century) Al-Hawi (The content, – i.e. of medicine), vol IX, sect 23 (epiphora) and 28 (night blindness). Xth cent
15. Casserius J (1609) Pentoestheseion. Venet
16. Wharton T (1658) Adenographia, sive glandularum totius corporis descriptio. Londini
17. Schneider CV (1661) De catharris. vol III. Cited in Duke Elder S (1961) System of ophthalmology, vol II, p 559. Kimpton, London
18. Steno N (Niels Stensen) (1662) De glandulis oculorum. In: Observationes anatomicae, Leyden
19. Krause C (1842) Handbuch der Anatomie des Menschen, T II. Hahm, Hannover, p 515
20. Sappey PC (1853) Recherches sur les glandes des paupières. Gaz Med Paris 33:515–517, 528–531, 543–544
21. Krause W (1854) Über die Drüsen der Conjunctiva. Z rat Med 4:337–341
22. Krause W (1862) Anatomie et physiologie de la conjonctive. Ann Ocul (Paris) 48:159–171
23. Béraud BJ (1859) Note sur les glandes lacrymales. Gaz Méd Paris 53:827–829
24. Wolfring K (1872) Untersuchungen über die Drüsen der Bindehaut des Auges. Zbl Med Wiss 10:852. Quoted by Terson [54]
25. Wicherkiewicz (1872) Centrabl Med Wiss. 54. Ref (1885) in Rev Gén Ophtalmol 4:255–256
26. Ciaccio GV (1874) Osservazioni interno alla struttura della congiuntiva umana. Mem Acad Sci, Bologna
27. Meibom H (1666) De vasis palpebrarum novis epistola. Müller, Helmstadt
28. Zeis (1835) v Ammon's Z Ophthalmol 4:231. Quoted by Duke Elder S (1961) System of ophthalmology, vol 2. Kimpton, London, p 526
29. Moll JA (1857) Bemerkungen über den Bau der Augenlider des Menschen. Graefes Arch Ophthalmol 3:258–268
30. Henle J (1862) Eingeweidelehre. Quoted by Nuel [32]
31. Stieda L (1867) Über den Bau der Augenlidbindehaut des Menschen. Arch Mikrosk Anat 3:357–365
32. Nuel JP (1882) Des glandes tubuleuses pathologiques dans la conjonctive humaine. Ann Ocul (Paris) 88:5–24
33. Aristotle (4th century B.C.) Perì aísthéseos kai aístheton (On sense and the sensible). Trad. Bekker E (1831–1870) Aristoteli Opera, vol I–II, p 438, lines a20–26. Academia Regia Borussica, Berlin
34. Janin J (1772) Mémoires et observations sur l'oeil. Paris

35. Martini F (1884) Von dem Einflusse der Sekretionsflüssigkeiten auf den menschlichen Körper, und insbesondere von dem Einflusse der Thränen auf das menschliche Auge. Leipzig
36. Arlt T (1855) Über den Tränenschlauch. Graefes Arch Ophthalmol 1:135–160
37. Hippocraticum Corpus (5th–4th centuries B.C.) Aphorismoí (Aphorisms), sect III, no 12
38. Hippocraticum Corpus (5th–4th centuries B.C.) Perì aérön, hydátön, tópön (Airs, waters, places), sects IV and X
39. Hippocraticum Corpus (5th–4th centuries B.C.) Prorrëtikón beta (Predictions II), sects 18 and 27
40. Celsus AC (ca. 20 A.D.) De Medicina (On medicine), liber VI, chapt VI
41. Voinot J (1981–1982) Inventaire des cachets d'oculistes gallo-romains. Conf Lyon Ophtalmol 150. Quoted by Liotet et al. [392] pp 3–8
42. Galen (2nd century A.D.) Ton morion logos K, chapt XI (Lacrimal anatomy)
43. Aëtius of Amida (5th century A.D.) Tetrabiblion, chap II (eye diseases), LXXVII (sclerophthalmia), LXXVIII (psorophthalmia) and LXXIX (xerophthalmia)
44. Erotianus (1st century A.D.) Vocum Hippocraticarum collectio, no 30. Edidit E. Nachmanson, Goteburg (1918)
45. Dioscorides (1st century A.D.) Perì yles iatrikés (On medical themes), I, sect 46. Edidit M. Wellman, Berlin (1906–1914)
46. Pavlos of Egina (7th century A.D.) Hypomnema, vol I, chap 21
47. Papyri Argentoratenses Graecae. Edidit C Kalbfleish (1901) Index Lectianum in Academia Rostockiensi
48. Hippocraticum Corpus (5th–4th century B.C.) Perì topön tou kat' anthrópou (On places in the human), chap 13, sect 2
49. Galen In: Kühnt CG (ed) (1821–1833) Galeni opera omnia. Lipsiae, 12, 731
50. Mackenzie W (1857) Xeroma conjonctival ou xérophthalmie. In: Traité des maladies des yeux, 4th edn, vol I. Masson, Paris, pp 109–110
51. Hubbenet Ch von (1986) Observations sur l'héméralopie. Ann Ocul (Paris) 44: 293
52. Leber T (1883) Über die Xerosis der Bindehaut und die infantile Hornhautverschwärung. Graefes Arch Klin Exp Ophthalmol 29:225–290
53. Parsons JH (1904) Pathology of the eye, vol 2. Hodder & Stoughton, London, pp 102, 546
54. Terson A (1892) Notes sur les glandes acineuses de la conjonctive et sur les glandes lacrymales orbito-palpébrales. Arch Ophtalmol (Paris) 12:745–770
55. Schirmer O (1903) Studien zur Physiologie und Pathologie der Tränenabsonderung und Tränenabfuhr. Graefes Arch Ophthalmol 56:197–291
56. Magnani C (1908) Contributo alla terapia dello xeroftalmo. Ann Ottalmol 37:483–486
57. Wolff E (1946) The mucocutaneous function of lid margin and the distribution of tear fluid. Trans Ophthalmol Soc UK 66:291–308
58. Wolff E (1948) Anatomy of the eye and orbit. Lewis, London
59. Ehlers N (1965) The precorneal film. Acta Ophthalmol (Suppl) (Copenh) 81: 5–136
60. Pfister RR (1973) The normal surface of corneal epithelium: A scanning electron microscopic study. Invest Ophthalmol Vis Sci 12:654–668
61. McEwen WK (1962) Secretion of tears and blinking in the eye. In: Dawson H (ed), vol 3. Academic Press, London, p 271
62. Adler FH (1965) Physiology of the eye. Mosby, St. Louis, Mo
63. Mishima S (1965) Some physiological aspects of the precorneal tear film. Arch Ophthalmol (Chicago) 73:233–241
64. Lemp MA, Holly FJ, Iwata S, Dohlman CH (1970) The precorneal tear film. I. Factors in spreading and maintaining a continuous tear film over the corneal surface. Arch Ophthalmol (Chicago) 83:89–94

65. Lemp MA, Dohlman CH, Kuwabara T, Holly FJ, Carroll JM (1971) Dry eye secondary to mucus deficiency. Trans Am Acad Ophthalmol Otolaryngol 75:1223–1227
66. Holly FJ, Lemp MA (1971) Surface chemistry of the tear film. Implications for dry eye syndromes, contact lenses and ophthalmic polymers. Contact Lens Soc Am 5:12–19
67. Holly FJ, Lemp MA (1971) Wettability and wetting of corneal epithelium. Exp Eye Res 11:239–250
68. Tiffany JM (1982) Separation of lipid classes by thin-layer chromatography on urea-silica gel plates. J Chromatogr 243:329–338
69. Wright P, Mackie IA (1972) Mucus in the healthy and diseased eye. Trans Ophthalmol Soc UK 97:1–7
70. Mérida Nicolich M (1919) Nuevas orientaciones terapéuticas del tracoma por la disminución de la secreción lacrimal. Arch Oftalmol Hisp-Am 19:705–727
71. Berger E (1894) Action des toxines sur la sécrétion lacrymale. Pathogénie de la kératomalacie survenant dans les maladies infectieuses. Rév Gén Ophtalmol 13:193–198
72. Shearn MA, Tu WH, Stephens BG, Lee JC (1970) Virus like structures in Sjögren's syndrom. Lancet 1:568–569
73. Burns JC (1983) Persistent cytomegalovirus infection. The etiology of Sjögren's syndrom. Med Hypotheses 10:451–460
74. Ziegler JL, Beckstead JA, Volberding PA, Abrams DI et al. (1984) Non-Hodgkin's lymphoma in 90 homosexual men. N Engl J Med 311:565–570
75. Anonymous (1984) The viral aetiology of rheumatoid arthritis. Lancet 1:772–774 (editorial)
76. Reymond C (1882) Della secrezione delle ghiandole di Meibomio e dei suoi rapporti col xerosi epiteliale. Rev Gén Ophtalmol 1:444–446
77. Elschnig A (1908) Beitrag zur Aetiologie und Therapie der chronischen Conjunctivitis. Dtsch Med Wochenschr 34:1133–1135
78. Hiwatari K (1918) On the conjunctivitis meibomiana (Elschnig). Am J Ophthalmol 1:645–646
79. Filatov VP (1922) Traitement opératoire de la conjonctivite et de la blépharite meibomienne. Klin Monatsbl Augenheilkd 69:657. Ref (1925) in Ann Ocul (Paris) 162:221
80. Bitot P (1863) Mémoire sur une lésion conjonctivale non encore décrite, coïncidant avec l'héméralopie, lu à l'Académie de médecine par le Dr Bitot de Bordeaux. Gaz Hebdom Med Clin 284–288
81. Mori S (1922) Primary changes in eyes of rats which result from deficiency of fat-soluble vit. A in diet. JAMA 79:197
82. Goldblatt H, Benischek M (1927) Vitamin A deficiency and metaplasia. J Exp Med 46:699–707
83. Venco L (1920) Un syndrome typique de xérophtalmie par avitaminose. España Oftalmol (Málaga) 5:161–167
84. Kreiker A (1930) Zur Klinik und Histologie der epithelialen Bindehautxerose. Graefes Arch Ophthalmol 124:191–205
85. Treacher Collins E (1931) The harderian gland; xerophthalmia; vitamin A deficiency; keratomalacia. Trans Ophthalmol Soc UK 50:201–230
86. García Miranda R (1948) Síndrome de Sjögren asociado a manifestaciones de rosácea ocular. Arch Soc Oftalmol Hisp Am 8:590–602
87. Lorente Buesa M (1943) Un nuevo caso de dacriocistitis y avitaminosis A. Arch Soc Oftalmol Hisp Am 3:43–46
88. Beitch I (1970) The induction of keratinization in the corneal epithelium. Invest Ophthalmol 9:827–843
89. Sullivan WR, McCulley JP, Dohlman CH (1973) Return of goblet cells after vitamin A therapy in xerosis of the conjunctiva. Am J Ophthalmol 75:720–725
90. Sommer A, Emran N (1978) Topical retinoic acid in the treatment of corneal xerophthalmia. Am J Ophthalmol 86:615–617

91. Alessandro F (1913) Sécrétion des larmes pendant le jeune. Arch Ottalmol 20:193–215, 1912. Abstract (1913) in Ann Ocul (Paris) 150:158
92. Trowell HC, Davies JNP, Dean RFA (1954) Kwashiorkor. Arnold, London
93. Boissin JP, Abbas L (1975) Variations de la sécrétion lacrymale en vol. Bull Soc Ophtalmol Fr 75:761–764
94. Malbrel P, Monbrun M (1977) Appareillage en lentilles souples dans les cas d'hyposécrétion lacrymale. Bull Soc Ophtalmol Fr 77:1045–1047
95. Friend J, Kiorpes T, Thoft RA (1983) Conjunctival goblet cell frequency after alkali injury is not accurately reflected by aqueous tear mucin content. Invest Ophthalmol Vis Sci 24:612–618
96. Velpeau AALM (1839) Médicine opératoire. Paris. Quoted by Bernard [208]
97. Carron Du Villards CJF (1838) Guide pratique pour l'étude et le traitement des maladies des yeux. Quoted by Bernard [208]
98. Textor C (1847) De l'extirpation de la glande lacrymale, comme moyen de guérir le larmoiement. J Chir Augenheilkd 6. Abstract (1847) in Ann Ocul (Belg) 18:218–221
99. Lawrence (1867) Recherches sur l'extirpation de la glande lacrymale pour la cure radicale des voies lacrymales. CR II Conc Ophthalmol Univ, Paris, p 35
100. Badal I (1885) Extirpation de la glande lacrymale en totalité: Portion orbitaire et portion palpébrale. Considérations anatomiques et physiologiques. Arch Ophtalmol (Paris) 5:386–401
101. Peyret (1886) L'extirpation de la glande lacrymale et ses indications. Doct thesis, University of Bordeaux
102. Wecker L de (1888) Traitement du larmoiement persistant. Rev Gén Ophtalmol 7:383–384
103. Truc H (1889) De l'extirpation des glandes lacrimales orbitaires dans les larmoiements incoercibles chez les granuleux. Arch Ophtalmol (Paris) 9:342–351
104. Wagenmann A (1902) Einiges über die Erkrankung der Tränenorgane, besonders auch der Tränendrüse. Münch Med Wochenschr 16:681
105. Friede R (1925) Zur Exstirpation der palpebralen Tränendrüse. Klin Monatsbl Augenheilkd 74:682–687
106. Avizonis P (1928) Über schädliche Folgen der Tränendrüsenentfernung. Ber Vers Dtsch Ophthalmol Ges (Heidelberg) 47:341–345
107. Engelking E (1928) Über Hornhaut- und Bindehautveränderungen infolge mangelnder Tränensekretion. Klin Monatsbl Augenheilkd 81:75–84
108. Sjögren H (1950) Quelques problèmes concernant la kératoconjonctivite sèche et le syndrome de K.C. sicca. Ann Ocul (Paris) 183:500–514
109. Axenfeld T (1899) Das <reflectorische Weinen> der Neugeborenen, nebst Bemerkungen über die angebliche besondere Drüse des psychischen Weinens. Klin Monatsbl Augenheilkd 37:259–270
110. McEwen WK, Kimura SJ, Freeney ML (1958) Filter-paper electro-phoresis of tears. Am J Ophthalmol 45:67–70
111. Herzenstein U (1868) Beiträge zur Physiologie und Therapie der Thränenorgane. Berlin
112. Goldzieher V (1876) Pester med.-chir. Presse. Quoted by Goldzieher V (1894) Un symptome jusqu'ici inconnu de la paralysie faciale complète. Arch Gén Ophtalmol 13:1–8
113. Hutchinson J (1876) Ophthalmol Hosp Rep 8:53. Quoted by Goldzieher [394].
114. Gardner WJ, Stowell A, Dutlinger R (1947) Resection of the greater superficial petrosal nerve in the treatment of unilateral headache. J Neurol Surg 4:105–114
115. Golding-Wood PH (1961) Observations on petrosal and vidian neurectomy in chronic vasomotor rhinitis. J Laryngol Otol 75:232–247
116. Ruskin SL (1928) The sensory field of the facial nerve. Arch Otolaryngol 7:351–358
117. Dubois Poulsen A (1937) Le ganglion sphéno-palatin et l'oeil. Ann Ocul (Paris) 174:217–284
118. Bourquin E (1920) Lähmung des Stirnastes des Gesichtsnervs. Beitrag zur Lehre der Tränendrüseninnervation. Klin Monatsbl Augenheilkd 65:105

119. Crespí Jaume G (1942) Síndrome secreto-motor ocular unilateral. Arch Soc Oftalmol Hisp Am 1:601–612
120. Riley CM, Day RL, Greeley DM, Langford WS (1949) Central autonomic dysfunction with defective lacrimation. Report of five cases. Pediatrics 3:468–478
121. Barraquer Moner JI, Hernández A (1977) Ein neues Syndrom: Hyposekretion der Tränendrüse, Hypotonie und mangelhafte Konvergenz. Klin Monatsbl Augenheilkd 171:859–862
122. Decker (1876) Contribution à l'étude de la kératite neuroparalytique. Thesis, University of Berne
123. Feuer N (1877) Wiener Med Presse, No 43 & 45. Quoted by Paton [393]
124. Gaule VJ (1891) Der Einfluss des Trigeminus auf die Hornhaut. Centralbl Physiol 15:409–415
125. Olsen T (1985) Reflectometry on the precorneal tear film. Acta Ophthalmol (Copenh) 63:432–438
126. Mulock Houwer AW (1927) Keratitis filamentosa and chronic arthritis. Trans Ophthalmol Soc UK 47:88–96
127. Duhring L (1884) Des rapports de la dermatite herpétiforme avec l'affection que l'on designe sous le nom d'impétigo herpétiforme. Am J Med Sci, p 391, and Dermatitis herpetiformis. JAMA 3:225. Quoted by Brocq [394]
128. Lortat Jacob E (1956) Le pemphigus oculaire: dermatite bulleuse muco-synéchiante et atrophiante. Bull Soc Ophtalmol Fr 56:503
129. Leoz de la Fuente G (1945) Pénfigo ocular. Arch Soc Oftalmol Hisp Am 5:1113–1121
130. Norn MS (1972) Vital staining of cornea and conjunctiva. Acta Ophthalmol Suppl (Copenh) 113:1–66
131. Arruga Liró H (1934) Conjuntivitis seca asociada a otras acrinias. An Acad Med Barcelona, Brochure, p 23
132. Adenis JP, Bonnetblanc JM, Cardoso M, De Laval M, Catanzano G, Rammaert B, Vallat M (1979) Dysplasie ectodermique idrotique. Etude anatomoclinique. Rév Méd Limoges 10:265–269
133. Fiessinger N, Wolff M, Thevenard A (1923) Ectodermose erosive pluriorificielle. Soc Méd Hopitaux 4:446–458
134. Rendu R (1917) Sur un syndrome caractérisé par l'inflammation simultaneé de toutes les muqueuses externes (conjonctivale, nasal, linguale, buccopharingée, orale et balanopréputiale) coexistant avec une éruption varicelliforme puis quatre membres. J Practiciens 30:351
135. Stevens AM, Johnson FC (1922) A new eruptive fever associated with stomatitis and ophthalmia. Report of two cases in children. Am J Dis Child 24:526–533
136. Curtius F (1925) Kongenitaler partieller Riesenwuchs mit endokrinen Störungen. Dtsch Arch Klin Med 147:310
137. Engman MF (1935) Congenital atrophy of the skin, with reticular pigmentation. JAMA 105:1252–1256
138. Cole HN, Rauschkolb JE, Toomey J (1930) Dyskeratosis congenita with pigmentation, dystrophia unguis and leukokeratosis oris. Arch Dermatol Syphil 21:71–95
139. Lyell A (1956) Toxic epidermal necrolysis; an eruption resembling scalding the skin. Br J Dermatol 68:355–361
140. De Haas EBH (1964) The pathogenesis of keratoconjunctivitis sicca. Ophthalmologica 147:1–18
141. Graefe A von (1857) Graefes Arch Ophthalmol 3:289. Quoted by Berger [142]
142. Berger E (1894) Névroses de sécrétion de la glande lacrymale. – Larmoiement et sécheresse de la conjonctive dans la goitre exophtalmique. Arch Ophtalmol (Paris) 14:101–110
143. Bey Handousa A (1952) Proptosis caused by lipoidosis. Br J Ophthalmol 36:20–25

144. Piper HF (1953) über Erkrankungen des äusseren Auges und deren Folgezustände. Klin Monatsbl Augenheilkd 122:129–141
145. Guzzinati GC (1954) Ricerche sulla secrezione lacrimale nei diabetici. Boll Ocul 33:754–760
146. Sipple JH (1961) The association of pheochromocytoma with carcinoma of the thyroid gland. Am J Med 31:163–166
147. Rötth A de (1941) On the hypofunction of the lacrimal gland. Am J Ophthalmol 24:20–25
148. Radnót M, Németh B (1955) Wirkung der Testosteronpräparate auf die Tränendrüse. Ophthalmologica 129:376–380
149. Ayala A, Canales ES, Karchmer S, Alarcón Segovia D, Zárate A (1979) Premature ovarian failure and hypothyroidism associated with sicca syndrome. Obst Gynecol 53:98–101
150. Hauer K (1931) Kasuistischer Beitrag zur Aetiologie der Tränendrüsenhypofunktion. Klin Monatsbl Augenheilkd 87:79–81
151. Fuchs A (1919) Funktionsstörung der Speichel und Tränendrüsen. Ophthalmol Ges Wien (7/7/1919). Ref (1920) in Arch Oftalmol Hisp Am 20:231
152. Schöninger L (1924) über Keratitis filiformis bei Hypofunktion der Tränendrüse. Klin Monatbl Augenheilkd 73:208–210
153. Axenfeld T (1929) Bemerkungen zu den Nebenwirkungen der Exstirpation der palpebralen Tränendrüse. Klin Monatsbl Augenheilkd 82:243–247
154. Hadden WB (1888) On "dry mouth" or suppression of the salivary and buccal secretions. Trans Clin Soc Lond 27:176–182
155. Wecker L de, Masselon (1891) Tumeurs symétriques des glandes lacrymales palpébrales et des parotides. Ann Ocul (Paris) 106:443–444
156. Fuchs E (1891) Gleichzeitige Erkrankung der Thränendrüsen und der Parotiden. Deutschmann's Beitr Augenheilkd 3:8, Abstract (1892) in Rev Gén Ophtalmol 11:323–324
157. Mikulicz J von (1892) Über eine eigenartige symmetrische Erkrankung der Thränen- und Mundspeicheldrüsen. Beitr Chirurg (Festschr Th Billroth) 2:610–630
158. Fraser (1893) Xerostomia (mouth dryness) with dryness of the nose and eyes. Edinburgh Hosp Rep, vol I. Abstract (1894) in Rev Gén Ophtalmol (Fr) 13:44–45
159. Haeckel H (1902) Beitrag zur Kenntnis der symmetrischen Erkrankung der Thränen- und Mundspeicheldrüsen. Arch Klin Chirurg 69:191–203
160. Gougerot H (1925) Insuffisance progressive et atrophie des glandes salivaires et muqueuses de la bouche, des conjonctives, (et parfois des muqueuses nasale, laringée, vulvaire): Sécheresse de la bouche, des conjonctives, vulvaire, etc. Bull Soc Franç Dermatol Syphil (Paris) 32:376–379
161. Sjögren H (1930) Keratoconjunctivitis sicca. Hygiea. Quoted by Sjögren [108]
162. Sjögren H (1940) Keratoconjunctivitis sicca. In: Modern Trends in Ophthalmology. Butterworth, London
163. Hippocraticum Corpus (5th–4th century B.C.) Köiakaì prognóseis (Cos' prenotions), sect 21, no 433
164. Isidorus Hispalensis (7th century A.D.) Ethimologiarum, liber IV, chap VII
165. Fischer E (1889) über Fädchenkeratitis. Graefes Arch Ophthalmol 35:201–215
166. Isakowitz J (1928) Die endocrine Periarthritis (Umber) und Keratitis filiformis. Klin Monatsbl Augenheilkd 81:85–86
167. Sjögren H (1933) Zur Kenntnis der Keratoconjunctivitis sicca (Keratitis filiformis bei Hypofunktion der Tränendrüsen) Acta Ophthalmol Suppl (Copenh) 2:1–151
168. Rothman S, Block M, Hauser FV (1951) Sjögren's syndrome associated with lymphoblastoma and hypersplenism. Arch Dermatol Syphilol 63:642–643
169. Talal N, Bunim JJ (1964) The development of malignant lymphoma in the course of Sjögren's syndrome. Am J Med 36:529–540
170. Fye KH, Terasaki PI, Moutsopoulos HM, Daniels TE, Michalski JP, Talal, N (1976) Association of Sjögren's syndrome with HLA-B8. Arthritis Rheum 19:883–886

171. Hinzowa E, Ivanyi D, Sula K, Horejs J, Dostal C, Drizhal I (1977) HLA-Dw3 in Sjögren's syndrome. Tissue Antigens 9:8–10
172. Anderson JR, Gondie RB, Gray KG, Buchanan WW (1961) Antibody to thyroglobulin in patients with collagen diseases. Scott Med J 6:449
173. Alspaugh MA, Talal N, Tan EM (1976) Differentiation and characterization of autoantibodies and their antigens in Sjögren's syndrome. Arthritis Rheum 19:216–222
174. Kassan SS, Akizuki M, Steinberg AD, Reddick RL, Chused TM (1977) Antibody to a soluble acidic nuclear antigen in the Sjögren's syndrome. Am J Med 63:328–334
175. Frost Larsen K, Isager H, Manthorpe R (1978) Sjögren's syndrome treated with bromhexine: a randomised clinical study. Br Med J 1:1579–1581
176. Gratwohl AA, Moutsopoulos HM, Chused TM, Akizuki M, Wolf RO, Sweet JB, Deisseroth AB (1977) Sjögren-type syndrome after allogeneic bone-marrow transplantation. Ann Intern Med 87:703–706
177. Lawley TJ, Peck GL, Moutsopoulos HM, Gratwohl AA, Deisseroth AB (1977) Scleroderma, Sjögren-like syndrome, and chronic Graft-versus-host disease. Ann Intern Med 87:707–709
178. Manthorpe R, Permin H, Tage Jensen U (1979) Auto-antibodies in Sjögren's syndrome with special reference to liver-cell membrane antibody (LMA). Scand J Rheumatol 8:166–172
179. Moutsopoulos HM, Webbe BL, Vlagopoulos TP, Chused TM, Decker JL (1979) Differences in the clinical manifestations of Sicca-Syndrome in the presence and absence of rheumatoid arthritis. Am J Ophthalmol 66:733–736
180. Fox RI, Robinson C, Curd J et al. (1986) First International Symposium on Sjögren's syndrome: Sugested criteria for classification. Scand J Rheumatol (Suppl) 61:28–30
181. Murube del Castillo J, Cortés Rodrigo MaD (1989) Eye parameters for the diagnosis of xerophthalmos. Clin Exp Rheumatol 7:145–150
182. Lutz A (1931) Über die nervösen Bahnen der Tränenabsonderung. Graefes Arch Ophthalmol 126:304–337
183. Baum JL, Feingold M (1973) Ocular aspects of Goldenhar's syndrome. Am J Ophthalmol 75:250–257
184. Bietti GB (1963) Irido-pupillare Anomalien und Xerosis conjunctivae. Klin Monatsbl Augenheilkd 143:321–331
185. Meyer HJ (1965) Dysgenesis mesodermalis und Xerosis conjunctivae. Klin Monatsbl Augenheilkd 147:26–31
186. Ullrich O (1949) Turner's syndrome and status Bonnevie-Ullrich. Am J Hum Gen 1:179
187. Holly FJ, Lemp MA (1977) Tear physiology and dry eyes. Surv Ophthalmol 22:69–87
188. Allen JC (1968) Congenital absence of the lacrimal punctum. J Pediatr Ophthalmol 5:176–178
189. Caccamise WC, Townes PL (1980) Congenital absence of the lacrimal puncta associated with alacrima and aptyalism. Am J Ophthalmol 89:62–65
190. Homer (8th century B.C.) Odyssey, cant 4, vers 219–230
191. Magaard H (1882) Über das Sekret und die Sekretion der menschlichen Thränendrüse. Virchows Arch Pathol Anat 89:258–271
192. Arruga Liró H (1943) La conjuntivitis seca. Arch Soc Oftal Hisp Am 2:68–71
193. Ridley F (1928) An antibacterial body present in great concentration in tears, and its relation to infection of the human eye. Proc R Soc Med 21:55–65
194. Ruprecht KW, Loch EG, Giere W (1976) Sandgefühl der Augen und hormonale Kontrazeptiva. Klin Monatsbl Augenheilkd 163:198–204
195. Buonfiglio Marabottini R (1978) Esame qualitativo del film precorneale in rapporto alla sintomatologia, etiopatogenesi e terapia delle sue alterazioni. Minerva Oftalmol 20:255–261

196. Carreras Matas M (1974) Mogadón, aspirina y secreción lagrimal: Observaciones clínicas. Arch Soc Españ Oftalmol 34:883–886
197. Sidi Y, Douer D, Pinkhas J (1977) Sicca syndrome in a patient with toxic reaction to busulfan. JAMA 238:1951. Abstract (1977) in Am J Ophthalmol 85:276–277
198. Turut P, Hache JC, François P, Arnott G (1977) Les complications ophtalmologiques du Pexid. Bull Soc Ophtalmol Fr 77:1003–1007
199. Brückner MR (1949) L'effect de la dihydro-ergotamine dans un cas d'hypersétion lacrymale. Ann Ocul (Paris) 182:464
200. Maes JE (1938) The effect of the removal of the superior cervical ganglion on lacrhymal secretion. Am J Physiol 123:359
201. Keller HH (1978) Nospilin, ein neues Präparat zur Lokaltherapie allergisches und entzündlicher Erkrankungen des äusseren Auges. Praxis (Switz.) 45:1661–1664
202. Vale J, Gibbs ACC, Phillips CI (1972) Topical propranolol and ocular tension in the human. Br J Ophthalmol 56:770–775
203. Sanz López A (1981) Historia de la Dacriología. Thesis Doctoralis, University of Madrid
204. Jaensch PA (1925) Ein Blastom der Orbita vom Habitus eines karzinomatösen Parotismischtumor. Klin Monatsbl Augenheilkd 74:716–723
205. Rollet J (1936) La couche de liquide pré-cornéenne. Arch Ophtalmol (Paris) 53:5–24, 111–134, 255–280
206. Barraquer Moner JI (1964) Etiología y patogenia del pterigion y de las excavaciones de la córnea de Fuchs. Arch Soc Am Oftalmol Optom 5:49–60
207. Fuchs E (1911) Über Dellen in der Hornhaut. Graefes Arch Ophthalmol 78:82–92
208. Bernard P (1843) Mémoire sur un nouveau moyen de guérir les fistules lacrymales et les larmoiements chroniques réputés incurables. Ann Ocul (Belg) 10:193–209
209. Hyrtl J (1847) Handbuch der topographischen Anatomie. Braumüller, Vienna
210. Bahr G von (1941) Könnte der Flüssigkeitsabgang durch die Cornea von physiologischer Bedeutung sein? Acta Ophthalmol (Copenh) 19:125–134
211. Maurice DM, Mishima S (1961) Evaporation from the corneal surface. J Physiol 155:49–50
212. Mishima S, Maurice DM (1961) The oily layer of the tearfilm and evaporation from the corneal surface. Exp Eye Res 1:39–45
213. Ehlers N (1967) A calculation of the average tear flow. Acta Ophthalmol (Copenh) 45:273–274
214. Iwata S, Lemp MA, Holly FJ, Dohlman CH (1969) Evaporation of water from the precorneal tear film and cornea in the rabbit. Invest Ophthalmol Vis Sci 8:613–619
215. Santos Fernández J (1903) Las enfermedades de los ojos en un pais cálido. Arch Oftalmol Hisp Am 3:153–192
216. Wyon NN, Wyon DP (1987) Measurement of acute response to draught in the eye. Acta Ophthalmol (Copenh) 65:385–392
217. Borel G (1894) Histéro-traumatismes oculaires. Rev Gén Ophtalmol (Fr) 13:227–229
218. García Mansilla S (1907) Manifestaciones secretorias del histerismo en el aparato de la visión. Arch Oftalmol Hisp Am 7:71–72
219. Kristensen EB, Norn M (1974) Benign mucous membrane pemphigoid. I. Secretion of mucus and tears. Acta Ophthalmol (Copenh) 52:266–281
220. Hamano H, Hamano T, Hamano T, Hori M, Kawabe H, Mitsunaga S (1980) Observations of the precorneal tear film of Sjögren's syndrome by bio differential interference microscope. Folia Ophthalmol Japon (Gan ki) 31:753–755
221. Kilp H, Schmid E, Vogel A (1982) Tränenfilmuntersuchungen im Spiegelbezirk. Klin Monatsbl Augenheilkd 80:49–52
222. Edmund J (1951) Photoelectric measurement of the corneal gloss. Danish Science, Copenhagen, p 136
223. Graves (1923) Trans Ophthalmol Soc UK 43:386. Quoted by Norn
224. Pflüger E (1882) Zur Ernährung der Cornea. Klin Monatsbl Augenheilkd 20:69–81

225. Straub M (1888) Fluoreszinlösung als ein diagnostisches Hilfsmittel für Hornhauterkrankungen. Centralbl Augenheilkd 12:75–77
226. Schirmer O: Quoted by Sjögren [167]
227. Römer P, Gebb, Löhlein W (1914). Quoted by Marx [232]
228. Kleefeld G (1920) Une nouvelle coloration des ulcères cornéennes. Quoted by Förster [230]
229. Stenstam T (1947) On occurrence of keratoconjunctivitis sicca in cases of rheumatoid arthritis. Acta Med Scand 127:139–148
230. Förster HW (1951) Rose bengal test in diagnosis of deficient tear formation. Arch Ophthalmol (Chicago) 45:419–424
231. Bijsterveld OP van (1969) Diagnostic tests in sicca syndrome. Arch Ophthalmol (Chicago) 82:10–14
232. Marx E (1924, 1926) Über vitale Färbungen am Auge und an der Lidern. Graefes Arch Ophthalmol 114:465–482, 116:114–125
233. Norn MS (1968) Bromo thymole blue. Acta Ophthalmol (Copenh) 46:231–242
234. Norn MS (1973) Lissamine green. Vital staining of cornea and conjunctiva. Acta Ophthalmol (Copenh) 51:483–491
235. Hess V von (1892) Graefes Arch Ophthalmol 38:1. Quoted by Mulock Houwer [126]
236. Nuel JP (1892) La kèratite filamentaire. Arch Ophtal (Paris) 12:593–623
237. Fraunfelder FT, Wright P, Tripathi RC (1977) Corneal mucus plaques. Am J Ophthalmol 83:191–197
238. Dohlman CH, Friend J, Kalevar V, Yagoda D, Balazs E (1976) The glycoprotein (mucus) content of tears from normal and dry eye patients. Exp Eye Res 22:359–365
239. Ollendorff A (1900) Über die Rolle der Mikroorganismen bei der Entstehung der neuroparalytischen Keratitis. Graefes Arch Ophthalmol 49:456–509
240. Marx E (1921) De la sensibilité et du déssèchement de la cornée. Ann Ocul (Paris) 158:774–789
241. Go Ing Hoen, Marx E (1926) Sur le déssèchement de la cornée. Ann Ocul (Paris) 163:334–358
242. Norn MS (1969) Desiccation of the precorneal film. I. Corneal wetting time. II. Permanent discontinuity and Dellen. Acta Ophthalmol (Copenh) 47:865–880, 881–889
243. Girard LG, Moore CD (1969) Dry spots of the cornea. In: Luntz MH (ed) Proc First S Afric Int Ophthalmol Symp. Butterworth, London, p 25
244. Brown SI (1970) Further studies on the pathophysiology of keratitis sicca of Rollet. Arch Ophthalmol (Chicago) 83:542–547
245. Lemp MA, Hamill JR (1973) Factors affecting tear film break-up time in normal eyes. Arch Ophthalmol 89:103–105
246. Marquardt R, Wenz FH (1980) Untersuchungen zur Tränenfilmstabilität. Klin Monatsbl Augenheilkd 176:879–884
247. Mengher LS, Bron AJ, Tonge SR, Gilbert DJ (1984–1986) Non-invasive assessment of tear film stability. In: Holly FJ (ed) The preocular tear film. Dry Eye Institute, Lubbock, p 64–75
248. Klein M (1949) The lacrimal strip and the precorneal film in cases of Sjögren's syndrome. Br J Ophthalmol 33:387–388
249. García Calderón A (1887) Afectos lagrimales. Rev Espec Oftalmol Sifil Dermatol Afec Urin 11:3–18
250. Demtschenko S (1872) Zur Innervation der Thraenendrüse. Pflügers Arch Ges Ophthalmol 6:191. Abstract (1873) in Ann Ocul (Paris) 69:65–66
251. Tepliachine (1894) Recherches sur les nerfs sércrétoires de la glande lacrymale. Arch Ophtalm (Paris) 14:401–413
252. Köster G (1900) Klinischer und experimenteller Beitrag zur Lehre von der Lähmung des Nervus facialis. Dtsch Arch Klin Med 68:343–382
253. Beetham WP (1935) Filamentary keratitis. Trans Am Ophthalmol Soc 33:413–435

254. Henderson JW, Prough W (1950) Influence of age and sex on flow of tears. Arch Ophthalmol (Chicago) 43:224–231
255. Jones LT (1966) The lacrimal secretory system and its treatment. Am J Ophthalmol 62:47–60
256. Jacobs HB (1959) Symptomatic epiphora. Br J Ophthalmol 43:415–434
257. Royer J, Deschamps F, Roth A (1979) Intérêt d'une notation échelonnée du test de Schirmer pour le diagnostic des syndromes secs. Bull Soc Ophthalmol Fr 79:665–667
258. Sjögren H: Quoted by De Rötth [147]
259. Hashimoto M, Otsuka H, Chinen Y, Azuma R (1963) A new Schirmer test using phenol-red paper strip. Folia Ophthalmol Japon (Gan Ki) 14:337–340
260. Casado González M (1971) Contribución al estudio de las correlaciones histofuncionales entre la glándula lagrimal y las glándulas salivales. Rev Clin Españ 122:211–216
261. Holly FJ, Beebe WE, Esquivel ED (1984) Lacrimation kinetics in humans as determined by a novel technique. In: Holly FJ (ed) The preocular tear film. Dry Eye Institute, Lubbock, Texas, p 76–78
262. Kupihashi K, Yanagihara N, Honda Y (1977) A modified Schirmer test: the fine-thread method for measuring lacrimation. J Pediatr Ophthalmol 14:390–397
263. Singh K, Jain IS (1973) Basic lacrimal secretion test. Ophthalmologica 166:306–310
264. Scherz W, Doane MG, Dohlman CH (1974) Tear volume in normal eyes and keratoconjunctivitis sicca. Graefes Arch Ophthalmol 192:141–150
265. Gruzdew VF (1939) Zur Methodik der funktionellen Diagnostik des Tränenapparats. Abstract in Zentralbl Ges Ophthalmol 43:566
266. Frieberg T (1941) Einige physiologische Gesichtspunkte zur Behandlung der Tränenwege. Acta Ophthalmol (Copenh) 19:93
267. Nover A, Jaeger W (1952) Kolorimetrische Methode zur Messung der Tränensekretion (Fluorescein-Verdünnungstest). Klin Monatsbl Augenheilkd 121:419–425
268. Kirchner C (1964) Untersuchungen über das Ausmaß der Tränensekretion beim Menschen. Klin Monatsbl Augenheilkd 144:412–417
269. Mishima S, Gasset A, Klyce SD, Baum JL (1966) Determination of tear volume and tear flow. Invest Ophthalmol 5:264–276
270. González de la Rosa M, Serrano García M, Cardona Guerra P, Hernández Calzadilla C (1981) Cuantificación de la lacrimación: nuevo método fluorofotométrico. Arch Soc Canar Oftalmol 6:32–39
271. Norn MS (1965) Lacrimal apparatus tests. A new method (lacrimal streak dilution test) compared with previous methods. Acta Ophthalmol (Copenh) 43:557–566
272. Norn MS (1966) Lacrimal apparatus test. Acta Ophthalmol (Copenh) 43:557–565
273. Bozóky L, Korchmáros I (1962) Über die Untersuchung der Tränenableitung mittels radioaktiver Isotope. 7th annual meeting Ophthalmol Ges, Vienna, pp 164–167
274. Rossomondo RM, Carlton WH, Trueblood JH, Thomas RP (1972) A new method of evaluating lacrimal drainage. Arch Ophthalmol (Chicago) 88:523–525
275. Sörensen T, Taagehoj Jensen F (1975) Determination of tear flow using a radiactive tracer. Acta Ophthalmol (Suppl) (Copenh) 125:43–44
276. Cabezas JA, Porto JV, Frois MD, Marino C, Arzua J (1964) Acide sialique dans les larmes humaines. Biochim Biophys Acta 83:318–325
277. McDonald JE (1968) Surface phenomena of tear films. Trans Am Ophthalmol Soc 66:905–939
278. Norn MS (1983) External eye. Methods of examination. Scriptor, Copenhagen, p 77
279. Rolando M, Fernández Refojo M (1983) Tear evaporimeter for measuring water evaporation rate from the tear film under controlled conditions in humans. Exp Eye Res 36:25–33
280. Fourcroy AF de, Vauquelin LN (1791) Examen chimique des larmes et de l'humeur des narines. Ann Chim (Paris) 9:113–130
281. Frerichs FT (1846) In: Wagner R: Handwörterbuch der Physiologie, vol III, p 617

282. Haeringen NJ van, Glasius E (1976) The origen of some enzymes in tear fluid, determined by comparative investigation with two collection methods. Exp Eye Res 22:267–272
283. Liotet S, Cohen N, Diatkine-Daumezon S, Chatellier P (1979) Determination d'un profil protéique des larmes humaines et son intérêt pratique. Contactologia 1F:38–51
284. Dartt DA, Knox I, Palau A, Botelho SY (1980) Proteins in fluids from individual orbital glands and tears. Invest Ophthalmol Vis Sci 19:1342–1347
285. Berta A (1982) A polyacrylamide-gel electrophoretic study of human tear proteins. Graefes Arch Klin Exp Ophthalmol 219:95–99
286. Setten GB van, Viinikka L, Tervo T, Pesonen K, Tarkkanen A, Perheentuppa J (1989) Epidermal growth factor is a constant component of normal human tear fluid. Graefes Arch Ophthalmol 227:184–187
287. Solé A (1955) Die Stagoskopie der Tränen. Klin Monatsbl Augenheilkd 126:446–451
288. Tabbara KF, Okumoto M (1982) Ocular ferning test. A qualitative test for mucus deficiency. Ophthalmology 89:712–714
289. Balík J (1952) The lacrimal fluid in keratoconjunctivitis sicca. A quantitative and qualitative investigation. Am J Ophthalmol 35:773–782
290. Holly FJ, Patten JT, Dohlman CH (1977) Surface activity determination of aequous tear components in dry eye patients and normals. Exp Eye Res 24:479–491
291. Wells PA, Ashur ML, Foster CS (1986) SDS gradient polyacrylamide gel electrophoresis of individual ocular mucus samples from patients with normal and diseased conjunctiva. Curr Eye Res 5:823–831
292. Rindello (1936) Ricerche sul Lysozim in rapporto ad alcune questioni interessanti dell'oftalmologia. Boll Ocul. Ref (1937) in Br J Ophthalmol 21:388
293. Massart J (1889) Sensibilité et adaptation des organismes a la concentration des solutions salines. Arch Biol 9:515. Quoted by Cantonnet [296]
294. Hamburger (1906). Quoted by Cantonnet [296]
295. Janssen PT, van Bijsterveld OP (1983) A simple test for lacrimal gland function: a tear lactoferrin assay by radial immunodiffusion. Graefes Arch Klin Exp Ophthalmol 220:171–174
296. Cantonnet A (1908) Formules de collyres isotoniques aux larmes. Arch Ophthalmol (Paris) 28:617–621
297. Mastman GJ, Baldes EJ, Henderson JW (1961) The total osmotic pressure of tears in normal and various pathological conditions. Arch Ophthalmol (Chicago) 65:509–513
298. Lecha Marzo A (1916). Quoted by Alvarez de Toledo [395]
299. Cerrano E (1909) Ricerche fisico-chimiche sulle lacrime in relazione alla prática dei collirii. Arch Farmacol Sper Sci Affin 8:347–358
300. Cifarelli PS, Bennett MJ, Zaino EC (1966) Sjögren's syndrome: A case report with an additional diagnostic aid. Arch Intern Med 117:429–431
301. Chisholm DM, Mason DK (1968) Labial salivary gland biopsy in Sjögren's disease. J Clin Pathol 21:656–660
302. Tarpley TM, Anderson LG, White CL (1974) Minor salivary gland involvement in Sjögren's syndrome. Oral Surg 37:64–74
303. Tanabe M, Hasegawa E, Matsuo N, Tamai T, Satoh K, Kojima K, Sato CH, Murakami TH (1984) Lacrimal gland accumulation of 67Ga citrate in patients with Sjögren's syndrome. Eur J Nucl Med 9:233–236
304. Egberg PR, Lambert S, Maurice DM (1977) A simple conjunctival biopsy. Am J Ophthalmol 84:798–801
305. Marner K (1980) Snake-like appearance of nuclear chromatin in conjunctival epithelial cells from patients with keratoconjunctivitis sicca. Acta Ophthalmol (Copenh) 58:849–853
306. Prause JU, Marner K (1986) Snake-like nuclear chromatin in imprints of conjunctival cells from patients with Sjögren's syndrome. In: Holly FJ (ed) The

preocular tear film in health, disease and contact lens wear. Dry Eye Institute, Lubbock, pp 167–161

307. Vergés Roger C, Pita Salorio D (1988) Estudio de la población de células caliciformes conjuntivales en los síndromes de ojo seco mediante un método citológico atraumático. Arch Soc Españ Oftalmol 55:525–530

308. Holm S (1949) Keratoconjunctivitis sicca and the sicca syndrome. Acta Ophthalmol (Suppl) (Copenh) 33:1–230

309. Martínez M (1775) Anatomía completa del hombre, con todos los hallazgos, nuevas doctrinas, y observaciones raras chap III: De las lágrimas. Escribano, Madrid, pp 441–446

310. Bernheim J (1893) Über die Antisepsis des Bindehautsackes und die bakterienfeindliche Eigenschaft der Thränen. Deutschmann's Beitr Augenheilkd 8:61

311. Kristensen HK, Zilstorff Pedersen K (1953) Acta Otolaryngol (Stockh) 43:537. Quoted by Boberg Ans J (1955) Corneal sensitivity and the naso-lacrimal reflex after retrobulbar anesthesia. Br J Ophthalmol 39:705–726

312. Giardini A, Roberts JRE (1950) Concentration of glucose and total chloride in tears. Br J Ophthalmol 34:737–743

313. Potts AM (1970) Tearing and smog. Sight Sav Rev 40:193–195

314. Allansmith MR, Drell D, Anderson RP, Newman L (1971) Comparison of electrophoretic mobility of tear lysozyme in 50 subjects. Am J Ophthalmol 71:521–529

315. Betsch A (1928) Die chronische Keratitis filiformis als Folge mangelnder Tränensekretion. Klin Monatsbl Augenheilkd 80:618–623

316. Hallauer C (1930) Clinical and experimental examination of the lysozyme content of the conjunctiva and lacrimal fluid. Arch Augenheilkd 103:199–214

317. Cordella M, De Caro G (1965) Primi tentativi di terapia della sindrome di Sjögren con Fisalemina. Atti Soc Oftalmol Lombarda 2:141–147

318. Impicciatore M, Moraini G, Bertaccini G (1973) Action of eledoisin on human lacrimal secretion in normal and pathological conditions. Naunyn-Schmiedebergs Arch Pharmacol 279:127–131

319. Bietti GB, Capra P, De Caro G (1973) Zur Anwendung eines neuen Medikamentes, des Eledoisins, zur Behandlung der Keratoconjunctivitis sicca. Ber Dtsch Ophthalmol Ges 73:399–407

320. Munoa Roiz JL (1973) Tratamiento del síndrome de Goujerot-Sjögren mediante la asociación de fisalemín-eledoisina y medroxiprogesterona. Arch Soc Españ Oftalmol 33:507–512

321. Dartt DA, Baker AK, Vaillant C et al. (1984) Vasoactive intestinal polypeptide stimulation of protein secretion from rat lacrimal gland acini. Am J Physiol 247:502–509

322. Diaz G, Orzalesi N, Testa Riva F (1980) Stereological investigation of the effects of metaproterenol, pilocarpine and atropine administration on the human lacrimal gland. Exp Eye Res 30:291–298

323. Pesonen K, Alfthan H, Stenman UH, Viinikka L, Perheentuppa J (1986) An ultrasensitive time-resolved immunofluorometric assay of human epidermal growth factor. Ann Biochem 157:208–211

324. Tiburtius H, Merker HJ (1973) Über eine neue Behandlungsmöglichkeit der herabgesetzten Tränenproduktion. Klin Monatsbl Augenheilkd 162:535–539

325. Dioscorides (3rd century A.D.) Euporista (Home remedies) II, 47 (Unauthentic?)

326. Garau Alemany J (1881) De la hemeralopía y su frecuencia en el soldado. Rev Espe Oftalmol Sifil Dermatol Afec Urin 4:282–297, 339–353

327. Viusa S (1920) Las enfermedades oculares por carencia (avitaminosis). España Oftalmol (Málaga) 5:161–167

328. Vaughan DG (1954) Xerophthalmia. Arch Ophthalmol (Chicago) 51:789

329. Pirie A (1977) Effects of locally applied retinoic acid on corneal xerophthalmia in the rat. Exp Eye Res 25:297–302

330. Sorsby A (1944) Discussion to the communication of Ridley F: The tears. Br J Ophthalmol 28:195–198
331. Paganoni C (1961) La cocarbossilasi nel trattamento della sindrome di Gougerot-Howers-Sjögren. Ann Ottalmol 87:663–668
332. Nover A (1954) Tierexperimentelle Untersuchungen über die Regenerations- und Transplantationsfähigkeit der Tränendrüse unter lokalem und allgemeinem Hormonreiz (Thyroxin). Graefes Arch Ophthalmol 156:98–118
333. Brückner MR (1945) Über einen erfolgreich mit Perandren behandelten Fall von Sjögren'schen Symptomenkomplex. Ophthalmologica 110:37–42
334. De Roetth A (1950) The dry eye. Acta XVI Conc Ophthalmol Univ, London. Br Med Assoc I:456–464
335. Calmettes L, Deodati F, Planel, Bec P (1956) Influence de la sécrétion hormonale génitale sur les glandes lacrymales. Ann Ocul (Paris) 189:729
336. Werb A (1971) Unusual causes of epiphora. Br J Ophthalmol 55:559–564
337. Tabbara KF, Frayha RA (1983) Alternate day steroid therapy for patients with Sjögren's syndrome. Ann Ophthalmol 15:358–361
338. Charleux J (1968) Traitement de la maladie de Gougerot-Sjögren. Com Soc Ophthalmol Lyon. Ref (1968) in Ann Ocul (Paris) 201:1164
339. Drossos AA, Skopouli FN, Costopoulos JS, Papadimitriou CS, Moutsopoulos HM (1986) Cyclosporin A (Cy A) in primary Sjögren's syndrome: a double blind study. Ann Rheum Dis 45:732–735
340. Alcoati of Toledo (1160 A.D., 554 A.Hg) Yamá sive liber de oculis: Quinta Maqäla. Sevilla. Edited (1973) by Univ Salamanca
341. Pérez Lorenzo V (1934) Tratamiento local de la xerosis corneal por las vitaminas en solución oleosa. Arch Oftalmol Hisp Am 34:159–160
342. Aguilar Bartolomé JM (1957) El empleo de la metil celulosa en Oftalmología. Arch Soc Oftalmol Hisp Am 17:203–214
343. Swan KC (1944) Reactivity of the ocular tissues to wetting agents. Am J Ophthalmol 27:1118. Abstract (1945) in Arch Soc Oftalmol Hisp Am 5:406–407
344. Mims JL (1951) Methylcellulose solution for ophthalmic use. Arch Ophthalmol (Chicago) 46:664
345. Krishna N, Brow F (1964) Polyvinyl alcohol as an ophthalmic vehicle. Effect on regeneration of corneal epithelium. Am J Ophthalmol 57:99–106
346. Marquardt R (1986) Die Behandlung des trockenen Auges mit einem neuen tropffähigen Gel. Klin Monatsbl Augenheilkd 189:51–54
347. Gifford S, Puntenney I, Bellows J (1943) Keratoconjunctivitis sicca. Arch Ophthalmol (Chicago) 30:207–216
348. Hamilton B (1940) Keratitis sicca, including Sjögren's syndrome. Trans Ophthalmol Soc Austral 2:63, 1940. Quoted (1942) in Br J Ophthalmol 26:280–281
349. Bisantis C (1976) Emploi d'un collyre fait d'auto-serum dans les affections conjonctivales liées à une sécrétion lacrymale alterée. Ann Ocul (Paris) 209:759–762
350. Liotet S, Perrin, D (1982) Amélioration spectaculaire d'un syndrome sec sévère par instillation de colostrum. Bull Soc Ophthalmol Fr 82:15–16
351. André B (1979) Etude clinique du collyre à la chondroitine sulfate dans le cadre des syndromes de sécheresse oculaire. Med thesis, University of Nancy
352. DeLuise VP, Scott Peterson W (1984) The use of topical healon tears in the menagement of the refractory dry-eye syndrome Ann Ophthalmol 16:823–824
353. Filatov VP, Chevalyev VE (1951) Surgical treatment of the parenchymal xerosis (in Russian). J Oftalmol (Odessa) 3:131–137
354. Murube del Castillo J (1986) Transplantation of salivary gland to the lacrimal basin. Scand J Rheumatol (Suppl) 61:264–267
355. Weve H (1928). Quoted by Sjögren [108]
356. Absolon MJ, Brown CA (1968) Acetyl-cysteine in keratoconjunctivitis sicca. Br J Ophthalmol 52:310–316
357. Michel J von (1884) Lehrbuch der Augenheilkunde, 1st edn. Wiesbaden, p 500

358. Charlton CF (1920) The function of the protein in the lacrimal secretion. Am J Ophthalmol 3:802–804
359. Sapse AT, Bonavida B, Stone FW, Sercarz EE (1969) Proteins in human tears. Immunoelectrophoretic patterns. Arch Ophthalmol (Chicago) 81:815–819
360. Liegl O (1965) Zur Therapie der Keratitis filiformis. Klin Monatsbl Augenheilkd 147:883–884
361. Johnson LV, Nosik WA (1951) Greater superficial petrosal neurectomy for relief of chronic bullous keratitis. Arch Ophthalmol (Chicago) 45:32–37
362. Wright RE (1927) Maladie de Mikulicz traitée par les rayons X. Am J Ophthalmol 10:903. Ref (1928) in Ann Ocul (Paris) 165:776
363. Montero Iruzubieta J, González Latorre M, Díaz Ruiz C, Montero Marchena J (1988) Modificaciones del test de Schirmer en la querato-conjuntivitis seca (QCS) tras tratamiento con láser He-Ne. Estudio a doble ciego. Arch Soc Españ Oftalmol 54:813–818
364. MacLean AL (1945) Sjögren syndrome. Bull Johns' Hopkins Hosp 76:179. Quoted by Sjögren [108]
365. Flynn F, Schulmeister A (1967) Keratoconjunctivitis sicca and new techniques in its management. Med J Austral 1:33–41
366. Trevor Roper PD (1967) The Frank Flynn tear-supplying spectacles. Trans Ophthalmol Soc UK 87:105–107
367. Dohlman CH, Doane MG, Reshmi CS (1971) Mobile infusion pumps for continuous delivery of fluid and therapeutic agents to the eye. Ann Ophthalmol 3:126–128
368. Charleux J, Brun P (1973) Glandes lacrymales artificielles. Bull Soc Ophtalmol Fr 73:5–6, 683–686
369. Rosen J, Brown SI (1974) A simple moist chamber. Am J Ophthalmol 78:859–860
370. Poirier RH, Ryburn MF, Israel ChW (1977) Swimmer's goggles for keratoconjunctivitis sicca. Arch Ophthalmol (Chicago) 95:1405–1406
371. Savar DA (1978) A new approach to ocular moisture chambers. J Pediatr Ophthalmol 15:51–53
372. Gasset AR, Kaufman HF (1971) Hydrophilic lens therapy of severe keratoconjunctivitis sicca and conjunctival scarring. Am J Ophthalmol 71:1185–1189
373. Buller F (1876). Quoted by Larena Gómez (396)
374. Römer P (1899) Experimentelle Untersuchungen über Infektion vom Conjunctivalsack aus. Z Hygiene 294–328. Cited in Záboj Bruckner (1924) Lacrimal passages in the guinea pig and rabbit. Br J Ophthalmol 8:158–165
375. MacMillan JA, Cone W (1937) Prevention and treatment of keratitis neuroparalytica by closure of the lacrimal canaliculi. Arch Ophthalmol (Chicago) 18:352–355
376. Rashid RC (1987) Rashid argon laser caniculoplasty. Abstracts 1st meeting Int Soc Dakryol Budapest, p 18
377. Foulds WS (1961) Intracanalicular gelatin implants in the treatment of keratoconjunctivitis sicca. Br J Ophthalmol 45:625–627
378. Freeman JM (1975) The punctum plug: Evaluation of a new treatment for the dry eye. Trans Am Acad Ophthalmol Otolaryngol 79:874–879
379. Adams AD (1978) Silicone plug for punctum occlusion. Trans Ophthalmol Soc UK 98:499–499
380. Bernard JA, Fayet B, Pouliquen Y (1989) Nouveaux modèles de clous méatiques et de pose-clous. Bull Soc Ophthalmol Fr 89:1131–1132
381. Patten JT (1976) Punctal occlusion with N-butyl-cyanoacrylate tissue adhesive. Ophthalmic Surg 7:24–26
382. Murube del Castillo J (1986) Ectropionization of the lacrimal punctum in Sjögren's syndrome. Scand J Rheumatol (Suppl) 61:268–269
383. Lamberts D (1987) Punctal occlusion. Int Ophthalmol 27:44–46
384. Murube del Castillo J (1988) Tratamiento del xeroftalmos con transplantes de glándula salival. Arch Soc Españ Oftalmol 54:151–164

385. Murube del Castillo J, Bahamón Caycedo M (1990) Transplante de glándula sublingual en pacientes con ojo seco. Estudio histológico postoperatorio. Tiempos Méd, Anuario 4:224–231
386. Herzog V, Sies H, Miller F (1976) Exocytosis in secretory cells of rat lacrimal gland. Peroxidase release from lobules and isolated cells upon cholinergic stimulation. J Cell Biol 70:692–706
387. Hann LE, Tatro JB, Sullivan DA (1989) Morphology and function of lacrimal gland acinar cells in primary culture. Invest Ophthalmol Vis Sci 30:145–158
388. Weil BA, Milder B (1985) Sistema lagrimal. Dacriología básica: diagnóstico y tratamiento de sus afecciones chap 13: El ojo seco. Med Panamericana, Buenos Aires, p 124
389. Milder B, Weil BA (1983) The lacrimal system. Appleton-Century-Crofts, Norwalk
390. Harris EK (ed) (1989) The Sjögren's syndrome handbook. USA
391. Wood CA (1917) The Am Encycl Diction Ophthalmol, vol XI. Cleveland Press, Chicago, pp 8576–8577
392. Liotet S, van Bijsterveld OP, Blétry O, Chomette G, Moulias R, Arrata M (1987) L'oeil sec. Masson, Paris
393. Paton L (1926) El trigémino y sus lesiones oculares. Br J Ophthalmol 10:305
394. Brocq L (1888) De la dermatite herpétiforme de Duhring. Ann Dermatol Syphilogr (2nd ser) 9:1–20
395. Alvarez de Toledo R (1917) Sobre el valor práctico del signo de Lecha Marzo, para el diagnóstico de la muerte real. Libr Guevara, Granada
396. Larena Gómez C (1982) Estudio histopatológico y ultraestructural secuencial del ojo seco experimental. Thesis, University of Barcelona

Chapter 2

Functional Morphology of the Conjunctiva

J.W. Rohen and E. Lütjen-Drecoll

1 Conjunctiva

The eyelids, which serve as a protective device for the eye (Fig. 1), moisten the surface of the cornea by producing a 10-μm-thick tear film. When this film is washed off in rabbits, the corneal thickness immediately decreases (Fig. 2). If the corneal surface is covered with lipids secreted by the meibomian glands, the thickness of the cornea remains unchanged, even if the lids stay open [2]. These experiments show that the precorneal tear film prevents desiccation of the cornea, and that its lipid layer plays a most essential role in maintaining this function.

When the lacrimal gland is removed in rabbits, keratinization of the corneal epithelium occurs. This shows that the aqueous layer is important for the maintenance of corneal transparency. The adherence of the lipid and aqueous layer of the corneal surface requires a mucous layer sticking to the epithelial cells of the corneal epithelium, whose surface is enlarged by microvilli and microplicae. If this mucous layer produced mainly by goblet cells is absent, the tear film no longer adheres and the cornea is damaged. Thus, the precorneal tear film consists of three layers which are produced by different glands of the conjunctiva (Fig. 3).

The conjunctiva represents a mucous membrane which is readily movable both against the eyeball and the eyelids due to its loose stroma containing a dense network of elastic fibers. An important prerequisite for this gliding movement between eyelids and eyeball, which may occur independently of each other, is the preocular tear film which covers the mucous membrane of the conjunctiva and prevents desiccation of the conjunctiva. Another essential task of the conjunctiva is immunological defense against antigens such as viruses, bacteria, or particles. The conjunctival epithelium not only possesses special cells involved in immunological reactions, such as Langerhans' cells, but also contains numerous lymphocytes penetrating the epithelial lining. In many places lymphatic follicles develop within the conjunctival tissue, which contains T and B lymphocytes, various subtypes of reticular cells, and macrophages. In contrast to the eye, the conjunctiva possesses its own lymphatic drainage system.

M.A. Lemp/R. Marquardt (Eds.) The Dry Eye
© Springer-Verlag Berlin Heidelberg 1992

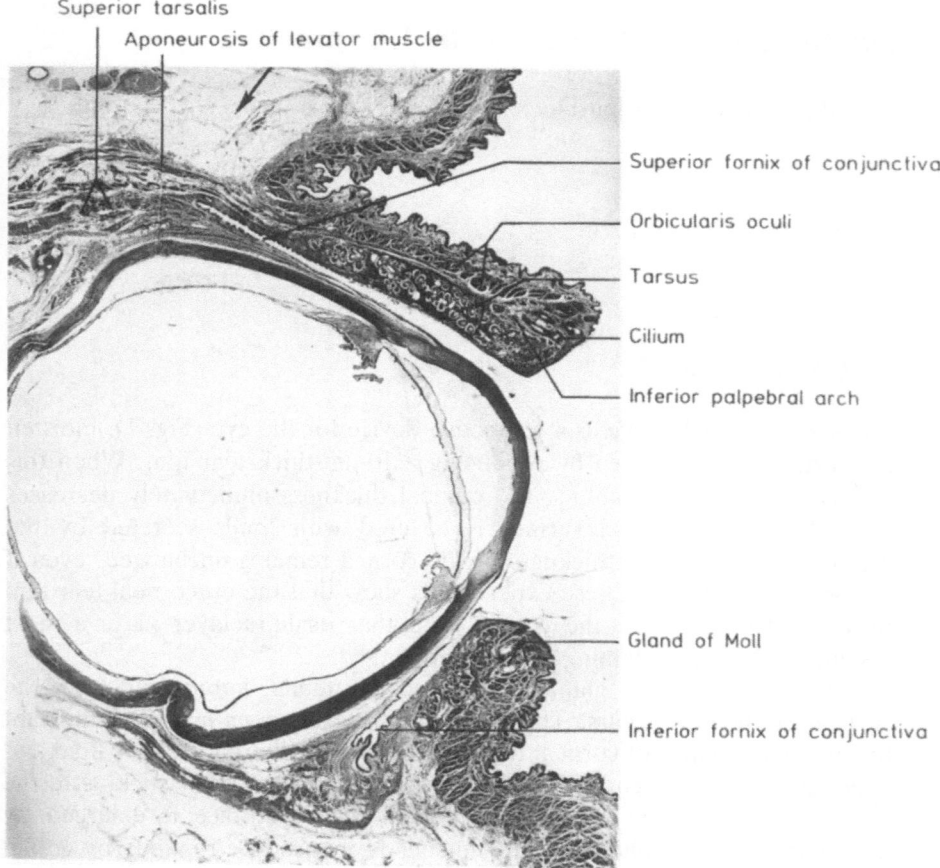

Fig. 1. Sagittal section through the bulb of the eye with upper and lower lids (35-year-old man). (Azan stain, ×4; from [1])

Finally, the conjunctiva is able to absorb a wide range of different substances, and its regenerative power is remarkable. Injuries to the cornea can be healed quickly using cell reserves from the bulbar conjunctival epithelium. Moreover, the conjunctiva is richly innervated so that it can protect the eye from damage due to environmental influence. It is the source of reflexes, including simple protective reactions (increase in lacrimal secretion), movements of eyeballs and lids, general body movements, escape mechanisms, and intentional actions.

1.1 Tear Film

The tear film of the conjunctiva can be subdivided into a smaller precorneal tear film which covers the corneal surface and a somewhat thicker preocular

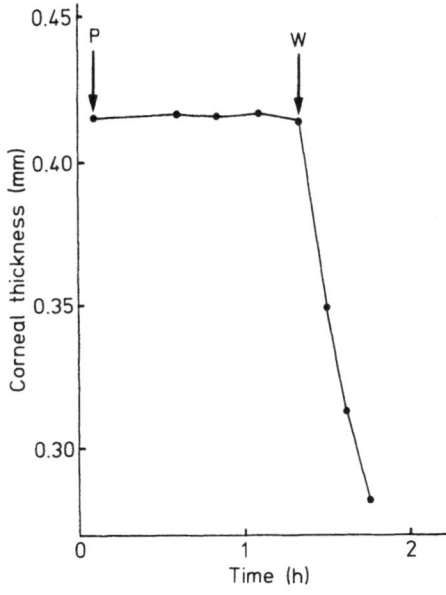

Fig. 2. Change in corneal thickness (rabbit). *P*, Eye proptosed; *W*, corneal surface washed with physiological saline. (From [2])

tear film covering the conjunctival epithelium. The thickness of the precorneal tear film varies between 4 and 10 μm, becoming thinner due to evaporation when the eyes are open (Fig. 3). Under normal conditions, the tear fluid comes from the palpebral glands (so-called basal secretion), which secretes about 1–2 μl liquid per minute (total volume 7–9 μl). Brandt and Fritsche [7] calculated an average secretion of 9.5 μl/day. In cases of corneal irritation, emotional excitement, or irritation by foreign bodies, the tear secretion (now coming mainly from the lacrimal gland) can increase 20–30 times (so-called reflex secretion). According to Jaeger [5] the precorneal tear film fulfills five tasks:

- It protects the cornea from desiccation.
- It maintains the refractive power.
- It plays a role in the immunological defense mechanisms against infections.
- It enhances the oxygen permeation into the cornea.
- It supports corneal dehydration due to its hyperosmolarity.

Basically, the precorneal tear film consists of three layers. The main part is the aqueous layer (thickness 8 μm), which is covered by a thin lipid layer (thickness 0.1 μm). The lipids, which represent a mixture of different lipids (phospholipids, cholesterol ester, neutral fat, etc.), are produced mainly by the meibomian glands of the upper and lower eyelid, but the glands of Zeis and Moll also contribute to this secretion. The lipid mixture would, however, not spread on the aqueous layer of the tear film if it did not contain a surface-active carbohydrate component, the hydrophilic terminal chains of which permit the formation of a monolayer on water. The tear film regenerates in two phases. First the aqueous fluid is spread when the lids

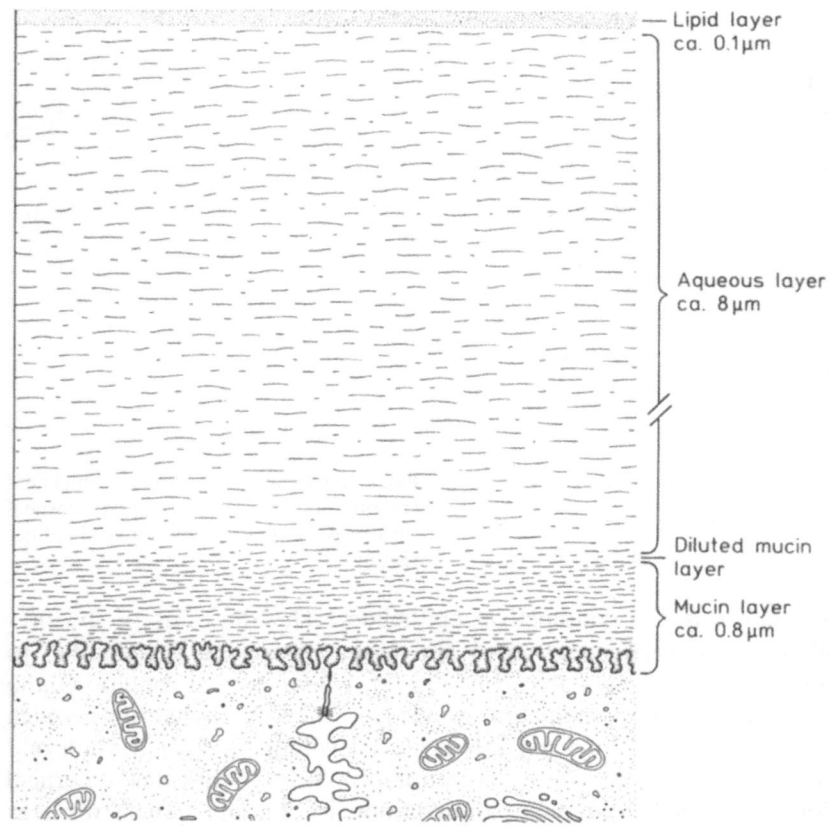

Fig. 3. Schematic diagram of the precorneal tear film. (From [4])

are closed; subsequently, when the lids are opened, the secretion of the meibomian glands is spread over the aqueous layer.

The aqueous layer of the tear film is approximately 8 μm thick and consists of water, electrolytes, and organic substances, among which there are about 30 different proteins [3,6]. Exfoliated epithelial cells, lymphocytes, and remnants of cells are also found within the aqueous layer. Tear-specific proteins are lactoferrin, lysozyme, prealbumin, and immunoglobulins. Normally a serum protein deriving from the conjunctival vasculature does not penetrate into the lacrimal fluid, but it is found in cases of conjunctivitis, sicca syndrome, and other pathological situations. Approximately one-third of the tear-specific proteins are prealbumins, which are of special importance for the stability of the film. During reflex secretion their production may be greatly increased. The immunoglobulins come mainly from the conjunctiva and consist basically of IgA and IgG (Table 1).

Table 1. Immunoglobulins in tear film compared to serum. (From [8])

Immunoglobulins	Tear film (mg/100 ml)	Serum (mg/100 ml)	Proportion tear film serum
Total protein	800	6.500	1:8
IgG	14	1.000	1:70
IgA	17	170	1:10
IgM	<5	100	<1:18
IgD	<1	11	1:11
IgE	250 ng/ml	2.000 g/ml	1:8

In pathological situations, an increased amount of immunoglobulins are secreted by the lacrimal gland, whose interstitium contains numerous lymphocytes and plasma cells. The lacrimal fluid also contains proteases and plasminogen activators as well as bactericidal proteins (lysozyme, β-lysine, lactoferrin) which are produced particularly in the lacrimal gland. The unspecific bacterolytic protein lysozyme is found in relatively high concentrations (1–2 g/l). Due to the fact that its concentration during reflex secretion can rise by 100%, lysozyme secretion was considered as a functional test for the lacrimal gland. Moreover, the lacrimal fluid is rich in other specific substances, such as histamine (approximately 10 mg/ml), prostaglandins, and catecholamines (dopamine, epinephrine, norepinephrine) [9]. From a functional point of view, the mucous layer of the tear film is of special importance. This layer measures about 0.8 µm in the precorneal tear film and about 1.4 µm in the preocular tear film [10]. The hydrophilic mucous is bound to the glycocalyx covering the surface of the corneal epithelial cells. It contains sialomucins (glycoproteins), which are generally thought responsible for the decrease in the surface tension [10,11]. By reducing the surface tension, an even distribution of liquid on the corneal surface is achieved. This is a prerequisite for the optical properties of the cornea. Together with the tear film lipids, the mucins reduce the surface tension to about 58 dyne/cm (Fig. 4), so that it becomes possible to moisten the otherwise hydrophobic corneal epithelial lining with water. Similar mechanisms play a role in other parts of the body as well in the respiratory or circulatory system.

1.2   Structure of the Conjunctival Epithelium

The conjunctival epithelium covers the conjunctival sac completely. It joins the corneal epithelium at the limbus and the epidermis at the lid margin (Fig. 1). Normally it is differentiated between a marginal conjunctiva (up to 2 mm away from the lid rim, near the area of the meibomian gland ducts), a tarsal conjunctiva covering the posterior surface of the upper and lower lids,

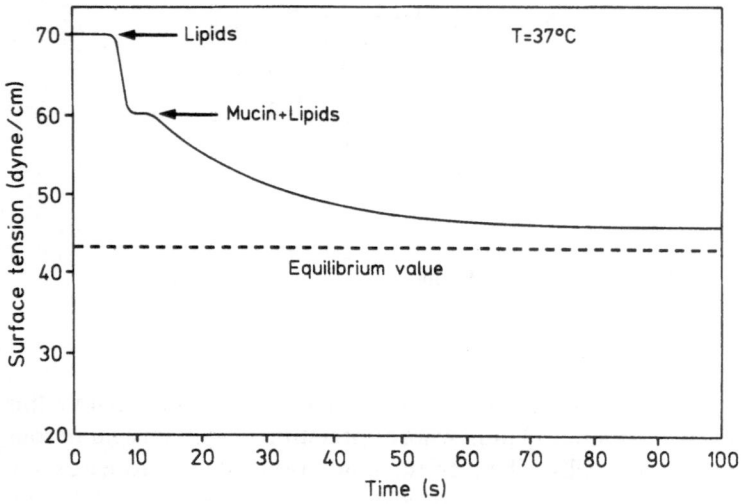

Fig. 4. Kinetics of spreading of a lipoid-mucin mixture. The distance between the spreading source and the tension sensor is 55 cm. (From [9])

a fornical conjunctiva, and a bulbar conjunctiva covering the eyeball. On the lid rim, the stratified, keratinized epithelium of the skin merges into the multilayered nonkeratinized squamous epithelium of the marginal conjunctiva. The epithelium of the tarsal conjunctiva consists of two or three rows of cells. The deeper (basal) layer is composed of cuboidal cells, and the superficial layer consists of tall cylindrical cells. In advanced age the epithelium flattens. In the bulbar conjunctiva the epithelium is gradually transformed into the five-layered, nonkeratinized squamous epithelium of the cornea. The total surface of the conjunctival sac measures 17.65 cm² in humans, whereas 1.04 cm² is apportioned to the corneal surface [12,13]. As a consequence of the corneal surface being larger in the rabbit, the relationship of the conjunctiva to cornea is only half of that in humans.

A varying number of mucus-producing goblet cells are dispersed in the conjunctival epithelium (Fig. 5). Within the tarsal conjunctiva, goblet cells often lie close to one another, thus forming into endothelial glands with small ductlike openings (so-called crypts of Henle; diameter 10–60 μm; Fig. 6). Using scanning electron microscopy, a polygonal pattern of cylindrical cells can be demonstrated, with goblet cells distributed randomly between them (Fig. 6). A kind of lawn consisting of microvilli (0.5–1 μm long and 0.4 μm thick) is found on the surface of the superficial cells. Dark, light, and medium-dark cells can be distinguished due to form and number of microvilli. The light cells carry a few, but relatively long microvilli whereas the dark ones possess short, thick microvilli [14,15].

The number of the goblet cells has often been examined, but with different methods. Marquardt and Wenz [16] found an average of 26–40 goblet cells per millimeter of conjunctival tissue in the fornix. According to

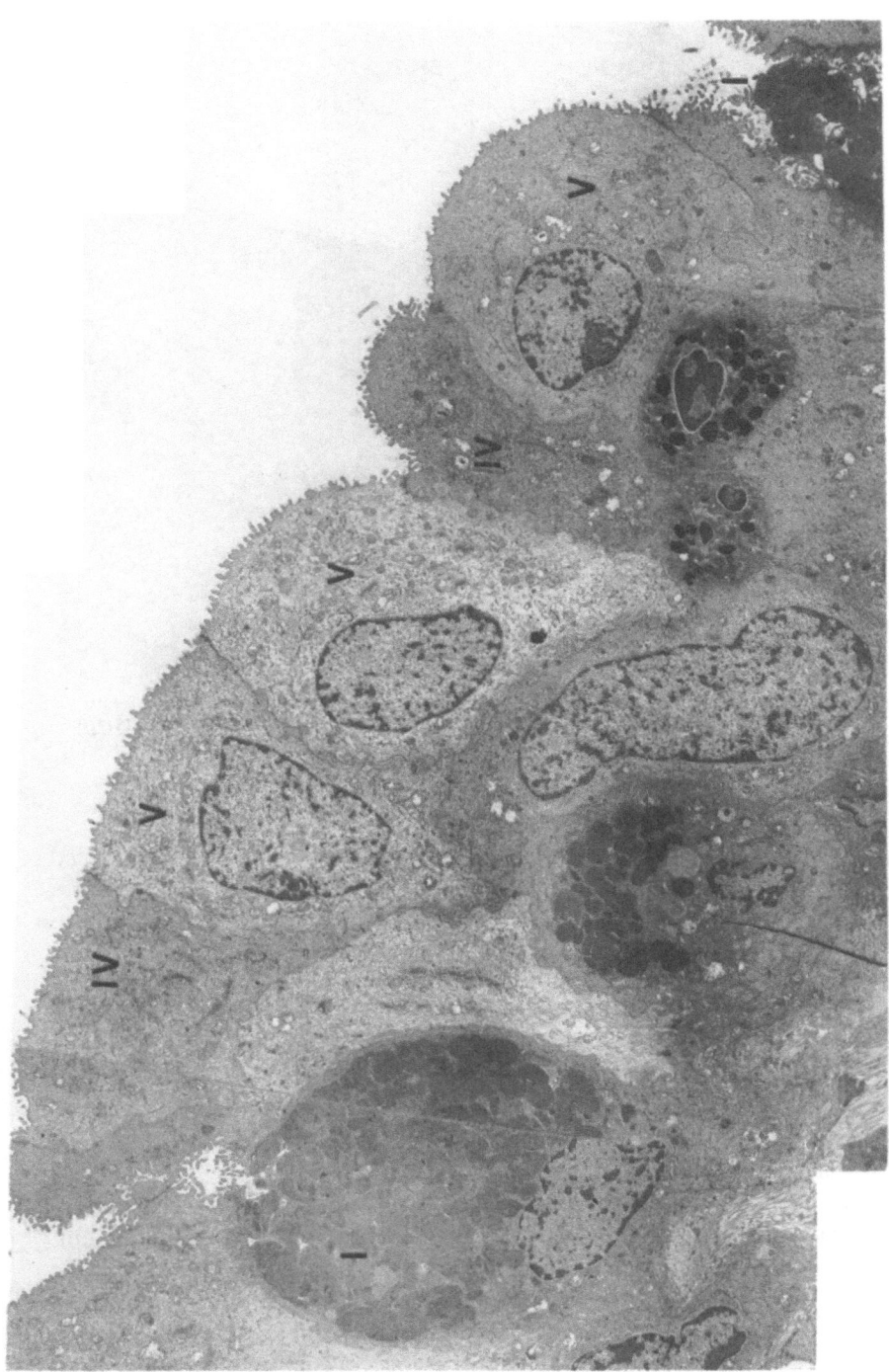

Fig. 5. Electron micrographs of the conjunctiva (composed figure, cynomolgus monkey). *I–V*, Different cell types (see Table 3). (×5000)

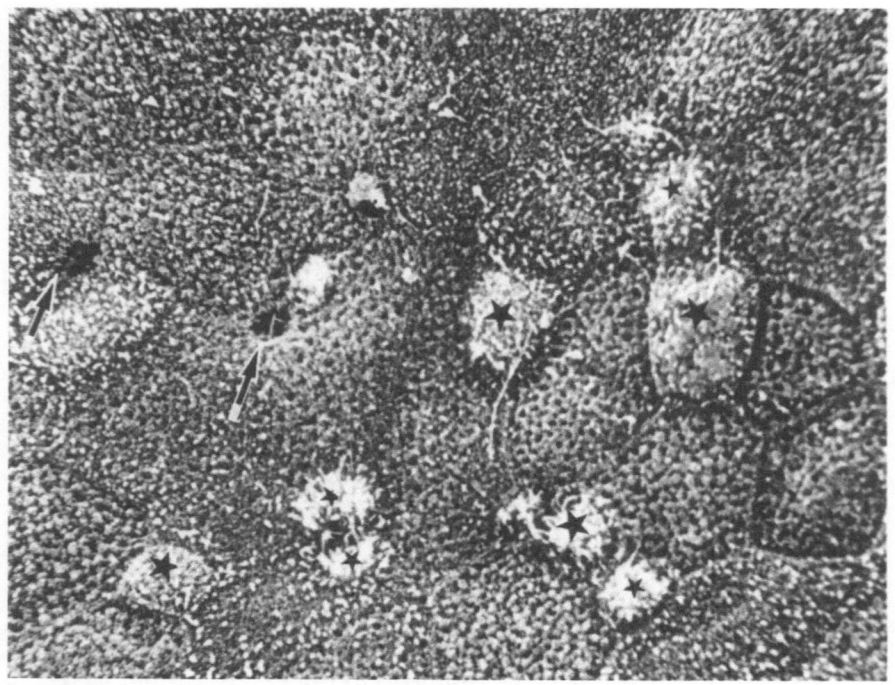

Fig. 6. Scanning electron micrograph of the surface of the human conjunctiva. *Arrows*, openings of Henle's crypts; *asterisks*, goblet cells. Note the numerous microvilli. (×950)

these authors, the number of goblet cells decreases only slightly in advanced age [16]. In places used mechanically (e.g., lid rims), goblet cells are rare, whereas in "quiet" areas (e.g., caruncula and plica semilunaris) their frequency is high. Goblet cells are found less frequently in the bulbar conjunctiva near the limbus than in the fornical or palpebral conjunctiva (Table 2). In case of radiation damage or inflammations, and particularly in the sicca syndrome, the number of goblet cells may be decreased considerably (Table 2). Using immunofluorescence techniques it has been demonstrated that the glycoproteins of the lacrimal fluid (GP_2 fraction, molecular weight approximately 1.3×10^6) are for the most part produced in the goblet cells and not in the lacrimal gland [18].

The regenerative capacity of the goblet cells is not completely clarified. When the corneal epithelium is experimentally removed, the bulbar epithelium grows from the limbus to the corneal surface and starts mitotic divisions. It is interesting to see that after 3–14 days goblet cells appear in the newly formed corneal epithelium although no goblet cells were found in this area before [19] (Fig. 7). Obviously, the regenerating stimulus must have triggered off capacities which could not be detected before. These

Table 2. Comparison of interpalpebral bulbar and inferior palpebral conjunctival goblet cell densities. (From [17])

	Density of goblet cells (cells/sq mm)	
	Interpalpebral bulbar ocular surface	Inferior palpebral ocular surface
Normal subjects	443 ($\pm$266)	1972 ($\pm$862)
KCS	102 ($\pm$139)	791 ($\pm$744)
Mild chemical burns	184 ($\pm$101)	1144 ($\pm$574)
Radiation KCS	45 ($\pm$46)	635 ($\pm$560)
Blepharitis and KCS (2nd degree)	138 ($\pm$110)	457 ($\pm$548)
COP	17 ($\pm$22)	99 ($\pm$130)
Stevens-Johnson syndrome	5 ($\pm$7)	43 ($\pm$96)
SLK	65 ($\pm$137)	140 ($\pm$192)
Atopic disease	82 ($\pm$11)	3 ($\pm$4)

KCS, keratoconjunctivitis sicca; COP, cicatricial ocular pemphigoid; SLK, superior limbic keratoconjunctivitis.

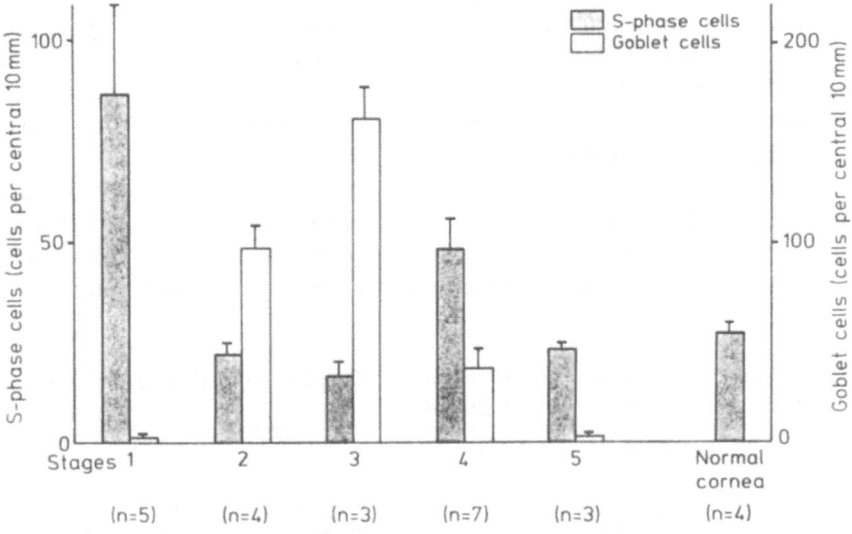

Fig. 7. S-phase cell and goblet cell frequency of regenerated conjunctival epithelium on cornea. *Bars*, standard error of the mean (*n*, number of samples). (From [18])

goblet cells disappear (after 6 weeks in rabbits) without the newly formed regeneration product of the cornea having cytologically taken over the characteristics of the previous corneal epithelium. This can also be confirmed by the changes occurring in the protein pattern, so that this phenomenon cannot be considered a metaplasia [20].

Cell types in the conjunctival epithelium: In older literature only two cells types are described: epithelial cells and goblet cells. There are, however, significantly more cell forms. Greiner et al. [21] were the first to describe a "second mucous secretory system;" Rohen and Steuhl [22] later characterized altogether five different cell forms which appear with a certain constancy in the conjunctival epithelium [23] (Table 3). Type I cells are goblet cells. They usually have numerous large mucin granules, a basal and often flattened nucleus, and a small basal cytoplasmic zone containing Golgi apparatus and endoplasmatic reticulum (Fig. 8A). Type II cells are seen as cells from secondary mucous-secretory system and are characterized by numerous small, electron-dense granules situated mostly in the apical cytoplasm. These granules contain predominantly acid glycosaminoglycans and proteins (Fig. 9B). Upon mechanical irritation, for example, by vehicles, the number of these cells increases, whereas the number of goblet cells decreases [24]. Type III cells are particularly rich in Golgi complexes, which are often situated near the nucleus. Specific granules are missing. The mitochondria are small and few in number. Type IV cells contain a large amount of rough endoplasmic reticulum, which fills most of the cytoplasm. These cells may produce various proteins normally found within the tear film (Fig. 8B). Type V cells stand out by their numerous mitochondria of the crista type, randomly distributed within the cytoplasm (Fig. 9A). Since mitochondria contain the enzymes of the respiratory chain and represent the ATP store, these cells are probably of special importance for the active energy-dependent ion transport of the epithelium.

Recently Lütjen-Drecoll et al. [25,26] have demonstrated by means of new histochemical methods that the stromal layer of the conjunctiva intensely stains for hyaluronic acid (Fig. 10), and that there is a continuous layer of hyaluronic acid on the surface of the conjunctiva. In addition, the

Table 3. Different cell types in the conjunctival epithelium, their morphological characteristics and possible functional significance

	Dominant characteristics	Products	Function
Type I (goblet cell)	Large mucin granula	Mucin, proteoglycans	Components of the tear film (mucin, etc.)
Type II	Small electron-dense granula	Acid glycosamino-glycans, glycoproteins	Components of the tear film (mucin, etc.)
Type III	Golgi complexes	?	Components of the tear film (mucin, etc.)
Type IV	Rough endoplasmic reticulum	Proteins, enzymes	Self-cleaning, defense
Type V	Mitochondria	–	Energy-dependent transport processes

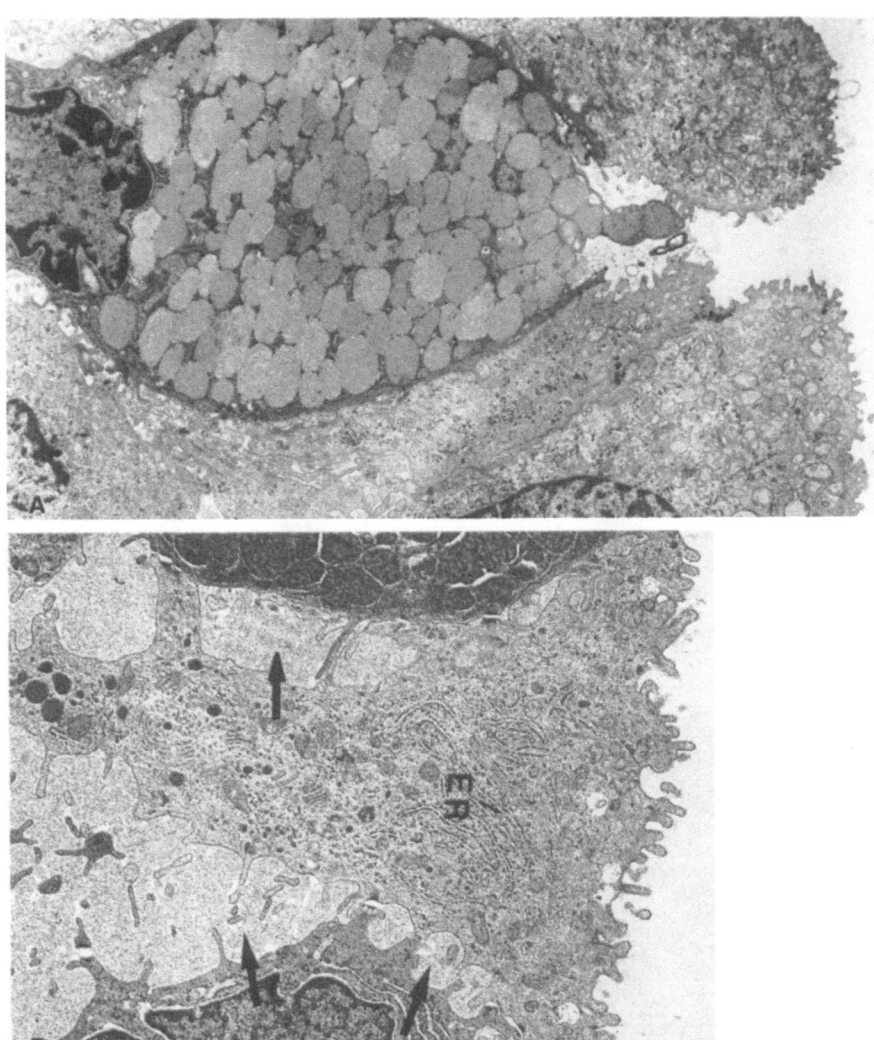

Fig. 8A,B. Electron micrographs of different cell types in the conjunctival epithelium of a cynomolgus monkey. **A** Type I cell (goblet cell; ×600); **B** Type IV cell (×12600). Note the great amount of rough endoplasmic reticulum (*ER*). The intercellular spaces (*arrows*) appear enlarged and filled with protein

related synthesizing enzyme hyaluronan synthase was found in the cell membranes of the bulbar, fornical, and palpebral conjunctiva. Only in the basal cuboidal cells near the basal lamina was no enzyme staining seen (Fig. 11). Another interesting finding was that the cornea epithelium also showed an intense positive staining for hyaluronan synthase, however only in the superficial and middle cell layers (Fig. 12). In the conjunctiva there

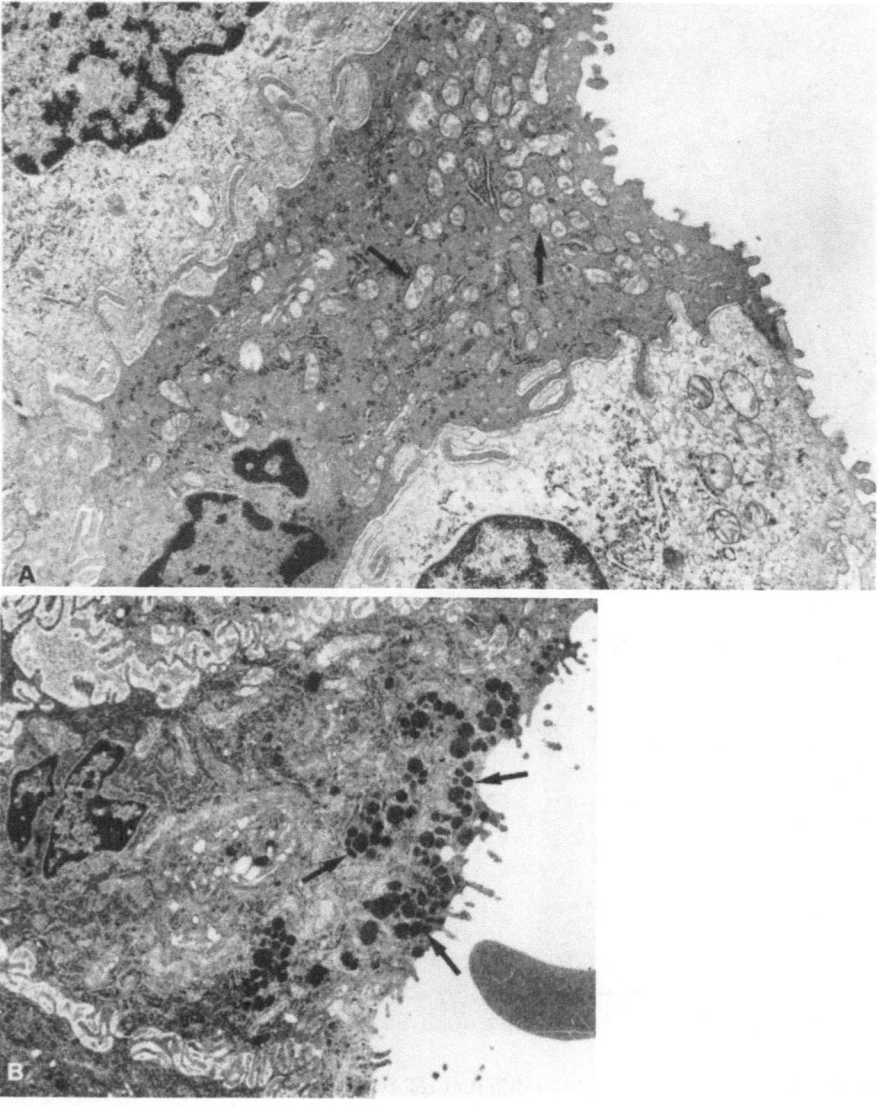

Fig. 9A,B. Electron micrographs of different cell types in the conjunctival epithelium of a cynomolgus monkey. **A** Type V cell (×8400). Note the great number of mitochondria (*arrows*). **B** Type II cell (×6000). Notice the electron-dense granules in the apical part of the cell (*arrows*)

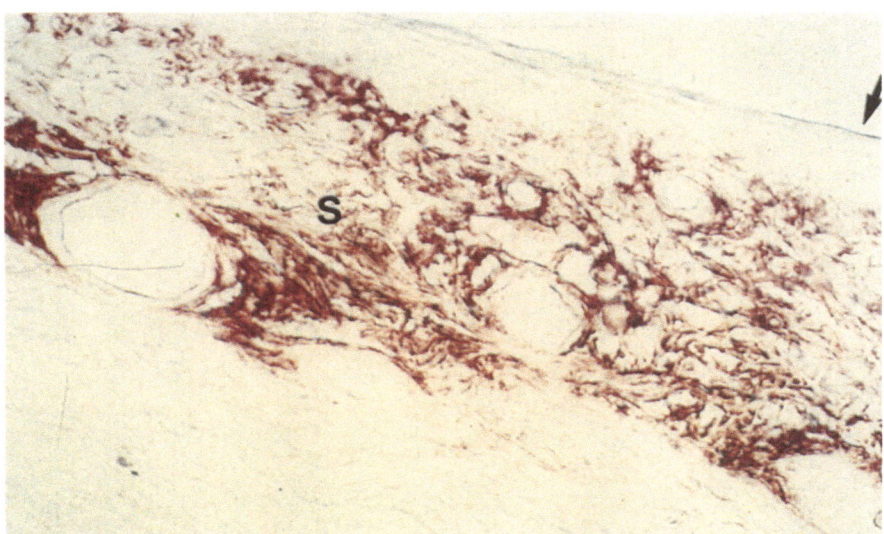

Fig. 10. Light micrograph of a paraffin section through the limbal conjunctiva of a rabbit eye, stained for hyaluronic acid (×160). The stroma of the conjunctiva shows an intense staining while the conjunctiva epithelium (*on top*) remains unstained. (From [25])

are two forms of goblet cells: those with and those without positive membrane staining for hyaluronan synthase [26]. Thus, a number of goblet cells may also be able to synthesize hyaluronic acid. The functional significance of hyaluronic acid in the conjunctiva and within the tear film is not clear. It may stabilize the tear film, impede desiccation of the mucous membrane, or fulfill mechanical functions.

1.3 Structure of the Limbal Region

In the transition zone of the bulbar conjunctiva to the cornea, the conjunctival epithelium becomes thicker and is gradually transformed into a stratified nonkeratinized squamous epithelium which, however, does not yet reveal the same regular pattern as the corneal epithelium (Fig. 13). The limbus epithelial cells are characterized by a well-developed cytoskeleton. They are connected to one another by numerous desmosomes. These structures may reflect the mechanical stress of the cells during eye movement. In contrast to the fornical conjunctiva, the epithelium of the limbal zone does not contain all five cell types described above; practically only types III and IV cells occur in this region. Goblet cells (type I) and cells rich in electron-dense granules (type II) are missing. Type IV cells containing large amounts of rough endoplasmic reticulum are rarely found, whereas cells of type V characterized by their large number of mitochondria occur very frequently

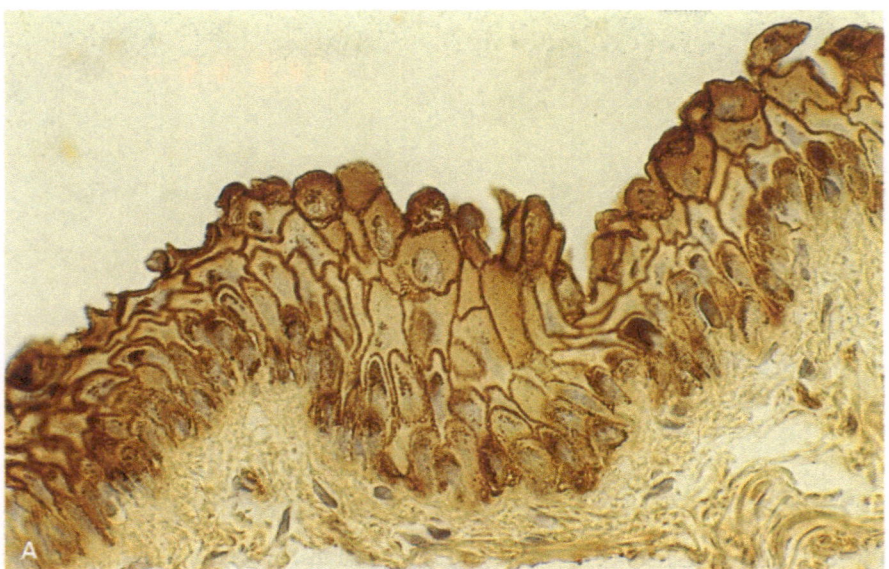

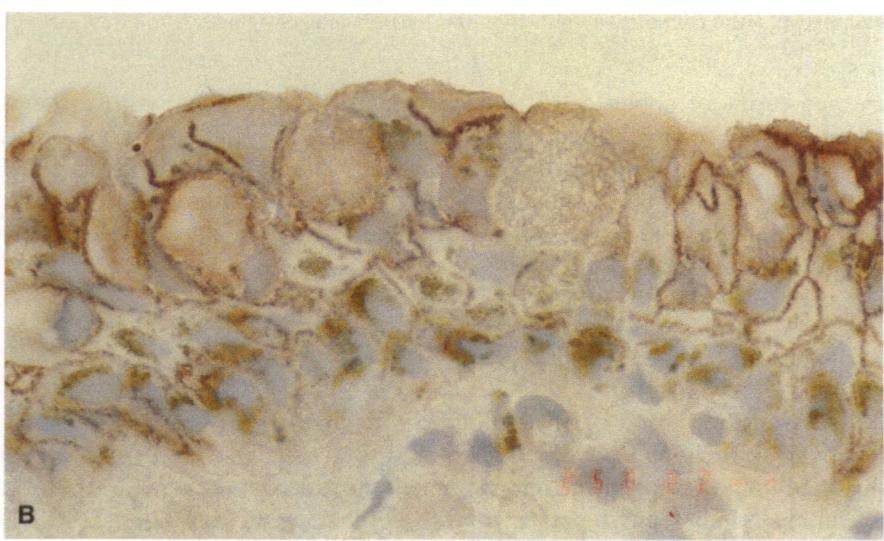

Fig. 11. A Light micrograph of the bulbar conjunctival epithelium. Immunohistochemical staining for hyaluronan synthase (cynomolgus monkey). The cell membranes of the epithelial cells reveal an intense positive staining for hyaluronan synthase. (×160; from [26]). **B** Light microcraph of the bulbar conjunctiva. Immunohistochemical staining for hyaluronan synthase (cynomolgus monkey). Notice that the conjunctiva epithelial cell membranes stain positively for hyaluronan synthase. The two goblet cells on the *left* also show a positive membrane staining, whereas the goblet cell on the *right* does not stain for this enzyme. (×250; from [26])

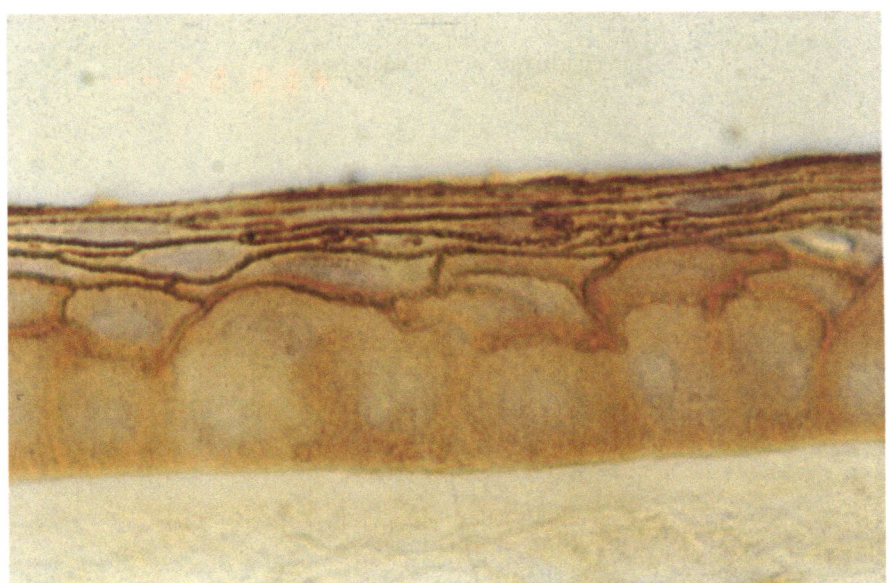

Fig. 12. Light micrograph of the cornea epithelium. Immunohistochemical staining for hyaluronan synthase (cynomolgus monkey). The cell membranes of the superficial and middle layer of the corneal epithelium reveal an intense staining for the enzyme; the basal cells remain unstained. (×400; from [26])

[27]. The energy delivered by the mitochondria is necessary for active energy-dependent ion or fluid transport in this region. Interestingly, the enzymes carbonic anhydrase and Na-K-ATPase, generally found in fluid transporting epithelia (e.g., renal tubules, ciliary epithelium, choroidal plexus epithelium), have also been demonstrated in the conjunctiva of the limbal zone. Membrane-bound Na-K-ATPase occurs in all cells of the limbus epithelium, whereas carbonic anhydrase could be detected only in the basal cells [27]. In the fornical and palpebral conjunctiva, carbonic anhydrase has been seen histochemically only in low concentrations or not at all. If present, the staining is also restricted to the basal cells [23,27,28]. In contrast, the enzyme hyaluronan synthase, which is clearly seen in the conjunctival epithelium, has not been found in the epithelium of the limbus, although hyaluronic acid is present here [25,26]. Hyaluronic acid is probably transported from the fornical conjunctiva to the limbus, but not produced there. The functional significance of ATPase and carbonic anhydrase found within the limbal epithelium is not clear. Raviola [29] observed a particularly high permeability of the limbus capillaries after injection of the tracer substances (e.g., horseradish peroxidase). Furthermore, the subconjunctival connective tissue is rich in lymphatic vessels which may drain fluid out of this region. The limbal conjunctiva is situated on the border of

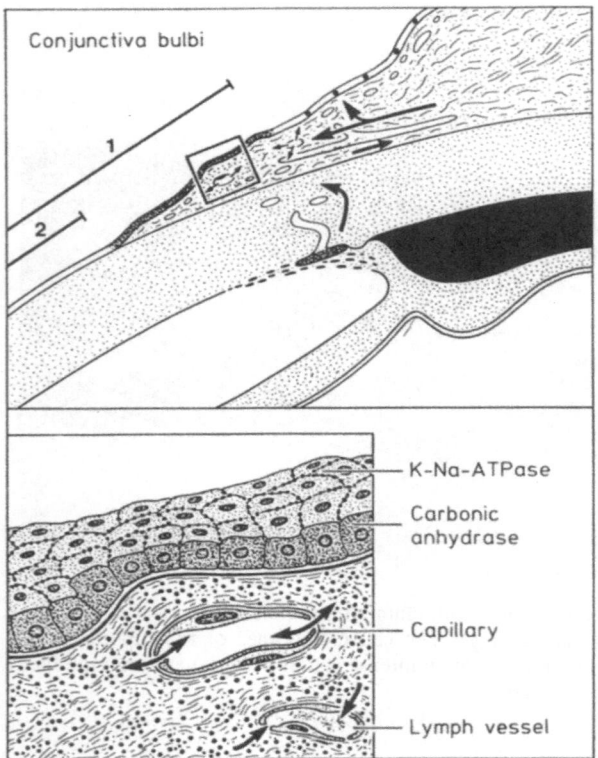

Fig. 13. Schematic diagram of the limbal conjunctiva. *Inset*, the distribution of K-Na-ATPase and carbonic anhydrase. *1*, Goblet cell free zone; *2*, zone of cornea epithelium; *arrows*, direction of flow. (From [27])

the dehydration zone of the cornea and might be involved in fluid transport, so that penetration of fluid into the cornea might be impeded effectively.

It is well known that the limbal conjunctiva is able to regenerate the corneal epithelium if it is damaged. This regeneration capacity is high and starts from the periphery. Recent experiments have shown that the regeneration takes place differently according to whether the distal part of the limbal epithelium (directly adjoined to the corneal epithelium) or the (proximal) bulbar zone is investigated. After the abrasion of the corneal epithelium of rabbits, the limbal epithelium grows rapidly onto the corneal surface. During the first days of regeneration, the enzyme carbonic anhydrase can be demonstrated only in the basal cells of the newly formed epithelial layer [4]. When the distal zone of the limbal epithelium is excluded from regeneration, vascularization of the cornea occurs, and goblet cells appear in the regeneration product [19,30].

1.4 Stroma of the Conjunctiva

The subepithelial connective tissue of the bulbar and fornical conjunctiva is wide-meshed, rich in tissue fluid, and well vascularized. It consists of a latticelike network of collagenous bundles and ground substance rich in hyaluronic acid [25,26]. Besides this, a dense network of elastic fibers exists within the stroma. The architecture of the different fiber systems can easily be explained by the mechanical stress during lid and eye movements. The palpebral conjunctiva is tightly bound to the tarsus and is hardly movable. Here, the collagenous and elastic fibers are radially orientated and more fixed within the tarsal plates.

1.5 Absorption Processes of the Conjunctiva

The bulbar and fornical conjunctiva possesses a high absorptive capacity. It has not yet been clarified whether the hyaluronic acid – present in abundance in the stroma – with its high water-binding capacity is functionally involved in the absorption processes. The superficial cells of the conjunctival epithelium possess numerous, low and irregularly distributed microvilli, often also microplicae, to which the tear film sticks. These organelles may play an important role in the absorption processes. The intercellular spaces are apically closed off by tight junctions (zonulae occludentes). In addition, two or three desmosomes are found here which connect the cells with one another to resist mechanical stress. In contrast to this, the middle and basal portion of the intercellular space is not closed off by junctional complexes so that it is easily able to dilate (Fig. 14). Often the intercellular spaces contain interdigitating cytoplasmic extensions or processes. This enlarges the surface of the interfaces and makes dilation easier. Using tracer substances it has been shown that the absorptive capacity of the conjunctiva is very high. Topically applied, labeled technetium is transported through the epithelium within 15 min of application [31,32]. When horseradish peroxidase, a relatively large molecule, is applied to the monkey conjunctiva, a few minutes later tracer-filled pinocytotic vesicles can be observed in the apical cytoplasm. The vesicles are transported to the gradually dilating intercellular spaces, where these tracer molecules accumulate (Figs. 15, 16). From the intercellular spaces the horseradish peroxidase can reach the stroma and the blood vessels unhindered [33] (Fig. 16). Latex particles can also be phagocytosed by the conjunctival epithelial cells and be transported via intercellular spaces to the stroma [34].

The ion exchange between conjunctiva, blood and potential changes has been measured by Maurice [35] using labeled ^{22}Na and ^{36}Cl.

Cations are moved to the outside; anions are normally moved to the inside of the mucous membrane. Theoretically, water should be absorbed, and by this the tear film would have to subside. But probably an outward-

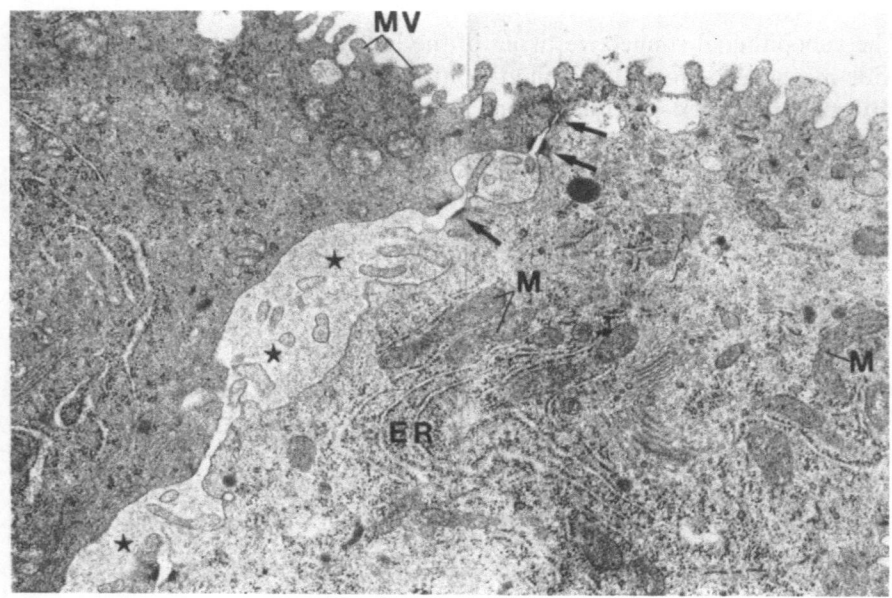

Fig. 14. Electron micrograph of the apical part of the conjunctival epithelium (cynomolgus monkey). Note the enlargement of the intercellular spaces (*asterisks*) and the site of junctional complexes (*arrows*). *ER*, Endoplasmic reticulum; *M*, mitochondria; *MV*, microvilli. (×22000)

directed chloride pump mechanism or the high water-binding capacity of the mucins and hyaluronic acid impedes a desiccation of the mucous membrane. Perhaps the type V cells rich in mitochondria [22,23], play also an important role in ion transport and in maintaining the ion balance between the membranes.

1.6 Vasculature and Innervation of the Conjunctiva

All parts of the conjunctiva are well vascularized. The palpebral conjunctiva receives its arterial supply by perforating branches of the arterial circle situated in the eyelids. A dense, generally elongated capillary network is formed immediately underneath the epithelium (Fig. 17A).

. The bulbar conjunctiva is supplied by the branches of the anterior ciliary arteries, which come from the region of the extraocular muscle tendons. They create a subepithelial wide-meshed, irregularly arranged capillary network (Fig. 17B). Electron-microscopically the capillary endothelium often shows fenestrations where the vessels adjoin the basal lamina of the epithelium. The fornical conjunctiva receives arterial branches from the palpebral and bulbar regions, which often anastomose with each other. The

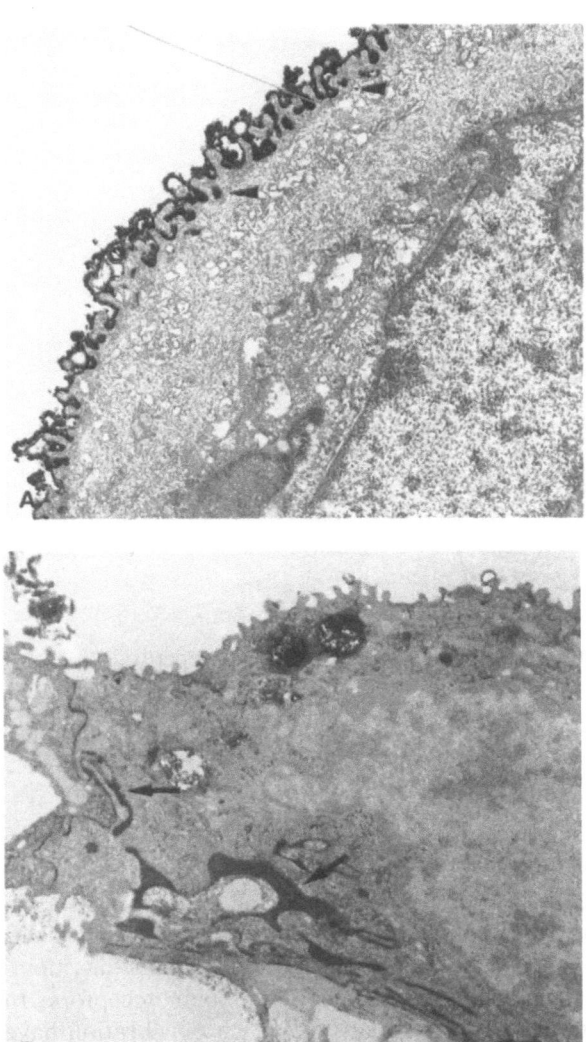

Fig. 15A,B. Electron micrographs of the conjunctival epithelium after application of horseradish peroxidase (HRP). **A** Cynomolgus monkey, 5 min after HRP treatment (×15 000). **B** Rabbit, 30 min after HRP treatment (×16 000). Note the location of the electron-dense reaction product. In **A** pinocytotic vesicles (*arrowheads*) are filled with HRP; in **B** the HRP is already found within the intercellular spaces (*arrows*)

arterial vessels are accompanied by veins, which are drained finally by the ophthalmic veins.

The innervation of the conjunctiva comes mainly from branches of the first branch of the trigeminal nerve. Their terminal branches come either from inside the eye or from episcleral nerves. The bulbar conjunctiva is

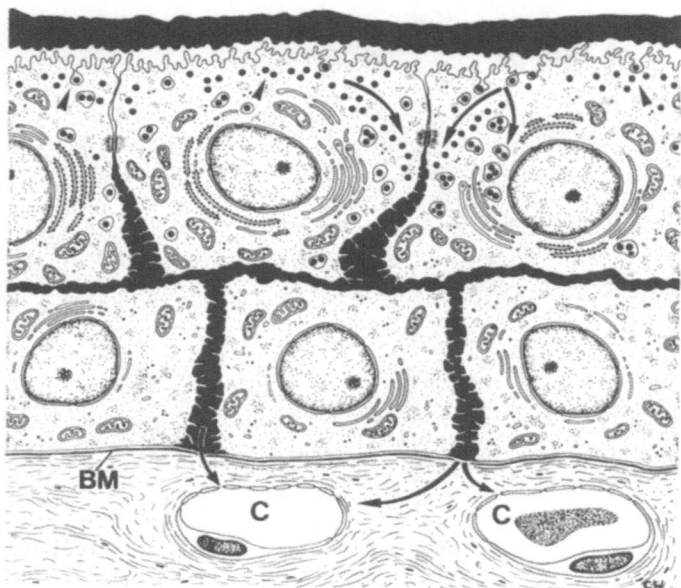

Fig. 16. Schematic drawing of the absorption pathways of horseradish peroxidase (*black*) through the conjunctival epithelium. The molecules are first transported through the apical portion of the epithelial cells, to bypass the apically located tight junctions. They reach then the expanding intercellular spaces and, from there the stromal layer. BM = Basement membrane; C = capillaries. (From [4])

supplied with branches of the long posterior ciliary nerves, which perforate the sclera in the limbus region and then run episclerally to the conjunctiva. In addition, nerves which come from the orbita reach the mucous membrane following the course of the anterior ciliary arteries. Sensory organs of different kinds have often been described in the conjunctival mucous membrane, and these have been classified as heat, cold, or pain receptors. In addition, mechanoreceptors and sensory organs for touch or vibration have been found [36].

1.7 Conjunctiva and Immunological Reactions

The conjunctiva, being a highly differentiated mucous membrane, is also involved in immunological defense mechanisms. Large dendritic cells (so-called Langerhans' cells) are found within the epithelium – just as in the epidermis – which probably originate from the bone marrow and migrate into the epithelium. They are able to present antigens of the mucous membrane to T-lymphocytes found near or within the mucous membrane. Normally, underneath the epithelium numerous small lymphatic follicles are developed, and lymphocytes can migrate from there into the epithelial

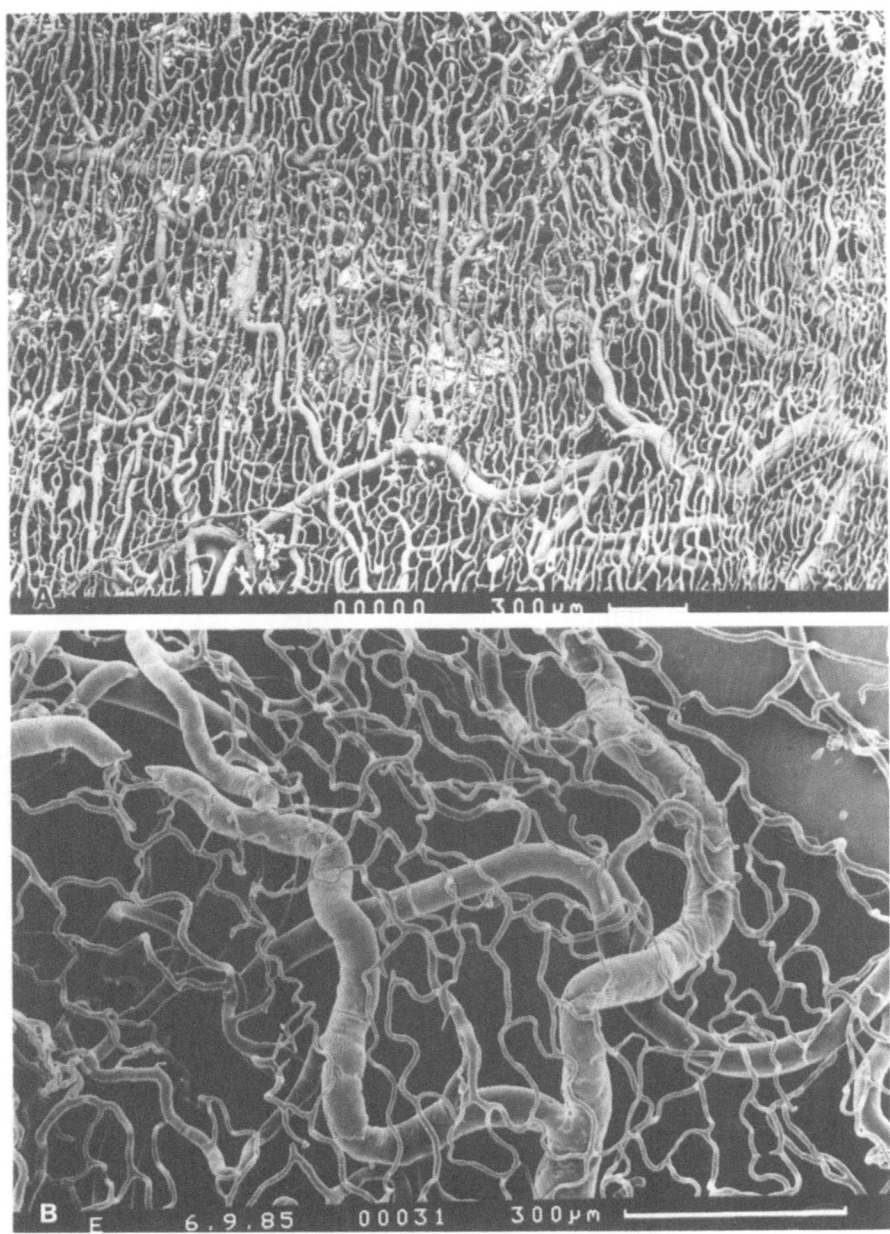

Fig. 17A,B. Scanning electron micrographs of corrosion casts of the conjunctival vasculature. **A** Palpebral conjunctiva of a cynomolgus monkey (*bar*, 300 µm). **B** Capillary network of the palpebral conjunctiva of a rabbit (*bar*, 300 µm)

layers. After antigen contact, T lymphocytes activate the B lymphocytes with the help of interleukins, so that these change into antibody-producing plasma cells. The conjunctiva always contains numerous plasma cells, which synthesize predominantly IgA and IgG. These immunoglobulins have been identified in the tear film (see Table 1). Especially the bulbar and fornical conjunctiva is rich in lymphocytes, which partially penetrate the epithelial layers and can be detected in the lacrimal fluid

2   Glands of Lids and Conjunctiva

2.1   Lid Glands

Normally, three morphologically and functionally different groups of lid glands can be distinguished (Fig. 18): the meibomian glands (glandulae tarsales), glands of Moll (glandulae ciliares), and glands of Zeis (glandulae ciliares accessoriae).

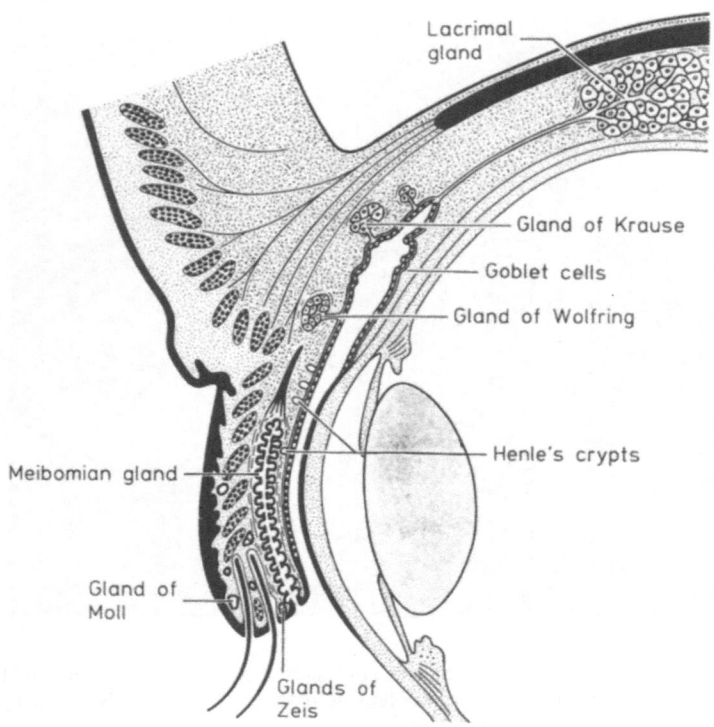

Fig. 18. Schematic drawing of site and distribution of accessory lacrimal glands

The meibomian glands are long sebaceous glands which during their development separate from the roots of the cilia or eyelashes. Their ducts terminate near the lid margin. The distal portion of the ducts is surrounded by muscle bundles which derive from the orbicularis oculi muscle of the lids (Riolan's muscle) [1,28]. The muscle bundles twist around the ducts and are able to squeeze the terminal portion of the ducts so that the sebaceous material is secreted onto the lid margin, preventing overflow of tears and leaving an oily film over the moistened cornea after blinking. The meibomian glands are the basic structure of the tarsal plates which otherwise consists of collagenous and elastic fibers surrounding the end pieces of the glands. The meibomian glands are arranged vertically parallel to one another, extending about 25 in number in the upper lid and 20 in the lower. Each consists of a central canal, into which open numerous rounded appendages that secrete the sebum. These appendages have a lobular or alveolar form. Their cells show all the characteristics of holocrine secretion, which contains mainly lipids and glycoproteins that are to be incorporated into the tear film.

The ducts consist of a stratified six-layered, squamous epithelium. Keratinization increases toward the lid margin, where the ducts are continuous with the epithelial lining of the lid margin. (For further details of secretory mechanisms and stimulation effect see the chapter by Dartt, this volume.)

The glands of Moll are considered to be specialized sweat glands, which differ from ordinary sweat glands in that their terminal portion is either straight or slightly coiled. The ducts, normally 1.5–2 mm in length, open into the follicles of the eyelashes. The epithelium of the terminal portion consists of two layers, an outer myoepithelial layer and an inner layer of pyramidal or cuboidal cells which contain a well-developed endoplasmic reticulum and numerous mitochondria. The glandular cells produce a secretion rich in proteins and lipoproteins the function of which is unknown. The type of secretory process is apocrine, where the lumen of the terminal portion appears considerably dilated, and the glandular cells are flattened after the apical portion of the cells have just been secreted into the duct.

The glands of Zeis are small, rudimentary sebaceous glands, morphologically comparable with the meibomian glands. They lie isolated within the distal portion of the eyelids near the lid margin. The number of these glands varies considerably. Their ducts open at the lid margin or into the follicle of the eyelashes. The ultrastructure of the holocrine glandular cells does not appear to be very different from that of the meibomian glands.

2.2 Accessory Lacrimal Glands

The accessory lacrimal glands are situated within the conjunctiva. They are usually named after the person who initially discovered them. The accessory lacrimal glands are believed responsible for the basal secretion of lacrimal fluid. Electron microscopy, immunohistochemistry, and histology have not shown essential, qualitative differences between the accessory glands and the lacrimal gland, although quantitative differences are present. However, there is one exception concerning S-100, the marker for derivatives of neural crest cells. Accessory glands were found to be positive for S-100 whereas lacrimal gland cells were negative for S-100. In addition, the number of myoepithelial cells is significantly smaller in accessory lacrimal glands than in the lacrimal gland proper. It is not known whether there are functional differences between these two groups of glands.

The glands of Krause are situated deep in the subconjunctival connective tissue. There are several fine ducts which unite into a rather long ductus which opens into the conjunctival fornix. The terminal portion of the duct can dilate, forming a little ampulla or sinus. Morphologically the acinus cells of the end pieces show the same structure as those of the lacrimal gland. Whether this is also true for their functional capacity is as yet undetermined.

The glands of Wolfring and Ciaccio are also accessory lacrimal glands but larger than Krause's glands. They are for the most part situated in the upper border of the tarsus or in the tarsus between the extremities of the meibomian glands or just above the tarsus. Normally there are two to five glands of Wolfring glands in the upper and two or three in the lower lid. They are tubuloalveolar glands with relatively large excretory ducts. The ducts are lined by a basal layer of cuboidal cells and a superficial layer of cylindrical cells. The epithelium of the ducts is continuous with that of the conjunctiva. Whether the accessory glands have specialized functions in addition to the basic secretion mentioned above is not clear.

Two further types of accessory glands are often described, namely those of Henle and Manz. Henle's glands are not considered to be true glands. They represent crypts or indentations of the conjunctiva which are covered by conjunctival epithelium, often containing many goblet cells. They are found most frequently in the palpebral conjunctiva between the tarsal plates and the fornix. The *glands of Manz* are small lobular thickenings or indentations of the epithelium in the limbus region which have been described in the pig, calf, and cow, but not normally in the human. They are also not glands in the true sense of the word.

3 Lacrimal Gland

The human lacrimal gland is a compound tubuloalveolar gland. Its end pieces appear to be relatively delicate and histologically uniform (Fig. 19). This is why they were referred to as "purely serous" earlier. But the *end pieces* do not consist of only one single cell population; quite a number of different cell forms have recently been found. Apart from the typical "serous" acinus cells – easily recognizable by their acidophilic, apically

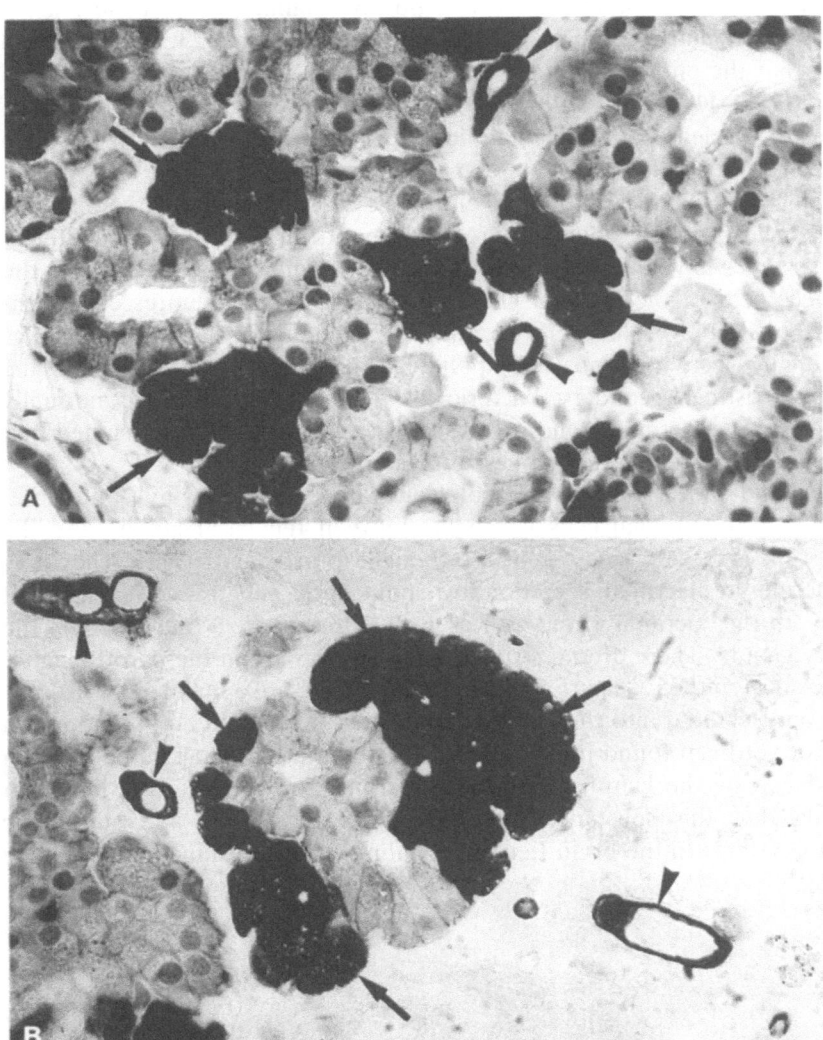

Fig. 19A,B. Light micrographs of the lacrimal gland (cynomolgus monkey). Histochemical demonstration of carbonic anhydrase in acinus cells (*arrows*) and in capillary endothelial cells (*arrowheads*). (**A** ×200; **B** ×400)

localized secretory granules, by the well-developed endoplasmic reticulum, and by the basolateral membrane infoldings – mucous-secreting cells containing mucinic granules and acid glycosaminoglycans are also apparent. In addition, within the end pieces, clusters of cells are found which stain positively for carbonic anhydrase (Fig. 19). Often the endothelium of the capillaries in the interstitial tissue also contain carbonic anhydrase.

Surprisingly, the endothelium shows a positive staining only at these areas where the capillary wall is adjacent to the epithelium [23,37]. It is well known that the enzyme carbonic anhydrase accelerates the reaction $CO_2 + H_2O \rightleftharpoons H^+ + HCO_3^-$ in both directions. This can lead either to a release of protons or a release of bicarbonate ions. It has not yet been clarified which of these reactions plays a role in tear secretion.

Using histochemical methods, end piece cells containing large amounts of sialic acid probably bound to proteins have been found [38]. Lactoferrin and lysozymes have also been localized by histochemical methods within the end piece cells of the lacrimal gland [39]. Using immunofluorescence techniques, interstitial cells were identified containing prolactin, which was occasionally seen in acinus cells [40]. The bactericidal lysozyme and the possibly existing secondary bactericidal factor β-lysozyme are normally secreted by the lacrimal gland in constant quantities [41]. It is assumed that the acinus cells are able to synthesize these substances.

The end pieces of the lacrimal gland are surrounded by contractile, branched myoepithelial cells which lie between the basal lamina and the acinus cells (Fig. 20). These cells are thought to produce ACTH. They may also accelerate lacrimal secretion by spontaneous contraction. The duct system of the lacrimal gland is less well differentiated than that of the salivary glands. There are no striated ducts such as are in the parotid gland. In the duct epithelia, apart from lysozymes, Leu-enkephalin may be produced and secreted into the lacrimal fluid. Met-enkephalin and β-endorphin have not yet been found in duct cells. The observation that Leu-enkephalin is produced by the lacrimal gland is surprising, for up to now it has been assumed that this substance is restricted to the central and autonomic nervous system. In the brain Leu-enkephalin acts on substance-P-containing

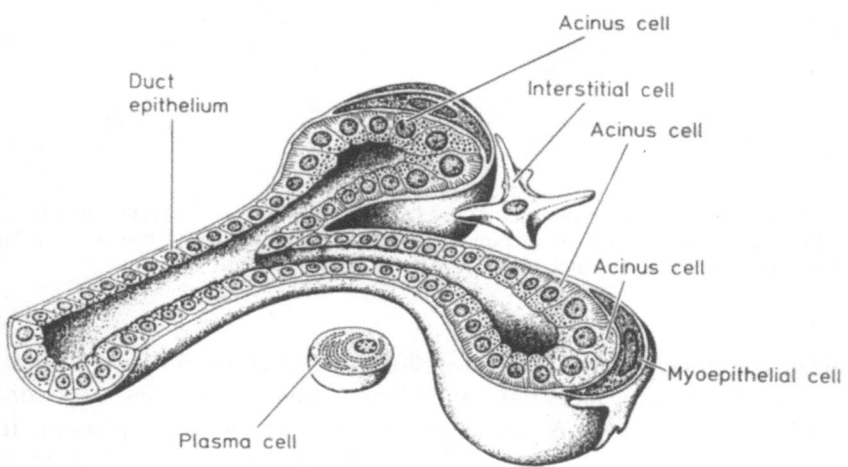

Fig. 20. Schematic drawing of different cell types in the lacrimal gland

neurons causing a decrease in pain sensitivity. In some mammals, such as the rat and guinea pig, substance-P-containing neurons have been found in certain nerve fibers of the lacrimal gland and are localized in the immediate vicinity of the ducts [40,41]. The palpebral fissure, with its mucous membranes covering the eye, might therefore be regarded as a "physiological wound;" thus, in the lacrimal fluid, the presence of a substance decreasing the sensitivity to pain might be important.

The interstitial tissue of the lacrimal gland is wide meshed and rich in free cells. It has a dense capillary network that contains many elongated capillaries surrounding the ducts, which are probably important for fluid adsorption. In the connective tissue of the human lacrimal gland, numerous free cells are often found, especially eosinophilic cells, lymphocytes, macrophages, and plasma cells. The plasma cells produce type A antibodies that occur in the lacrimal fluid. Normally, IgG and IgM are secreted only by the lacrimal gland in small quantities [3,6,41]. However, the largest portion of antibodies demonstrable in the tear film originates from the conjunctiva [18,41].

It is now well established that the secretory immunoglobulin IgA is excreted by the acinus cells into the lacrimal fluid. IgA is synthetized by plasma cells in a preliminary form that is bound to a glycopeptide (J-chain) before being incorporated into the acinus cells where the final polymeric molecule is produced. These molecules are transported to secretory granules in the apical cytoplasm where the immunoglobulins are secreted into the acinus lumen by exocytosis.

The secretion of proteins by the lacrimal gland can be stimulated by vasoactive intestinal peptide, α-melanocyte-stimulating hormone, adrenocorticotropic hormone, and to some extent by β-adrenergic agonists. Met-enkephalin, however, inhibits the secretory activity of the lacrimal gland (for more details, see the chapter by Dartt, this volume.)

The end pieces do not produce the lacrimal fluid in its final form. The concentration of water and solutes are changed by the lacrimal ducts by absorbing water from and by transporting potassium ions into the "primary lacrimal fluid." In addition, proteins and other substances can be secreted by the duct cells. The final composition of the lacrimal fluid is, however, not reached until the secretion of the accessory glands and the mucous membrane itself have joined the product of the lacrimal gland.

References

1. Rohen JW (1964) Das Auge und seine Hilfsorgane. In: Oksche A, Vollrath L (eds) Handbuch der mikroskopischen Anatomie des Menschen, vol 3, part 4. Springer, Berlin Heidelberg New York
2. Mishima S (1965) Some physiological aspects of the precorneal tear film. Arch Ophthalmol 73:233–241

3. Janssen PT, van Bijsterveld OP (1982) Immunochemical determination of human tear lysozyme (muramidase) in keratoconjunctivitis sicca. Clin Chim Acta 121:251–260
4. Steuhl KP (1989) Ultrastructure of the conjunctival epithelium. Dev Ophthalmol 19:1–104
5. Jaeger W (1981) Der präkorneale Film und seine Bedeutung für die Therapie des trockenen Auges. In: Hanselmayer H (ed) Neue Erkenntnisse über Erkankungen der Tränenwege. pp 39–53
6. Janssen PT, van Bijstervel OP (1983) Origin and biosynthesis of human tear fluid proteins. Invest Ophthalmol Vis Sci 24:623–630
7. Brandt, Fritsche (1967) Acta Ophthalmol (Copenh) 45:166
8. McClellan BH, Whitney CR, Newman LP, Allansmith MR (1973) Immunoglobulins in tears. Am J Ophthalmol 76:89–101
9. Holly FJ (1973) Formation and rupture of the tear film. Exp Eye Res 15:515–525
10. Nichols BA, Chiappino ML, Dawson CR (1984) Demonstration of the mucous layer of the tear film by electron microscopy. Invest Ophthalmol Vis Sci 26:464–473
11. Holly FJ, Lemp MA (1977) Tear physiology and dry eyes. Surv Ophthalmol 22:69–87
12. Ehlers N (1965) The precorneal film. Biomicroscopical, histological and chemical investigations. Acta Ophthalmol 81:1–136
13. Watsky MA, Jablonski MM, Edelhauser HF (1988) Comparison of conjunctival and corneal surface areas in rabbit and human eyes. Curr Eye Res 7:483–486
14. Pfister RR (1975) The normal surface of conjunctiva epithelium. A scanning electron microscopic study. Invest Ophthalmol Vis Sci 14:267–279
15. Greiner JV, Covington HI, Allansmith MR (1977) Surface morphology of the human upper tarsal conjunctiva. Am J Ophthalmol 83:892–905
16. Marquardt R, Wenz FH (1979) Histologische Untersuchungen zur Becherzellzahl der menschlichen Bindehaut. Klin Monatsbl Augenheilkd 175:692–696
17. Nelson JD, Wright JC (1984) Conjunctival goblet cell densities in ocular surface disease. Arch Ophthamol 102:1049–1051
18. Moore JC, Tiffany JM (1979) Human ocular mucus origins and preliminary characterisation. Exp Eye Res 29:291–301
19. Kinoshita S, Kiorpes TC, Friend J, Thoft RA (1982) Limbal epithelium in ocular surface wound healing. Invest Ophthalmol Vis Sci 23:73–80
20. Harris TM, Berry ER, Pakurar AS, Sheppard LB (1985) Biochemical transformation of bulbar conjunctiva into corneal epithelium: an electrophoretic analysis. Exp Eye Res 41:597–605
21. Greiner JV, Kenyon KR, Henriquez AS, Korb DR, Weidman TA, Allansmith MR (1980) Mucus secretory vesicles in conjunctival epithelial cells of wearers of contact lenses. Arch Ophthalmol 98:1843–1846
22. Rohen JW, Steuhl P (1982) Specialized cell types and their regional distribution in the conjunctival epithelium of the cynomolgus monkey. Graefes Arch Clin Exp Ophthalmol 218:59–63
23. Rohen JW (1986) Zur funktionellen Morphologie der Conjunctiva. Fortschr Ophthalmol 83:13–24
24. Steuhl KP, Rohrbach JM (1988) Ultrastrukturelle Veränderungen der Konjunktiva von Cynomolgusaffen nach Pilocarpin-Applikation? Klin Monatsbl Augenheilkd 192:672–676
25. Lütjen-Drecoll E, Schenholm M, Tamm E, Tengblad A (1990) Visualization of hyaluronic acid in the anterior segment of rabbit and monkey eyes. Exp Eye Res 51:55–63
26. Rittig M, Lütjen-Drecoll E, Prehm P (1991) Immunohistochemical localization of hyaluron-synthetizing cells in the primate cornea and conjunctiva. Exp Eye Res (in press)
27. Lütjen-Drecoll E, Steuhl P, Arnold WH (1982) Morphologische Besonderheiten der Conjunctiva bulbi. In: Marquardt R (ed) Chronische Conjunctivitis – trockenes Auge. Springer, Vienna New York, pp 25–34

28. Rohen JW, Steuhl KP, Arnold WH (1982) Zur funktionellen Morphologie der Conjunctiva. In: Marquardt R (ed) Chronische Conjunctivitis – trockenes Auge. Springer, Vienna New York, pp 5–24

29. Raviola G (1983) Conjunctival and episcleral blood vessels are permeable to blood-borne horse-radish peroxidase. Invest Ophthalmol Vis Sci 24:725–736

30. Tseng SCG, Hirst LW, Farazdaghi M, Green WR (1984) Goblet cell density and vascularization during conjunctival transdifferentiation. Invest Ophthalmol Vis Sci 25:1168–1176

31. Sørensen T, Taagehøj-Jensen F (1979) Conjunctival transport of technetium-99^m pertechnetate. Acta Ophthalmol 57:691–699

32. Ursing J (1967) On the disappearance of radiosodium ions from conjunctival and subconjunctival deposits in the rabbit. Berlinska Boktryckeriet, Lund

33. Steuhl KP, Rohen JW (1983) Absorption of horse-radish peroxidase by the conjunctival epithelium of monkeys and rabbits. Graefes Arch Clin Exp Ophthalmol 220:13–18

34. Latkovic S, Nilson SEG (1979) Phagocytosis of latex microspheres by the epithelial cells of the guinea pig conjunctiva. Acta Ophthalmol 57:582–590

35. Maurice DM (1973) Electrical potential and ion transport across the conjunctiva. Exp Eye Res 15:527–532

36. Ruskell GL (1985) Innervation of the Conjunctiva. Trans Ophthalmol Soc UK 104:390–395

37. Lütjen-Drecoll E, Eichhorn M, Bárány EH (1985) Carbonic anhydrase of epithelia and fenestrated juxtaepithelial capillaries of *Macaca fascicularis* Acta Physiol Scand 124:295–307

38. Jensen OA, Falbe-Hansen I, Jacobsen T, Michelsen A (1969) Mucosubstances of the acini of the human lacrimal gland (orbital part). Acta Ophthalmol 47:605–619

39. Gilette TE, Allansmith MR (1980) Lactoferrin in human ocular tissues. Am J Ophthalmol 90:30–37

40. Nikkinen A, Lehtosalo JI, Uusitalo H, Palkama A, Pranula P (1984) The lacrimal glands of the rat and the guinea pig are innervated by nerve fibers containing immunoreactivities for substances P and vasoactive intestinal peptide. Histochemistry 81:23–27

41. Dartt DA (1989) Signal transduction and control of lacrimal gland protein secretion: a review. Curr Eye Res 8:619–636

Chapter 3

Physiology of Tear Production

D.A. Dartt

1 Introduction

The tear film consists of three layers: an outer lipid layer, a middle aqueous layer, and an inner mucous layer. The numerous glands that surround the eye – various types of orbital glands – each contribute to the tear film. The meibomian glands and to a lesser extent the glands of Zeis and Moll secrete the lipids of the outer layer. The main lacrimal gland secretes the middle aqueous layer with an additional minor contribution from the accessory lacrimal glands (the glands of Kraus and Wolfring). The goblet cells and to some extent the crypts of Henle and the glands of Manz secrete the inner mucous layer. This chapter will focus mainly on two aspects of tear production: the neuroendocrine regulation of secretion from the orbital glands and the cellular mechanism of secretion.

The epithelia that line the ocular surface, including the corneal and conjunctival epithelia, are also electrolyte- and water-transporting tissues and can contribute to the tear film. Changes in permeability of the conjunctival blood vessels may also modify the tear film. The possible contribution of these structures to the tear film, usually overlooked when tear secretion is described, is also discussed here.

Classically, two types of tear secretion, basic and reflex, were postulated [1]. Basic secretion was thought to be a constant, slow secretion by glands such as the accessory lacrimal glands and the goblet cells, which were not known to have innervation. Reflex secretion was defined as an increased rate of secretion caused by neural stimulation and was thought to apply primarily to the main lacrimal gland. A general principle of homeostasis is that all cellular processes are regulated, or controlled, and usually very tightly. It is unlikely that a process as complex as secretion of the three essential layers of tears from several different glands would not be regulated. Furthermore, even a gland not directly innervated might be subject to paracrine control (diffusion of stimulatory chemicals from a nearby nerve or endocrine cell) or hormonal control. Arguing against the concept of basic versus reflex secretion was the demonstration that tear flow declined as

M.A. Lemp/R. Marquardt (Eds.) The Dry Eye
© Springer-Verlag Berlin Heidelberg 1992

sensory input was decreased, suggesting that secretion by all the orbital glands is probably regulated at some level [2]. However, only secretion by the main lacrimal gland, the largest and most accessible of the orbital glands, has been studied in any detail and that only recently.

Secretion from the individual orbital glands has not been well characterized. Many of the earlier investigations, especially of the main lacrimal gland, used tear fluid as this can be collected easily. Except for the main lacrimal gland, most of the orbital glands are small, and it is difficult to collect the secretory product, a prerequisite for study of secretion. A second problem is that studies on secretion by any of the orbital glands cannot be performed in humans to any extent. Even the main lacrimal gland cannot be studied as the many lacrimal gland secretory ducts are inaccessible. Thus, most of the knowledge of tear secretion comes from animal studies.

The first method developed to study secretion by individual orbital glands used an in vivo preparation in which the excretory duct of the main lacrimal gland of anesthetized cats, and later rabbits, was cannulated, and uncontaminated lacrimal gland fluid collected [3]. The arterial supply to the gland was isolated to allow injection of agonists or experimental drugs or manipulation of the extracellular ionic environment. This preparation was subsequently modified to investigate secretion from the rat exorbital lacrimal gland. In vivo preparations have also been developed to study meibomian gland secretion by collection of meibum directly from the excretory ducts [4], to study secretion indirectly from the accessory lacrimal glands in a rabbit model for keratoconjunctivitis sicca [5], and to measure goblet cell secretion after topical application of drugs and subsequent histochemical staining of mucin [6].

As in vivo preparations contain many uncontrolled variables, in vitro preparations have also been developed. For the main lacrimal gland these include rat exorbital gland pieces, isolated acini, cultured acini – the preparations of choice to study protein secretion and the intracellular mechanisms of secretion [7]. Culturing cells from individual orbital glands, which would allow investigation of secretion on a pure preparation of cells, and the use of specific antibodies and cDNA probes to study individual cells in a biopsy of the entire gland, the eyelid, or the conjunctiva are also on the horizon.

2 Overview of the Secretory Process

An overview of the general principles of the secretory process includes functional anatomy, functional innervation, signal transduction, and the cellular mechanism of protein, electrolyte/water, and lipid secretion.

2.1 Functional Anatomy

Secretory systems can be classified anatomically into two groups, single cells and epithelial "sheets," the latter containing exocrine glands. The type of secretion from each group may be polarized or nonpolarized [8]. The site of secretion can be regulated. Secretion from single cells may be nonpolarized; then, for example, the extracellular matrix molecules or the secretory vesicles can be released anywhere on the cell surface (Fig. 1). Mast cells in the conjunctiva and plasma cells in the main lacrimal gland are ocular examples

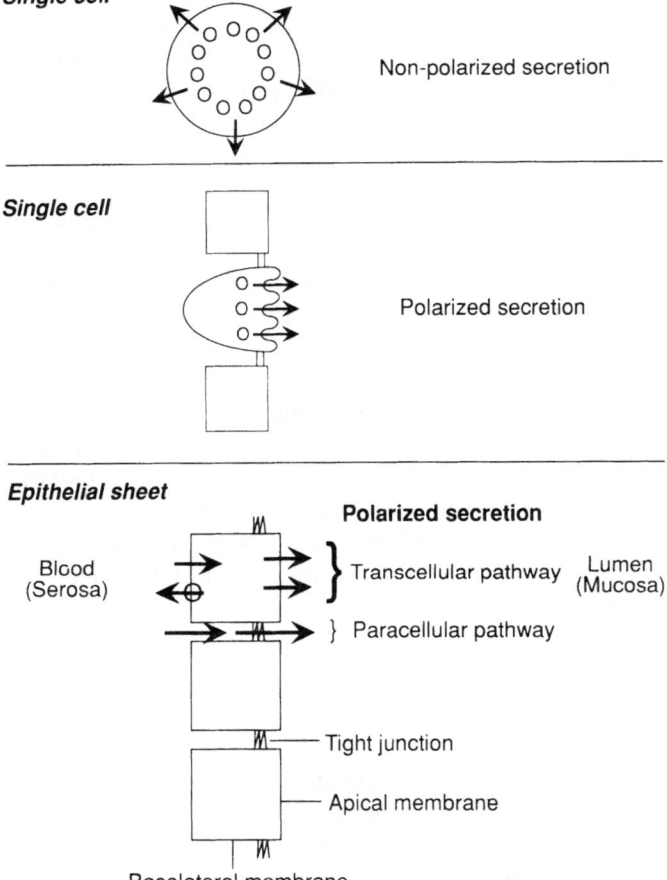

Single cell

Non-polarized secretion

Single cell

Polarized secretion

Epithelial sheet

Polarized secretion

Blood (Serosa)

Transcellular pathway

Lumen (Mucosa)

} Paracellular pathway

Tight junction

Apical membrane

Basolateral membrane

Fig. 1. Types of secretion. *Above,* single cell with secretory granules (*small circles*) that are released anywhere on the cell surface as indicated by the *arrows. Middle,* single cell joined above and below by tight junctions to two adjacent cells in an epithelium. Secretory granules (*small circles*) are released on one side of the cell as indicated by the *arrows. Below,* three cells joined by tight junctions to form an epithelium. *Arrows,* ion transport: *small circle at left with the arrow,* an ion pump

of nonpolarized single cells. Ion transport from these cells is also non-polarized. Because of this, these cells can regulate their ionic composition and volume but cannot transport or secrete large volumes of ions and water as can polarized epithelia. There is no net transport of fluid in a single, nonpolarized epithelial cell. Secretion from single cells may also be polarized; then, for example, the secretory granules are released from only one side of the cell. Goblet cells occurring as single cells embedded in the apical side of the conjunctiva is an ocular example of polarized single cells; they release mucus from only the apical side of the cell.

The multicellular glands of the eye can be considered as complex, involuted epithelial sheets as their tight junctions separate apical from basolateral membranes. Because of this, secretion can be directed to one side or the other, that is, the secretion is polarized. An example is the main lacrimal gland which directs extracellular matrix molecules to one side (basolateral) and secretory granules to the other (apical). There is no direct evidence yet that epithelial sheets also have nonpolarized secretion, although this might occur [8]. The separation of basolateral and apical membranes is important for fluid secretion. Different ion channels and ion transport proteins are located on the basolateral and apical membranes, a localization that is crucial for the polarized secretion of fluid by epithelia in general and the orbital glands in particular, and this is the basis for the secretion of large amounts of ions and water by these tissues. The tight junctions also connect cells and provide the basis for the separation of transcellular and paracellular transport. Transcellular transport, ion and water movement *through* cells, is caused by the transport proteins in the cell membrane and is dependent upon active transport of ions (Fig. 1). Para-cellular transport, ion and water movement *between* cells, depends upon the characteristics of the tight junction and is passive. Fluid secretion by the multicellular orbital glands is a combination of transcellular and paracellular transport of ions and water.

2.2 Functional Innervation or Neuroendocrine Control

Glandular secretion can be controlled by a broad spectrum of nerves and hormones. We classify neuroendocrine control here into the following cat-egories: neural, neurocrine, endocrine, paracrine, and autocrine. The same molecule may act by any of these routes depending on how it is transmitted; the effect depends on the receptors on the target tissue. It is likely that all these mechanisms of controlling secretion are present in the orbital glands although not all have been described to date.

2.2.1 Neural Control

In neural control of secretion, nerves upon depolarization release neuro-transmitters that interact with specific receptors on the cell membrane. For secretory glands there are three levels of control: the type of nerves that innervate the gland and the transmitters they contain, the type of receptors on the secretory cells, and the type of receptors on the vasculature. Neural stimulation which activates the receptors on the secretory cell is necessary to activate secretion, but secretion – in particular, electrolyte and water secretion – can be modified by vasoconstriction or vasodilation (see Sect. 3.1).

The neural control of secretion was limited classically to the parasympathetic and sympathetic nervous system and to cholinergic and α- and β-adrenergic receptors, respectively. In the late 1960s, investigators discovered that parasympathetic and sympathetic nerves contain biologically active peptides in addition to the classical neurotransmitters acetylcholine and norepinephrine. Many of the peptides were originally identified in the endocrine cells of the gastrointestinal tract but were later found in nerve endings throughout the body. Peptides found in nerve endings in or near the orbital glands to date include vasoactive intestinal peptide (VIP) [9], substance P [9], a family of enkephalins derived from proenkephalin A including Met-enkephalin and Leu-enkephalin [10], neuropeptide Y, and calcitonin gene related peptide. The peptides are released along with acetylcholine or norepinephrine and can stimulate or inhibit secretion by affecting receptors on secretory cells directly or modify secretion by affecting receptors on the vasculature. As is discussed in more detail below (Sect. 2.3), the classical neurotransmitter and the peptide, although released together, can have different cellular mechanisms of action and can activate different cellular second messenger pathways. Thus, their combined effects on secretion may be additive, inhibitory, or synergistic.

2.2.2 Neurocrine Control

The classical neurotransmitters and peptide neurotransmitters can also have neurocrine functions by being released from a nerve ending, traveling through the bloodstream, and acting directly on secretory cells or the vasculature. Candidates for this type of action are adrenocorticotropic hormone (ACTH) and α-melanocyte stimulating hormone (α-MSH), which are secreted by the anterior and intermediate lobes of the pituitary gland and stimulate protein secretion from the main lacrimal gland [11]. However, whether ACTH or α-MSH function physiologically to stimulate the lacrimal gland in vivo, whether the source of the ACTH and α-MSH is the pitutitary gland, and whether either is present in the lacrimal gland itself are not known.

2.2.3 Endocrine Control

Glandular secretion can also be regulated by hormones – endocrine control. Hormones are synthesized in endocrine glands, travel via the bloodstream, and act on a distant target cell, the secretory cell. An example of endocrine control of secretion by the orbital glands is the stimulatory effect of androgens on IgA and on secretory component secretion from the plasma cells and acinar cells, respectively, of the main lacrimal gland [12].

2.2.4 Paracrine and Autocrine Control

Classical neurotransmitters, biologically active peptides, and hormones can also have paracrine or autocrine actions. Cells release these molecules locally and the molecules act on other cells (paracrine effect) or on the same cell that secreted the molecule (autocrine effect). A candidate for the paracrine mode of stimulation is histamine release from conjunctival mast cells which could stimulate any of the glandular tissue in the conjunctiva, such as goblet cells or accessory lacrimal gland cells. Histamine in the autocrine mode could affect secretion from the mast cell that secreted it. Other compounds that could exert paracrine or autocrine control are growth factors, such as epidermal growth factor, recently identified in the main lacrimal gland of rodents, and inflamatory mediators, such as prostaglandins and leukotrienes, which can be produced by the conjunctival epithelium.

In addition to the several types of neuroendocrine control, agonists can have different time courses for their action. Classical neurotransmitters, biologically active peptides, and peptide hormones have a relatively rapid time course, on the order of seconds or minutes. These compounds stimulate release of preformed products, in the case of protein secretion, or activate ion channels or transport mechanisms already present in the membrane, in the case of electrolyte secretion. In contrast, steroid hormones and growth factors have a relatively longer time course, on the order of hours or days. These compounds stimulate synthesis of secretory proteins, ion channels, or ion transport proteins.

The concept of functional innervation of orbital glands has become more complex than nerves stimulating glands to secrete (reflex tears). One must consider several additional types of stimulation (neurocrine, endocrine, paracrine, autocrine), several target tissues (secretory cells, vasculature), and different time dependencies (short- and long-term).

2.3 Signal Transduction

Four separate cellular pathways can be activated to transduce the neuroendocrine extracellular signal to an intracellular signal for stimulation or inhibition of secretion. Three of the pathways are designated by the second messengers utilized: Ca^{2+}, diacylglycerol (DAG), cGMP; cAMP; and tyrosine kinase. The fourth pathway is activated by steroid hormones and involves induction or suppression of protein synthesis.

2.3.1   Ca^{2+}/DAG/cGMP-Dependent Pathway

Neuroendocrine stimuli that activate the Ca^{2+}/DAG/cGMP-dependent pathway first bind to specific receptors in the plasma membrane (Fig. 2) [13]. This interaction activates a guanine nucleotide-binding protein (G protein). This G protein increases the activity of phosphatidylinositol-4,5-bisphosphate (PIP$_2$) phosphodiesterase (also known as phospholipase C) to break down PIP$_2$ into 1,4,5-inositol trisphosphate (1,4,5-IP$_3$) and DAG. 1,4,5-IP$_3$ releases Ca^{2+} from an intracellular store that is nonmitochondrial. The released Ca^{2+} may, in conjunction with calmodulin, activate Ca^{2+}/calmodulin-dependent protein kinases to phosphorylate specific protein substrates. The DAG produced concomitantly with 1,4,5-IP$_3$ causes a translocation of protein kinase C (C kinase) to the plasma membrane where, in conjunction with minimal amounts of Ca^{2+} and the phosphatidylserine present in the membrane, it phosphorylates specific protein substrates. Both types of kinases phosphorylate proteins on serine and threonine residues and the newly phosphorylated proteins are thought to cause secretion directly.

The DAG produced from PIP$_2$ can also be converted to arachidonic acid. Arachidonic acid can also be produced by activation of phospholipase A$_2$ and phospholipase D. Arachidonic acid can be metabolized to form the eicosanoids, including the prostanoids (prostaglandins and thromboxanes), leukotrienes, and epoxides [14]. Prostaglandins, thromboxanes, and leukotrienes can be secreted and have a paracrine or autocrine effect. These eicosanoids are thought to interact with specific receptors on the cell membrane. In turn, activation of the receptor activates a G protein. Eicosanoids have many different cellular actions, including stimulating adenylate cyclase activity, inhibiting adenylate cyclase activity, and activating phospholipase C to release intracellular Ca^{2+}. Interaction with the G protein causes different cellular responses depending on the cell and the eicosanoid.

Stimuli that activate PIP$_2$ phosphodiesterase may also activate guanylate cyclase activity, usually located in the cytosol, to produce cGMP from GTP (Fig. 2) [15]. The increased cytosolic cGMP levels activate cGMP-dependent protein kinases (G kinase) to phosphorylate specific protein substrates on serine and threonine residues. The phosphorylated proteins are thought to stimulate secretion directly.

2.3.2   cAMP-Dependent Pathway

Neuroendocrine stimuli that activate the cAMP-dependent pathway first interact with specific receptors in the plasma membrane (Fig. 3) [15]. This interaction activates a stimulatory G protein which increases adenylate cyclase activity to produce cAMP from ATP. The increased cellular level of cAMP activates cAMP-dependent protein kinases (A kinase) to phosphorylate specific proteins on serine and threonine residues. It is thought that the phosphorylated proteins stimulate secretion directly.

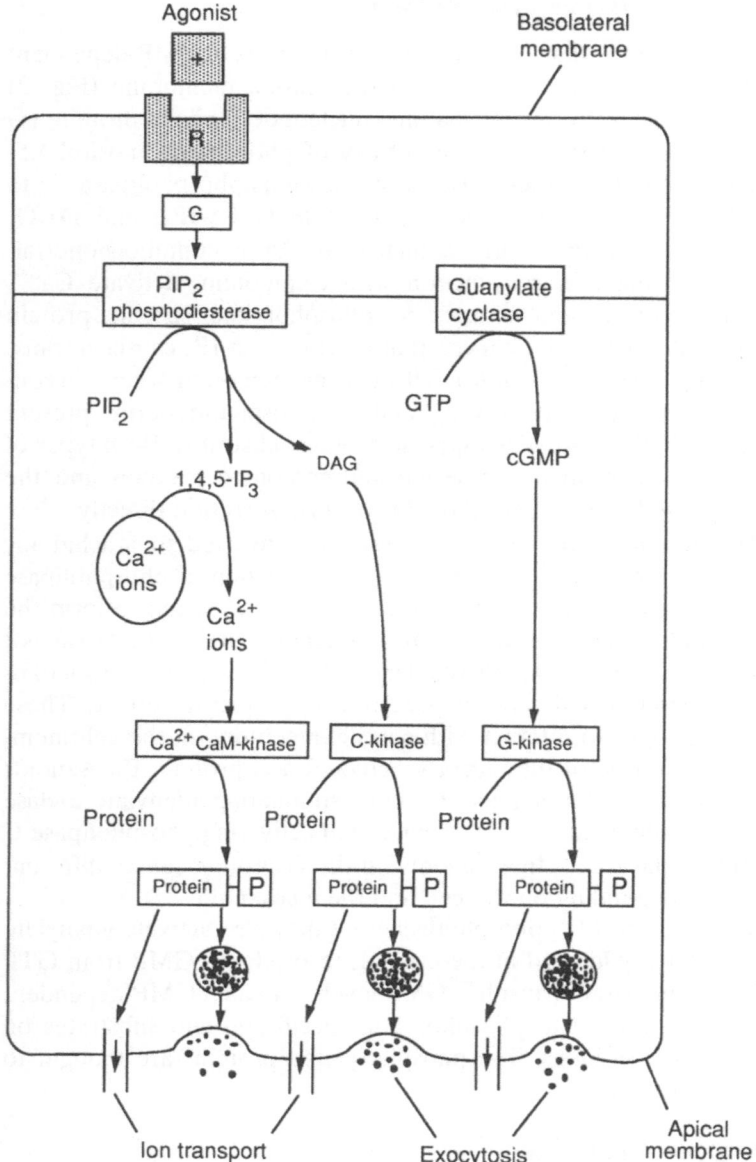

Fig. 2. Ca^{2+}/diacylglycerol/cGMP-dependent pathway for secretion. *R*, Receptor; *G*, guanine nucleotide binding protein (G protein); *PIP₂*, phosphatidylinositol bisphosphate; *1,4,5-IP₃*, 1,4,5 isomer of inositol trisphosphate; *DAG*, diacylglycerol; *CaM*, calmodulin; *Protein-P*, phosphorylated protein; *GTP*, guanosine triphosphate; *cGMP*, cyclic guanosine monophosphate; *circles*, secretory granules

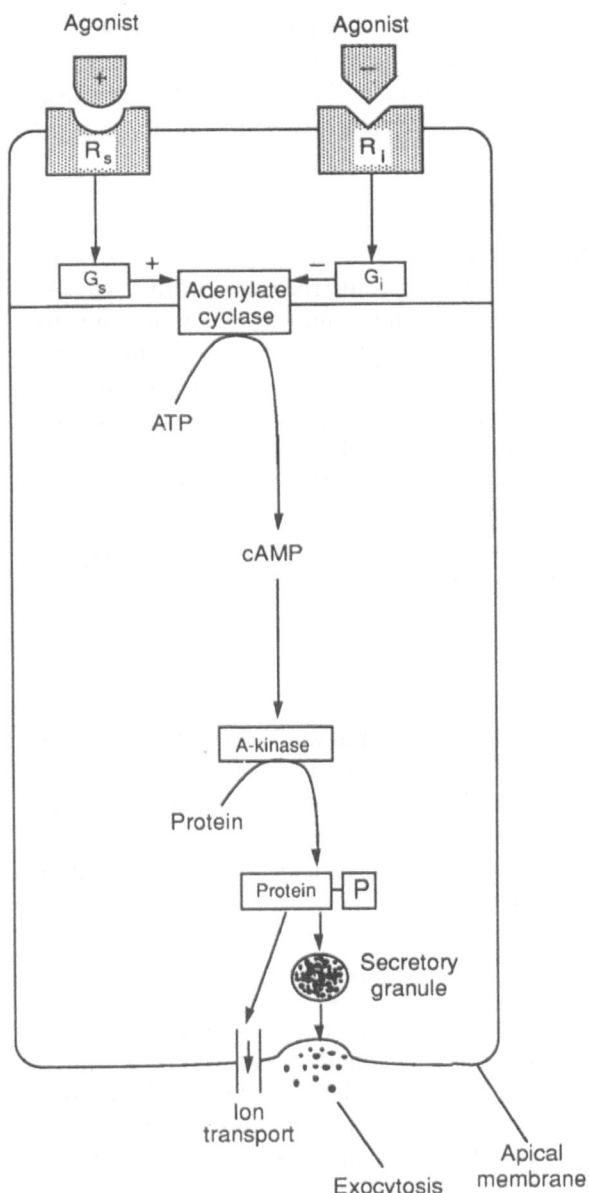

Fig. 3. cAMP-dependent pathway for secretion. s, +, Stimulation; i, −, inhibition; R, receptor, G, guanine nucleotide binding protein (G protein); ATP, adenosine triphosphate; $cAMP$, cyclic adenosine monophosphate; *Protein-P*, phosphorylated protein

Stimuli that inhibit the cAMP-dependent pathway first interact with specific receptors in the plasma membrane. This interaction activates an inhibitory G protein which binds to adenylate cyclase and prevents its activation by a stimulatory G protein. Stimulation of adenylate cyclase activity and the subsequent increase in cAMP levels are prevented.

2.3.3 Steroid Hormone-Activated Pathway

In contrast to the signal transduction pathways described above, steroid hormones enter the target cell and bind to specific receptors in the cytosol. This interaction activates the hormone-receptor complex, which migrates to the nucleus. There the activated steroid-receptor complex combines with acceptor proteins bound to the nuclear matrix. The entire complex interacts with the promoter elements of the target DNA molecule. In the case of secretion these newly synthesized proteins may be secretory proteins, ion channels, or ion pumps destined for insertion in the cell membrane. The stimulation of protein synthesis accounts for the longer time course of effects of steroid hormones compared with peptide hormones, biologically active peptides, and classical neurotransmitters.

2.4 Protein Synthesis

There are two types of protein secretion, regulated and constitutive [8]. For both types, proteins are synthesized in the rough endoplasmic reticulum and transported to the Golgi apparatus where the proteins are enzymatically modified by addition of oligosaccharides. In the *trans*-Golgi compartment, the proteins are packaged into membrane-bound vesicles that are segregated into regulated and constitutive pathways.

2.4.1 Regulated Protein Synthesis

For the regulated pathway, secretory proteins are stored in secretory granules adjacent to the site of release [8]. Regulated secretory granules have a long half-life and fill the secretory cell. The granules are prevented from fusing with the cell membrane until the level of the appropriate second messenger (Ca^{2+}, cAMP, cGMP, or DAG) is increased by interaction of stimuli with their receptors as described above (Sect. 2.3). With stimulation, the secretory granule membrane fuses with the cell membrane, and secretory proteins are released onto the cell surface. Compound exocytosis, the fusion of several secretory granules, may also occur before ultimate fusion with the membrane. Regulated secretory cells are thus able to release large amounts of protein at a rate higher than the rate of protein synthesis. Regulated proteins can be secreted in a polarized or a nonpolarized fashion.

2.4.2 Constitutive Protein Secretion

For the constitutive pathway, the secretory granules are short-lived [8]. The granule membranes fuse with the plasma membrane shortly after the granules are formed, and the secretory protein is released from the cell. The secretory granules are rarely visualized by electron microscopy. Control of constitutive protein secretion is effected by altering the rate of protein synthesis, and proteins are secreted as they are synthesized. There is no external stimulus for exocytosis, and change in the level of second messengers does not change the rate of exocytosis but may change the rate of protein synthesis. Constitutive proteins can be secreted in a polarized or a nonpolarized fashion.

2.5 Electrolyte and Water Secretion

The net movement of water across an epithelium is driven by the active transport of electrolytes. Physiologically, the most important actively transported electrolytes are Na^+ and Cl^-; the metabolic energy for their transepithelial transport is derived from Na,K-ATPase. Na,K-ATPase is present in cell membranes and transports Na^+ out of and K^+ into the cell. For secretory epithelia the cellular distribution of Na,K-ATPase is polarized, with most of the plasma membrane enzyme located on the basolateral membrane [16]. This orientation is opposite to the direction of net Na^+ flux. To resolve this problem, the following mechanism of secretion was proposed (Fig. 4) [16]: (a) A Na^+-Cl^- coupled transport mechanism located in the basolateral membrane allows Cl^- to enter the cell against its electrochemical gradient coupled to Na^+ entry along its electrochemical gradient. (b) The favorable electrochemical gradient for Na^+ is driven by the Na,K-ATPase in the basolateral membrane. (c) A passive Cl^- transporter, as yet unidentified, in the apical membrane allows Cl^- to exit from the cell into the secretory fluid with its electrochemical gradient producing a large, lumen-negative electrical potential. (d) The Na^+ that enters the cell by the Na^+-Cl^--coupled transport mechanism is pumped out of the cell into the basolateral space by the Na,K-ATPase. (e) The lumen-negative potential drives the movement of Na^+ from the basolateral space across the tight junction into the lumen. (f) The K^+ pumped into the cell by the Na,K-ATPase is recycled across the basolateral membrane by a passive K^+ transporter.

The passive K^+ transporter is responsible for the K^+ transient that can accompany stimulation of secretory cells. Patch clamp studies have described a Ca^{2+}- and voltage-sensitive K^+ channel (also known as the BK channel) in the basolateral cell membrane. This channel has a large conductance and can be activated by an increase in intracellular Ca^{2+}, by depolarization, or by an increase in the cellular cAMP level [17].

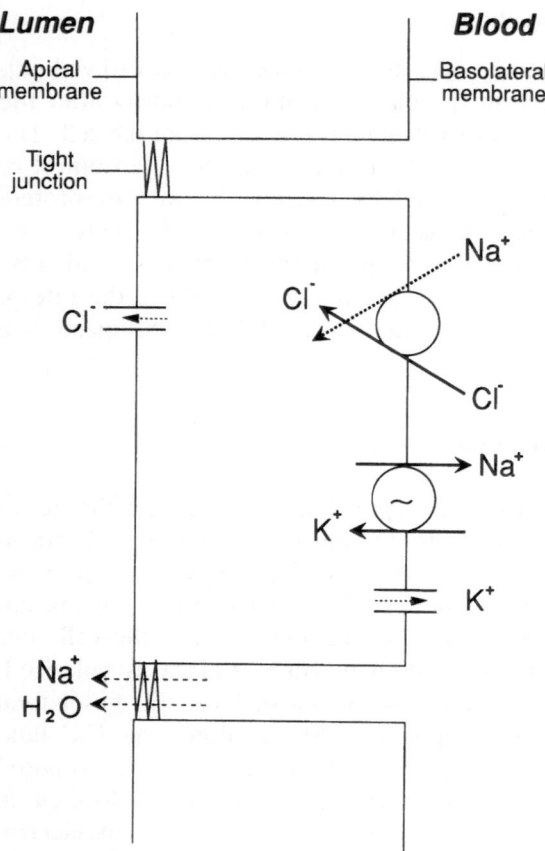

Fig. 4. Mechanism of electrolyte and water secretion. *Broken lines*, ion transport along an electrochemical gradient; *solid lines*, ion transport against an electrochemical gradient; *top circle*, ion cotransport protein; *bottom circle*, Na, K-ATPase.

As studied in the basolateral membrane, the passive Cl^- transporter has a smaller conductance than does the BK channel. Like the BK channel, it is activated by an increase in intracellular Ca^{2+} concentration and by depolarization. This Cl^- channel can also be activated by some stimuli of secretion. Cl^- channels present in the apical membrane permit the efflux of Cl^- from the cell into the lumen.

The Na^+-Cl^--coupled transporter in the basolateral membrane could be one or a combination of three mechanisms: Ca^{2+}-dependent Cl^- and Na^+ channels activated by stimuli, a $NaKCl_2$-coupled transporter, and a parallel array of Na^+/H^+ and Cl^-/HCO_3^--coupled transporters [18].

To stimulate secretion, stimuli could activate any of these transport mechanisms, although evidence suggests that it is the ion channels that are activated. Activation is by receptor-mediated changes in the level of second messengers as described above (Sect. 2.3).

2.6 Lipid Secretion

Lipids, including phospholipids, triacylglycerol, and cholesterol, are synthesized in the endoplasmic reticulum [19]. Glycolipids, including gangliosides, are synthesized in the endoplasmic reticulum, and oligosaccharides are added on in the Golgi apparatus. The lipids must then be segregated, sorted, and transported to the correct ultimate location in the cell. Secreted lipids are packaged within membrane-bound vesicles and stored until secretion. Within the vesicle, the mode of storage of nonpolar and polar lipids is different, and some lipids are bound to and transported with proteins.

3 Secretion by the Orbital Glands

3.1 Main Lacrimal Gland

3.1.1 Functional Anatomy

The lacrimal gland is a tubuloacinar exocrine gland with acini, intercalated ducts, and interlobular ducts. The acini consist of pyramidal acinar cells that surround a central lumen. The acinar cells make up about 80% of the glandular mass. For secretion to occur, secretagogues interact with receptors on the basolateral membrane of secretory cells. This interaction causes an increase in cellular second messenger levels resulting in release of secretory proteins by exocytosis and release of electrolytes and water into the acinar lumen (Fig. 5). The fluid secreted by acinar cells, termed primary fluid, consists of regulated proteins, such as lysozyme and lactoferrin, and electrolytes in the following millimolar concentrations (values for interstitial fluid are in parentheses): Na^+ 139 (134), Cl^- 105 (116), and K^+ 9 (6) [20]. The ionic composition of primary fluid is plasmalike, and the electrolyte concentrations do not change with stimulation but the volumes increase. The protein composition of primary fluid is, however, strikingly different from that of plasma; the former does not contain plasma proteins and contains its own secreted proteins. Primary fluid also contains constitutive proteins such as secretory IgA, which will be discussed below. As the primary secretion flows along the duct system, it is modified by duct cell secretion. Secretagogues interact with receptors on the cell membrane of duct cells to increase the level of second messengers. The second messengers cause electrolyte and water secretion from the duct cells which modifies the primary fluid. The duct cells secrete K^+ and water to increase the volume of secretion and the

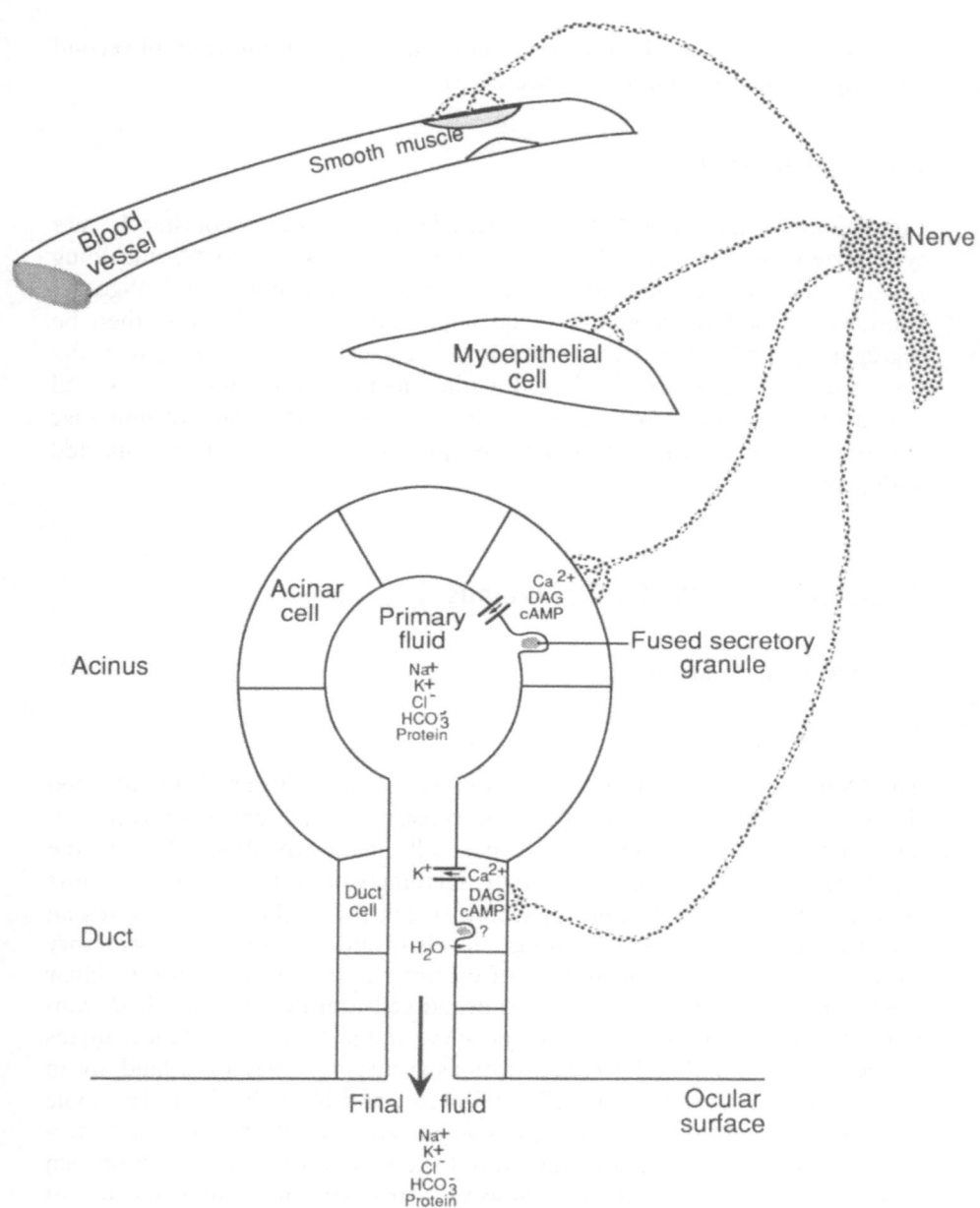

Fig. 5. Functional anatomy of the lacrimal gland. In this schematic illustration of the role of nerves, blood vessels, myoepithelial cells, acinar cells, and duct cells in lacrimal gland secretion, the lacrimal gland is represented by a single acinus with several acinar cells connected to a single duct lined with duct cells and opening onto the ocular surface. The second messengers used in acinar cells are Ca^{2+}, DAG, and cAMP. Increases in the level of the second messengers cause ion transport (*small arrows*) and protein secretion indicated by the fused secretory granule. In duct cells the same second messengers may stimulate K^+ secretion, water reabsorption, and protein secretion

K^+ concentration [20]. Under nonstimulated conditions (low flow rate) the duct cells can also reabsorb water. It is not known whether duct cells secrete regulated proteins, although they contain epidermal growth factor in the species measured (rat and rabbit) and secrete the constitutive protein secretory IgA. The final lacrimal gland fluid is hypertonic at low flow rates and becomes isotonic as the flow rate increases. At low flow rates the millimolar composition of final fluid is as follows (values for interstitial fluid are in parentheses): Na^+ 140 (134), Cl^- 86 (116), and K^+ 95 (6), and at stimulated flow rates: Na^+ 135 (134), Cl^- 123 (116), K^+ 46 (6), and HCO_3^- 20 (22) [20]. These values show that lacrimal gland fluid and thus tears have a higher K^+ concentration than does plasma, and that the K^+ concentration is dependent upon the level of stimulation. The final fluid protein concentration is approximately constant at all flow rates, that is, protein secretion increases as flow rate increases.

The lacrimal gland also contains myoepithelial cells that surround the acini in a basketlike layer (Fig. 5). Their function in lacrimal gland secretion is unknown, but in other tissues they contract, squeezing out presecreted fluid upon the appropriate neuroendocrine stimulus. Another important component of the lacrimal gland is the vasculature. Changes in blood flow can modify (but not activate) lacrimal gland secretion [21]. Vasodilation increases and vasoconstriction decreases prestimulated secretion. Plasma cells are also present in the lacrimal gland [12]. They are scattered throughout the gland in a nonrandom fashion and secrete the IgA portion of secretory IgA.

3.1.2 Functional Innervation

The final component of the lacrimal gland is the neural innervation (Fig. 5). Parasympathetic fibers are in close contact with acinar cells, duct cells, myoepithelial cells, and blood vessels [22]. Sympathetic nerves innervate the blood vessels and in some species are in close contact with secretory and myoepithelial cells [22]. The parasympathetic nerves are the major control of both electrolyte/water and protein secretion. Stimulation of the parasympathetic lacrimal nerve or intraarterial injection of cholinergic agonists stimulates both types of secretion [3]. Receptors for cholinergic agonists are located on acinar cells and presumably on ductal cells, although the latter have not been directly demonstrated. The receptor is a muscarinic receptor of the M_3 glandular type and is antagonized by atropine. Cholinergic receptors are also present on the vasculature. Cholinergic agonists cause vasodilation, which increases the rate of prestimulated secretion.

In addition to containing the parasympathetic neurotransmitter acetylcholine, the parasympathetic nerve endings also contain at least one biologically active peptide, VIP [9]. Intraarterial injection of VIP stimulates lacrimal gland electrolyte/water and protein secretion, as do cholinergic agonists [7]. In the submaxillary salivary gland, stimulation of the parasympathetic nerves releases VIP along with acetylcholine. Although this has not been demonstrated for the lacrimal gland, it is likely to occur. VIP also can affect the vasculature. In salivary glands VIP causes vasodilation and increases secretion. It is possible that VIP also causes lacrimal gland vasodilation, increasing the rate of stimulated secretion.

VIP is present in the human lacrimal gland, as shown by immuno-histochemistry [9]. VIP can stimulate human tear secretion, as demonstrated by the report of a patient with pancreatic cholera who had high serum VIP levels, epiphora, a significantly higher Schirmer test score, and significantly lower tear osmolarity values than normal controls [23].

The sympathetic nervous system primarily innervates the lacrimal gland vasculature, although in some species (dog, cat, guinea pig, monkey, human) sympathetic nerves also surround the acinar cells [7]. In vivo stimulation of sympathetic nerves causes a small increase in fluid secretion [3]. This stimulation is mediated by a β_1-adrenergic agonist interacting with β-adrenergic receptors on acinar cells [24]. It is not known whether there are β-adrenergic receptors on duct cells. If secretion has been stimulated by a cholinergic agonist, stimulation of the superior cervical ganglion or injection of sympathetic agonists causes vasoconstriction that inhibits electrolyte and water secretion [21]. The effect is via an α-adrenergic receptor on the blood vessels. In addition, there are α_1-adrenergic receptors on lacrimal gland acinar cells that stimulate protein secretion [7]. Circulating catecholamines, as well as neural stimulation, may activate these receptors. Whether activation of these receptors causes electrolyte and water secretion is not known, as there is no preparation in which fluid secretion can be measured independently of effects on the vasculature.

In addition to acetylcholine, norepinephrine, and VIP, lacrimal gland nerves also contain other neurotransmitters including substance P, a family of enkephalins, calcitonin gene related peptide, and neuropeptide Y [7,9,10]. These peptides could be present in the sympathetic or parasympathetic nerves and be released with norepinephrine or acetylcholine, respectively. Other peptides are likely to be discovered in lacrimal gland nerves. Of the peptides identified in the lacrimal gland, only the enkephalins have a known physiological function: they inhibit protein secretion stimulated by cholinergic agonists or VIP [26]. Other agonists stimulate lacrimal gland secretion, but they have not yet been localized to the lacrimal gland. Stimuli of electrolyte and water secretion include cholecystokinin and porcine histidine isoleucine containing peptide [28]. Stimuli of regulated protein secretion include α-MSH and ACTH [11].

3.1.3 Signal Transduction

Cholinergic, muscarinic agonists interact with a specific receptor on the plasma membrane (Fig. 6) [13]. The interaction activates phospholipase C to break down PIP_2 into 1,4,5-IP_3 and DAG [7]. Upon stimulation, the 1,4,5-

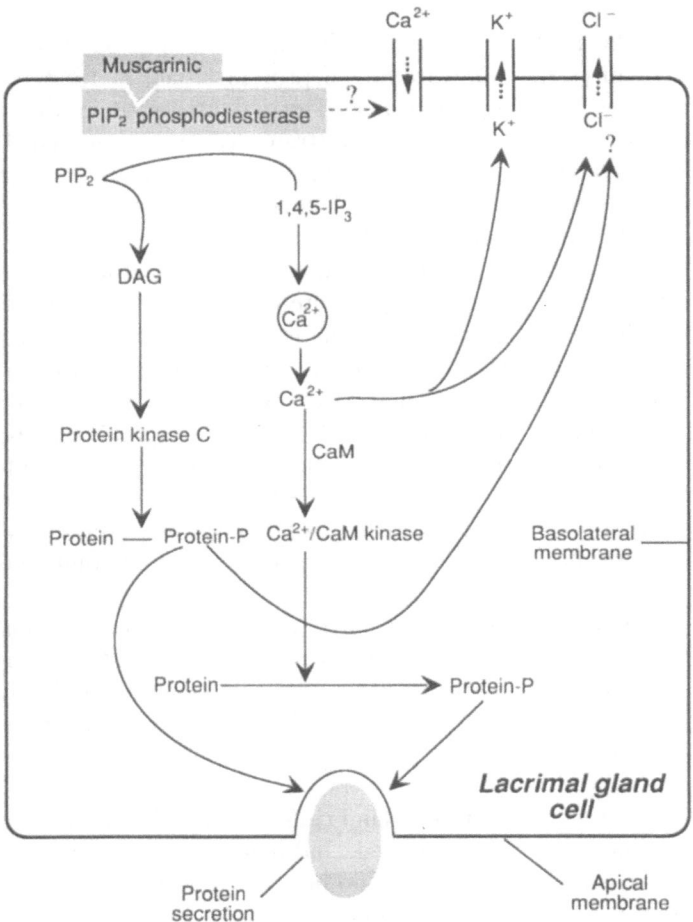

Fig. 6. Muscarinic agonist-stimulated pathway for lacrimal gland secretion. *PIP₂*, Phosphatidylinositol bisphosphate; *1,4,5-IP₃*, 1,4,5 isomer of inositol trisphosphate; *DAG*, diacylglycerol; *CaM*, calmodulin; *Protein-P*, phosphorylated protein; *broken lines*, ion transport along an electrochemical gradient. K^+ and Cl^- represent the first steps activated for electrolyte and water secretion

IP_3 level increases rapidly, and the levels of $1,3,4\text{-}IP_3$ and inositol 1,3,4,5-tetrakisphosphate ($1,3,4,5\text{-}IP_4$), which are metabolic products of $1,4,5\text{-}IP_3$, increase more slowly. It is not known whether $1,3,4\text{-}IP_3$ and $1,3,4,5\text{-}IP_4$ play a physiological role in secretion, but $1,4,5\text{-}IP_3$ causes a rapid release of Ca^{2+} from an intracellular store. This rapid increase in Ca^{2+} initiates secretion. The sustained phase of secretion is maintained by an influx of Ca^{2+} from an extracellular store. The increase in Ca^{2+} causes secretion either by activating ion channels such as K^+ and Cl^- channels directly or in conjunction with the Ca^{2+}-binding protein calmodulin. Together, the Ca^{2+} and calmodulin activate Ca^{2+}/calmodulin-dependent protein kinases that phosphorylate as yet unidentified specific protein substrates. The DAG also produced by cholinergic agonists causes the translocation of protein kinase C from the cytosol to the membrane where it is activated. The activated protein kinase C works by phosphorylating specific protein substrates as yet unidentified. It is the translocated, activated protein kinase C that could stimulate transport proteins directly by phosphorylation to cause electrolyte and water secretion or activate exocytosis to cause protein secretion.

In most tissues α_1-adrenergic agonists use the same signal transduction mechanism as cholinergic agonists to activate secretory cells. In the lacrimal gland, however, α_1-adrenergic and cholinergic agonists use separate cellular pathways. α_1-Adrenergic agonists do not activate phospholipase C to produce 1,4,5-IP_3 and DAG; they increase only DAG (Fig. 7) [7]. The enzyme activated to produce DAG has not yet been identified, although this may be phospholipase D. Like the cholinergic agonists, the increase in DAG resulting from α_1-adrenergic agonist action translocates and activates protein kinase C, which phosphorylates protein substrates to stimulate secretion. α_1-Adrenergic agonists also increase Ca^{2+} but to a very small extent compared with cholinergic agonists.

No agonists are known to activate guanylate cyclase in the lacrimal gland, and an increase in the cellular cGMP level does not stimulate regulated or constitutive lacrimal gland protein secretion [7]. Thus, it is unlikely that cGMP plays a major role in stimulating lacrimal gland secretion, although the effect of cGMP on electrolyte and water secretion has not been tested.

The levels of prostanoids in lacrimal gland cells after application of any stimulatory agonists has not been measured. Indirect evidence, however, shows that arachidonic acid and prostanoids do not affect regulated lacrimal gland protein secretion. They may play a role in electrolyte and fluid secretion as prostaglandin E_1 has been shown to stimulate lacrimal gland fluid secretion, and the effect involved β-adrenergic receptors [25]. The role of leukotrienes in the regulation of lacrimal gland secretion is unknown.

β-Adrenergic agonists, VIP, α-MSH, and ACTH stimulate lacrimal gland cells by activating adenylate cyclase, which increases cellular levels of cAMP (Fig. 8) [7]. This increase activates cAMP-dependent protein kinase, which acts by phosphorylating specific protein substrates, substrates probably different from those phosphorylated by protein kinase C and Ca^{2+}/calmodulin-dependent protein kinase, but not yet identified.

Activation of each second messenger pathway, Ca^{2+}/protein kinase C and cAMP, is an equally potent stimulus of electrolyte and water secretion. Thus, there are at least two separate pathways for stimulating lacrimal gland electrolyte and water secretion.

As both acetylcholine and VIP are present in parasympathetic nerves and probably released together upon neural stimulation, both these agonists

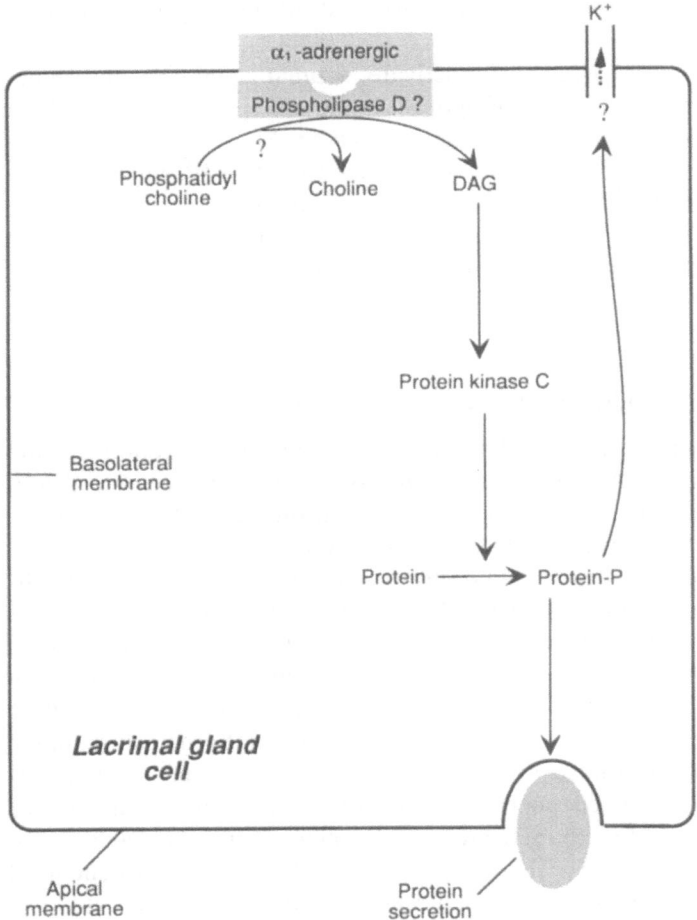

Fig. 7. α_1-Adrenergic agonist-stimulated pathway for lacrimal gland secretion. *DAG*, diacylglycerol; *Protein-P*, phosphorylated protein; *broken line*, ion transport along an electrochemical gradient. K^+ represents the first step activated for electrolyte and water secretion

could interact with lacrimal gland cells simultaneously [7]. The two agonists activate different cellular pathways, so one would expect that secretion in response to their simultaneous addition to be additive. This appears to be the case for fluid secretion but not for protein secretion, which is potentiated (synergistic). The interaction of the two pathways in the latter case occurs after the receptor-mediated increase in cAMP and intracellular Ca^{2+} levels, that is, at protein kinase activation or at exocytosis itself. Similar interactions between agonists using different intracellular pathways could occur upon activation of sympathetic nerves or in the presence of circulating catecholamines and hormones, as the simultaneous addition of α_1-adrenergic agonists and VIP or of cholinergic agonists and ACTH potentiate protein secretion.

All the agonists discussed so far activate lacrimal gland cells and stimulate secretion. Only one family of agonists – the enkephalins – that inhibit secretion have been identified in the lacrimal gland. Met-enkephalin inhibits protein secretion stimulated by cholinergic agonists or VIP but not by α_1-adrenergic agonists [26]. VIP-induced secretion is inhibited by the inhibition of adenylate cyclase activity (probably via an inhibitory G protein; Fig. 8), but the mechanism of inhibition of cholinergic agonist-induced activation is not known.

3.1.4 Cellular Mechanism of Electrolyte and Water Secretion

The cells responsible for electrolyte, water, and protein secretion are the acinar and duct cells. Agonists activate receptors on acinar cells to stimulate electrolyte, water, and protein secretion and on duct cells to stimulate electrolyte and water secretion. The effect of agonists on cellular electrolyte and water transport has been studied only in vivo and in isolated acinar cells because a pure population of duct cells is difficult to obtain. The following mechanism has been suggested for muscarinic stimulation of electrolyte and water secretion [16,18]. Activation of muscarinic receptors causes an increase in the intracellular Ca^{2+} concentration and activates protein kinase C which stimulates the secretion of Na^+, K^+, and Cl^- into the acinar lumen in plasmalike concentrations. Protein kinase C may stimulate ion transport by phosphorylating ion channels or transport proteins either directly or indirectly. Ca^{2+} can directly activate ion channels. It first activates apical Cl^- channels, which cause the outwardly directed Cl^- electrochemical potential gradient to drive Cl^- into the acinar lumen (Fig. 9). Ca^{2+} also activates the basolateral K^+ channels, which compensate for the depolarizing effect of Cl^- channel activation, by increasing K^+ efflux from the cell into the basolateral extracellular space. The K^+ efflux activates the Na,K-ATPase, which pumps K^+ into the cell to maintain the intracellular K^+ concentration and pumps Na^+ out of the cell into the basolateral intercellular spaces. The Na^+ then diffuses through the paracellular pathway into the acinar lumen. The increased flux of Cl^- into the acinar lumen causes a negative electrical potential in the lumen, further increasing the driving force for the flux of Na^+ into the lumen. To replenish the intracellular Cl^-, Na^+/H^+, and Cl^-/HCO_3^- cotransport proteins on the basolateral membrane increase in activity. Cholinergic stimulation also recruits additional Na,K-ATPase molecules to the basolateral membranes to ensure that Na^+ efflux and influx are equal during prolonged stimulation. K^+ is also secreted into the acinar lumen. It has been suggested that Ca^{2+} increases the K^+ flux into the acinar lumen by activating K^+ channels in the apical membrane.

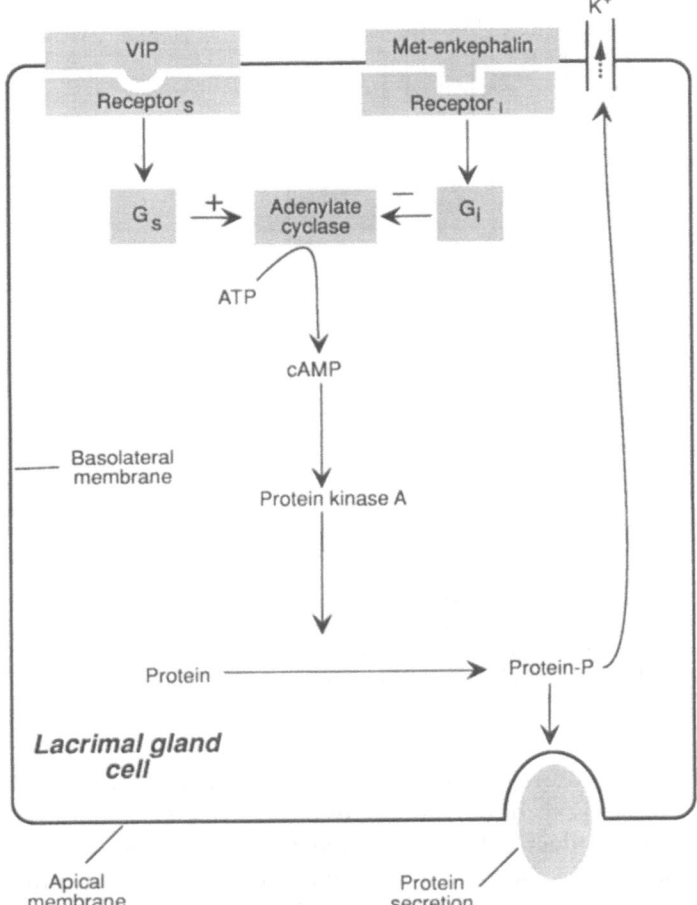

Fig. 8. cAMP-dependent pathway for lacrimal gland secretion. *s*, +, Stimulation; *i*, −, inhibition; *VIP*, vasoactive intestinal peptide. β-Adrenergic agonists, adrenocorticotropic hormone, and α-melanocyte stimulating hormone also interact with receptors in the lacrimal gland. *G*, Guanine nucleotide binding protein (G protein); *Protein-P*, phosphorylated protein; *ATP*, adenosine triphosphate; *cAMP*, cyclic adenosine monophosphate; *broken line*, ion transport along an electrochemical gradient. K^+ represents the first step activated for electrolyte and water secretion

The net flux of Na^+, K^+, and Cl^- into the acinar lumen causes an osmotic flux of water resulting in an isotonic primary fluid in the acinar lumens.

The ductal cells in the rat exorbital lacrimal gland are estimated to contribute about 30% of the volume of stimulated electrolyte and water secretion by the whole gland. In vivo studies indicate that lacrimal gland duct cells modify primary fluid by secreting K^+ so that the K^+ concentration in the lacrimal gland fluid secreted onto the eye is higher than in plasma

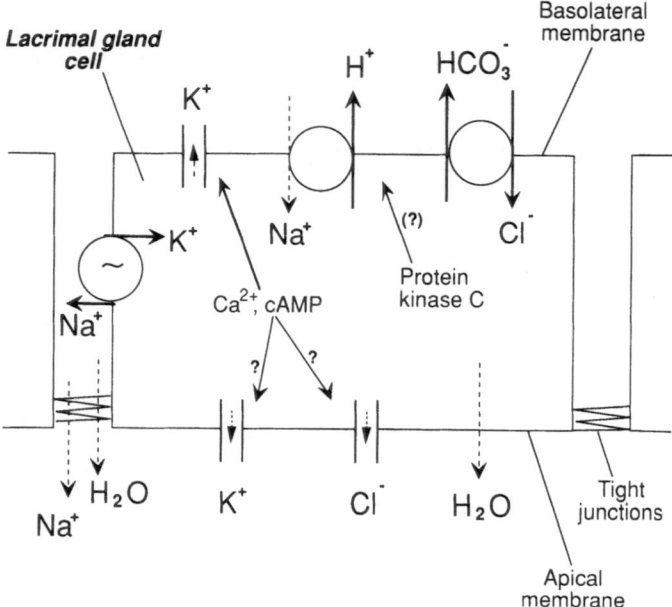

Fig. 9. Mechanism of lacrimal gland electrolyte and water secretion. Ca^{2+}, cAMP, and protein kinase C are the second messengers that activate lacrimal gland electrolyte and water secretion. *Broken lines*, ion transport along an electrochemical gradient; *solid lines*, ion transport against an electrochemical gradient; *top circles*, ion cotransport protein; *circle at left*, Na, K-ATPase

[20]. Duct cells can also reabsorb water making lacrimal gland fluid hypertonic as flow rate decreases [27]. In the absence of direct evidence about the mechanism of secretion in duct cells, one speculation is that the ductal epithelium contains apical K^+ channels responsible for K^+ secretion into ductal lumens and Na,K-ATPase in the basolateral membrane to provide the energy for ion transport. In addition, the water permeability of the duct apical membrane must be limited under certain conditions (e.g., low flow rate) so that water reabsorption occurs. Cholinergic agonists thus cause acinar and ductal secretion of lacrimal gland final fluid that contains relatively plasmalike Na^+ and Cl^- concentrations and a K^+ concentration higher than plasma level.

VIP, which increases intracellular levels of cAMP and does not increase the intracellular Ca^{2+} concentration, stimulates lacrimal gland fluid secretion as effectively as do cholinergic agonists [28]. cAMP-dependent protein kinase activates the Ca^{2+}-dependent K^+ channels located in the basolateral membrane (Fig. 9) [17]. These are the same K^+ channels activated by cholinergic agonists to stimulate lacrimal gland electrolyte and water secretion. This suggests that VIP, by increasing cAMP levels and activating cAMP-dependent protein kinase, stimulates fluid secretion by the same ion transport mechanisms as described for cholinergic agonists.

β-Adrenergic agonists also work via cAMP but produce only a small volume of secretion [24]. This is consistent with the weak effect of β-adrenergic agonists on protein secretion. These data imply that there are either few β-adrenergic receptors on lacrimal gland cells or no β-adrenergic receptors on lacrimal gland cells and β-adrenergic agonists interact non-specifically and weakly with another type of receptor.

3.1.5 Cellular Mechanism of Protein Secretion

Activation of several different second messenger pathways cause regulated protein secretion (Figs. 6–8). Cholinergic agonists work via Ca^{2+} and protein kinase C to increase protein secretion by the lacrimal gland. α_1-Adrenergic agonists stimulate protein secretion in the lacrimal gland by translocation and activation of protein kinase C [7]. α_1-Adrenergic agonists cause only a small increase in Ca^{2+} and do not increase inositol phosphates. VIP, α-MSH, ACTH, and to a lesser extent β-adrenergic agonists stimulate protein secretion by increasing cAMP levels. Thus, an increase in Ca^{2+} either directly or by activating Ca^{2+}/calmodulin-dependent protein kinases, an increase in the activation of protein kinase C, or an increase in the activation of cAMP-dependent protein kinase causes protein secretion from lacrimal gland acinar cells. Activation of each pathway causes the same magnitude of secretion. Thus, there are three separate intracellular pathways to stimulate lacrimal gland protein secretion [7]. For protein secretion to occur, the secretory granule membrane must fuse with the apical membrane and release the granule contents (secretory proteins) into the acinar lumen (exocytosis). Activation of the three kinds of protein kinases accelerates the rate of fusion of granule and apical membranes to cause the rapid, almost explosive phenomenon of exocytosis.

The rate of secretion of constitutive proteins by the lacrimal gland is also controlled. The major protein constitutively secreted by the lacrimal gland is secretory IgA, which defends the ocular surface against antigenic threat. Secretory IgA consists of polymeric IgA coupled to a glycopeptide called J chain and to secretory component. IgA and J chain are synthesized by plasma cells in the lacrimal gland parenchyma, and secretory component is secreted by lacrimal gland acinar and duct cells. IgA and J chain join to form a dimer (polymeric IgA) before leaving the plasma cell [12]. Polymeric IgA binds to secretory component which, after being synthesized (see Sect. 2.4), is incorporated into the basolateral membrane as the receptor for polymeric IgA. Once polymeric IgA has bound to secretory component, the complex is incorporated into vesicles or secretory granules that traverse the cytoplasm, bind to the apical membrane, and release secretory IgA into the acinar primary fluid or ductal final fluid. The rate of secretory IgA secretion is determined not by the rate of fusion of secretory granule membrane with apical membrane as is the case for regulated protein secretion but by the rate of synthesis of IgA, J chain, and secretory component. That is, the control is at the rate of gene transcription and RNA translation. It is not surprising then that the compounds that stimulate secretory IgA secretion differ from those that stimulate regulated protein secretion. What is surprising is that some of the stimuli and second messengers that stimulate electrolyte and water secretion, as well as regulated protein secretion, also stimulate constitutive protein secretion.

Sex steroids are the major controllers of secretory IgA synthesis and secretion [12]. Men have a higher level of IgA and secretory component than do women, and androgens (testosterone), but not estrogens, increase the levels of IgA and secretory component in orchiectomized male rats and in female rats. Estrogens do not affect stimulation by testosterone. The hypothalamic-pituitary axis controls such stimulation. Hypophysectomy completely inhibits the stimulation by testosterone of IgA and secretory component levels in the tears.

In addition to testosterone, several other compounds stimulate secretory IgA synthesis. Surprisingly, secretory component secretion is stimulated by an increase in cellular cAMP levels by VIP, β-adrenergic agonists (but only in the presence of testosterone), a permeable cAMP analog, activating adenylate cyclase activity with cholera toxin and inhibiting cAMP breakdown by 3-isobutyl-1-methylxanthine (only in the presence of testosterone) [29]. Not all agonists that increase cellular cAMP levels in lacrimal gland acinar cells stimulate secretory component secretion; α-MSH is not effective.

Cholinergic agonists inhibit secretory component secretion, in contrast to their effect on regulated protein secretion and electrolyte and water secretion. Thus, the second messengers cAMP and Ca^{2+}, previously thought to have only short-term effects localized to the plasma membrane and cytosol, appear also to affect protein synthesis via an effect in the nucleus, a long-term effect.

3.2 Accessory Lacrimal Glands

The accessory lacrimal glands (the glands of Krause and Wolfring), located in the conjunctival mucosa, are small glands with the same structure as the main lacrimal gland. In humans there are 4–42 accessory lacrimal glands in the upper conjunctival tissue and 6 or fewer in the lower conjunctiva [30]. Their weight is about 10% of the weight of the main lacrimal gland. By histochemical and immunohistochemical techniques, the main and accessory lacrimal glands are virtually indistinguishable. They have similar staining for three different cytokeratin markers and for vimentin. Both types of glands contain the regulated secretory proteins lysozyme and lactoferrin and the constitutive secretory protein secretory component [31]. The immunoglobulins IgG, IgA, IgM, IgD, and IgE have similar localization in both types of glands [32]. Finally, both types have myoepithelial cells, but the main lacrimal gland has more than the accessory glands. The only known difference between the glands is that the main lacrimal gland stains positively for S-100, a marker of nervous tissues and cells of neural crest origin, and the accessory glands do not [31].

Traditionally the accessory lacrimal glands, together with the other glands located in the conjunctiva, have been termed basic secretors. That is, they continuously secrete the protein, electrolytes, and water of the middle aqueous layer of the tear film and are not controlled by nerves or other stimuli. It has not yet been determined whether the accessory lacrimal glands contain nerve terminals, although the presence of nerve terminals has been correlated with the presence of myoepithelial cells in other tissues. The presence of regulated and constitutive secretory proteins in the glands, however, is consistent with neuroendocrine control of secretion.

Indirect evidence suggests that the accessory lacrimal glands can be stimulated to secrete fluid. In a dry eye rabbit model for studying accessory lacrimal gland fluid secretion, the main lacrimal gland excretory duct was closed by cautery and the harderian and nictitans glands removed. This results in an increase in tear osmolarity to about 310 mosmol/l, similar to the level seen in dry eye in humans [5]. The only source for the aqueous layer of tears is the accessory lacrimal glands. An increase in tear film osmolarity and an increase in tear volume in response to topical application of stimuli were interpreted as indicating an increase in accessory lacrimal gland secretion. As is for main lacrimal gland protein, electrolyte, and water secretion, compounds that increased the cellular level of cAMP stimulated accessory lacrimal gland secretion [5]. These compounds included the agonists VIP; α-, β-, and γ-MSH; glucagon; a permeable cAMP analog; an activator of adenylate cyclase, forskolin; and an inhibitor of cAMP breakdown, 3-isobutyl-1-methylxanthine. Unlike the findings in the main lacrimal gland, cGMP stimulated accessory lacrimal gland secretion. Furthermore, cholinergic agonists did not stimulate accessory lacrimal gland secretion by a muscarinic receptor mediated effect. Cholinergic agonists, however, stimulated accessory lacrimal gland secretion that was blocked by local anesthetic, suggesting stimulation by a neurally mediated but sensory effect. These results suggest that accessory lacrimal glands can be stimulated to secrete, and that regulation of their secretion may be neuroendocrine. There has been no research on the mechanism of electrolyte, water, and protein secretion by the accessory lacrimal gland cells, but it is likely that the mechanisms are the same as those of the main lacrimal gland cells.

3.3 Goblet Cells

Goblet cells, located in the apical, surface layer of the conjunctiva, are the primary secretors of the inner mucous layer of the tear film. Mucus consists of an extremely heterogeneous group of O-linked glycoproteins. The protein portions of goblet cell glycoproteins are synthesized in the endoplasmic reticulum, and the extensive number and complicated branches of saccharides are added in the Golgi apparatus and the *trans*-Golgi network (Fig. 10). The newly synthesized glycoproteins are condensed and stored in membrane-bound secretory granules at the apical side of the cell. Mucus from goblet cells in nonconjunctival tissue is thought to be secreted by a regulated mechanism. The mucus secretory granules are stored in the cytoplasm until the arrival of the appropriate stimulus to secrete, at which time the mucus granule membrane fuses with the apical membrane, and mucus is released onto the ocular surface.

The conjunctiva is innervated by sensory, parasympathetic, and sympathetic nerves. VIP is present in the conjunctiva of the rabbit but not the human [33]. The nerves innervate blood vessels, are present in the subepithelial layer and are sparsely present in the epithelium. There are no nerve endings in apposition to goblet cells, nor are nerve endings found in areas of increased goblet cell density. Thus, goblet cells do not appear to be innervated. There are, however, other stimulatory mechanisms, including paracrine stimulation (release of a stimulus from nearby nerve endings or

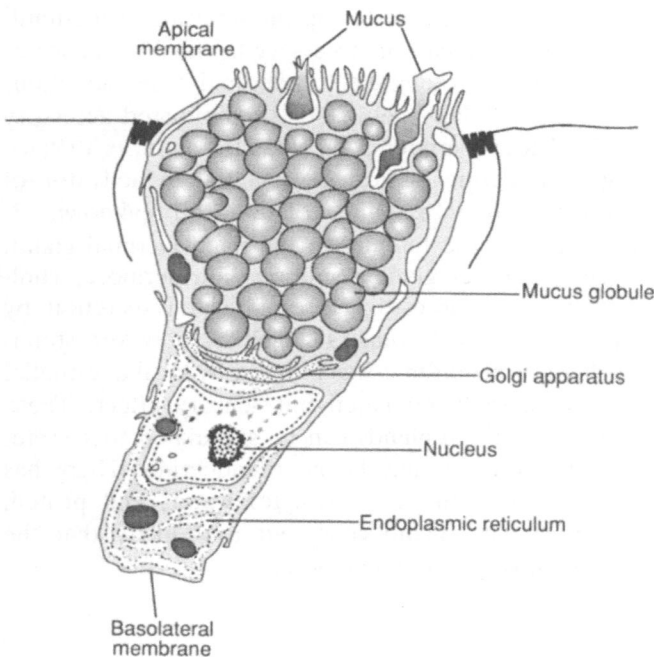

Fig. 10. Schematic representation of mucous synthesis and secretion by a conjunctival goblet cell. The cell is connected by tight junctions to the apical cells on the conjunctival epithelium. Mucus is released onto the ocular surface

other cells), autocrine stimulation (release of a stimulus from self-stimulating goblet cells), and hormonal stimulation (release of a stimulus from a distant or nearby site into the blood supply). In support of the latter mechanism, the suggestion has been made that goblet cell transdifferentiation may be controlled by a factor in the blood [34]. Finally, compounds present in tears could also stimulate goblet cell secretion. For example, epidermal growth factor is secreted by lacrimal gland duct cells into the tears.

The control of goblet cell mucus secretion has been studied primarily in nonconjunctival epithelia. In the intestine, goblet cells in the crypts can be stimulated to secrete by parasympathetic agonists and by histamine, and goblet cells on the villi can be stimulated by chemical irritants [35]. In the stomach, goblet cell secretion can be stimulated by cholinergic agonists, by increasing the cellular cAMP level with forskolin, by prostaglandin E_2, and by increasing protein kinase C activity with phorbol esters [36]. In airways, goblet cell mucus secretion is stimulated by a broad spectrum of proteinases (for example, elastase, thermolysin, and pronase) [37]. This evidence suggests that goblet cells can be stimulated to secrete mucus by receptor-mediated mechanisms similar to those described for the main lacrimal gland. The mechanisms, however, vary between tissues, and no consistent pattern of goblet cell stimuli has emerged.

There is some evidence that conjunctival goblet cell mucous secretion can be stimulated. A stable analog of prostaglandin E_2 has been reported to stimulate mucus secretion from rabbit goblet cells, and prostaglandin D_2 and its metabolite prostaglandin J_2 to stimulate guinea pig goblet cell secretion [6,38]. It is possible that goblet cell secretion of the mucous layer of the tear film can be stimulated and is controlled, and that goblet cells are not basic secretors as previously thought.

3.4 Meibomian Glands

The meibomian glands are sebaceous glands that secrete a complex mixture of lipids onto the edge of the eyelid. The glands lie in a row at the edge of the upper and lower eyelids, and their ducts open directly onto the inner margin of the eyelids. The lipids secreted by the meibomian glands overspread the aqueous layer to form the outer layer of the tear film [39]. Meibum (the meibomian gland secretion) contains hydrocarbons, sterol esters, wax esters, triacylglycerols, free cholesterol, free fatty acids, and polar lipids [40,41]. Meibomian glands consist of alveolar units, or lobules, of secretory cells that empty into a duct (Fig. 11). A single outside layer of germinal basal cells in the lobules do not contain lipid droplets [42]. As the cells move toward the duct, the endoplasmic reticulum develops, as do the lipid-containing secretory droplets synthesized by the endoplasmic reticulum and stored in the cell. The cells in the center of the alveolus contain abundant endoplasmic reticulum and secretory droplets. Secretion occurs by

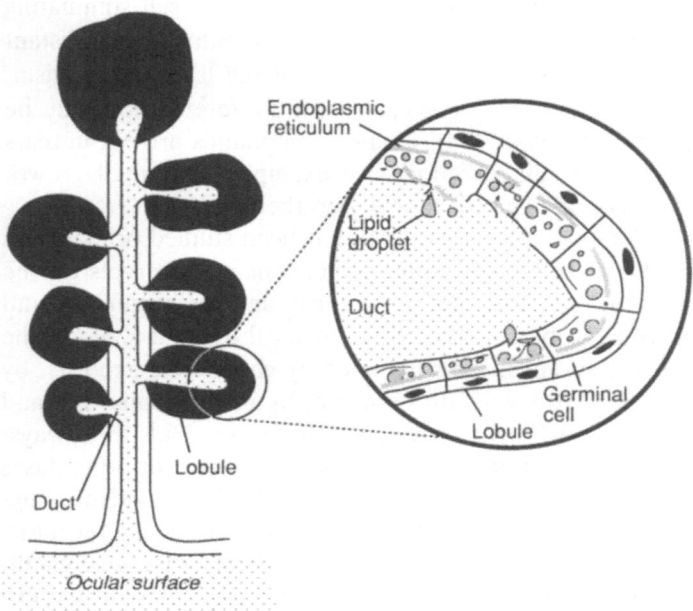

Fig. 11. Schematic representation of meibomian glands. *Left,* meibomian gland with lobules (*black*) emptying into a duct system that opens onto the ocular surface; *right,* detail of lobule showing the mechanism of lipid secretion

the disintegration of the lipid droplet-containing cells in the center of the alveolus into the ducts.

During blinking the meibomian glands are milked by contraction of the pars palpebrae of the orbicularis oculi, and secretion occurs by relaxation of the pars marginalis muscles that surround the duct orifice allowing the release of the meibum accumulated in the duct [43]. Between blinks the pars marginalis muscles are contracted preventing meibum from leaving the ducts and the pars palpebrae are relaxed allowing secretion to move into the duct.

In marmosets and some primates there are nerve fibers around the meibomian glands [44]. In rabbits early studies suggested sympathetic control of meibomian gland secretion as sectioning of cervical sympathetic nerves increased secretion. There may also be parasympathetic control of secretion as the nerves surrounding the meibomian glands are reactive for cholinesterase, and the anticholinesterase physostigmine, which prolongs the action of acetylcholine, also stimulates secretion [45]. Thus, there may be neural control of meibomian gland secretion in addition to the mechanical effects of blinking.

Another type of control of secretion is also possible, that is, control of the rate of synthesis of the lipids in meibum. This would be similar to the

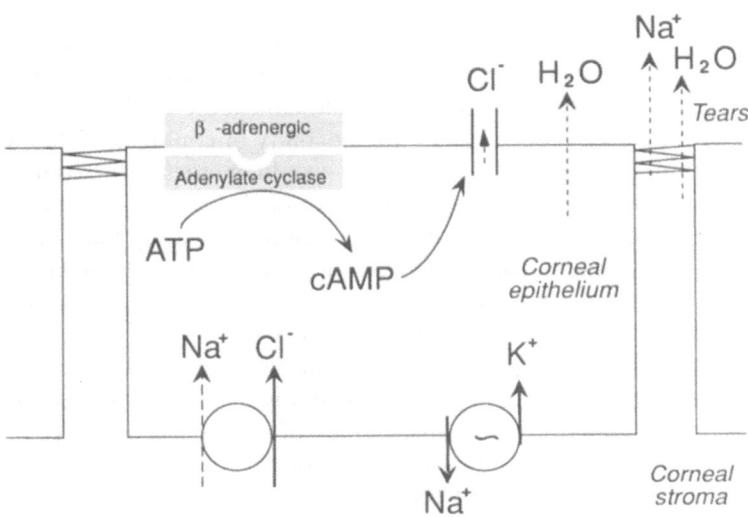

Fig. 12. β-Adrenergic pathway for stimulation of corneal epithelium electrolyte and water secretion. The corneal epithelium is represented by a single cell layer. *ATP*, Adenosine triphosphate; *cAMP*, cyclic adenosine monophosphate; *broken lines*, ion transport along an electrochemical gradient; *solid lines*, ion transport against an electrochemical gradient; *left circle*, ion cotransport protein; *right circle*, Na, K-ATPase. (From [46])

control of secretory IgA secretion in the main lacrimal gland and would involve long-term control of DNA transcription or RNA translation.

3.5 Nonglandular Epithelium

In addition to the orbital glands, there are several epithelia in the ocular surface that may contribute to tears. These include the corneal epithelium, the conjunctival epithelium, and the conjunctival blood vessels. The corneal epithelium and endothelium control corneal thickness by regulating Na^+, Cl^-, and water transport. Although the corneal epithelium actively transports Na^+ and water from the tears to the stroma, an increase in the cellular cAMP level in corneal epithelial cells stimulates Cl^- secretion from the stroma to the tears (Fig. 12) [46]. The Cl^- secretion can be stimulated by β-adrenergic agonists, a permeable cAMP analog, and an inhibitor of cAMP breakdown theophylline. Increased Cl^- secretion causes increased movement of Na^+ and water from stroma to tears, dehydrating the cornea and contributing to the aqueous layer of tears.

Little is known about the transport of ions and water by the conjunctival epithelium; it may also contribute to the aqueous layer. In rabbits the conjunctival epithelium was found to be permeable to Na^+ and Cl^-, about ten times more permeable than the cornea [47]. The electrical potential across the conjunctiva indicates a rate of transport of Na^+, Cl^-, and water from tears to blood that under certain conditions could diminish the tear film to dryness. As this does not occur, additional factors must be operating.

A second way in which the conjunctiva could contribute to the aqueous layer of the tear film is by changes in the permeability of conjunctival blood vessels. An increase in vascular permeability would increase the volume of the tear film; a decrease in permeability would decrease the volume. Evidence about such changes under normal conditions is lacking, but during ocular allergy an antigen-mediated increase in conjunctival blood vessel permeability increases the aqueous layer of the tear film [48]. Histamine release from ocular mast cells causes similar changes.

The conjunctival epithelium may also contribute to the mucous layer. In giant papillary conjunctivitis and vernal conjunctivitis there is an increase in the number of small vesicles in the apical sides of the apical conjunctival cells [49]. These vesicles contain mucuslike glycoproteins; mucous secretion from these vesicles might account for the increased mucus found in the tear film in these diseases.

4   Development of New Treatments for Dry Eye

Investigation of the normal stimuli of secretion and the normal mechanism of secretion of the individual orbital glands and the epithelia that line the ocular surface provides a scientific basis for the development of new treatments for dry eye. Two examples, still in the early stages of investigation, are described. First, Gilbard and I have used our findings on the stimuli of fluid secretion from the in vivo rabbit lacrimal gland to develop topical treatments for aqueous-deficiency dry eye [50]. We used stimuli of main lacrimal gland secretion in an experimental rabbit model for dry eye (no functioning main lacrimal, harderian, or nictitans glands) to determine the stimuli of accessory lacrimal gland secretion. We then used one of the stimuli, 3-isobutyl-1-methylxanthine, a compound that prevents breakdown of cAMP, as a topical drop in a preliminary 4-week human trial with ten female dry-eye patients [50]. Tear osmolarity was significantly decreased in all ten patients. This result could provide the basis for development of a series of new topical drugs to stimulate tear secretion.

Fig. 13. Schematic representation of stimulation of secretion by each of the orbital glands that contribute to the tear film. *Solid arrows* indicate that there is substantial evidence to support stimulated secretion; *dotted arrows* indicate that there is some evidence to support stimulated secretion; *solid arrows with question marks* indicate hypothetical mechanism of stimulated secretion. The meibomian glands secrete the lipid layer of the tear film; the lacrimal gland, accessory lacrimal glands, corneal epithelium, conjunctival epithelium, and conjunctival blood vessels secrete the aqueous layer; and the conjunctival goblet cells and conjunctival epithelium secrete the mucous layer

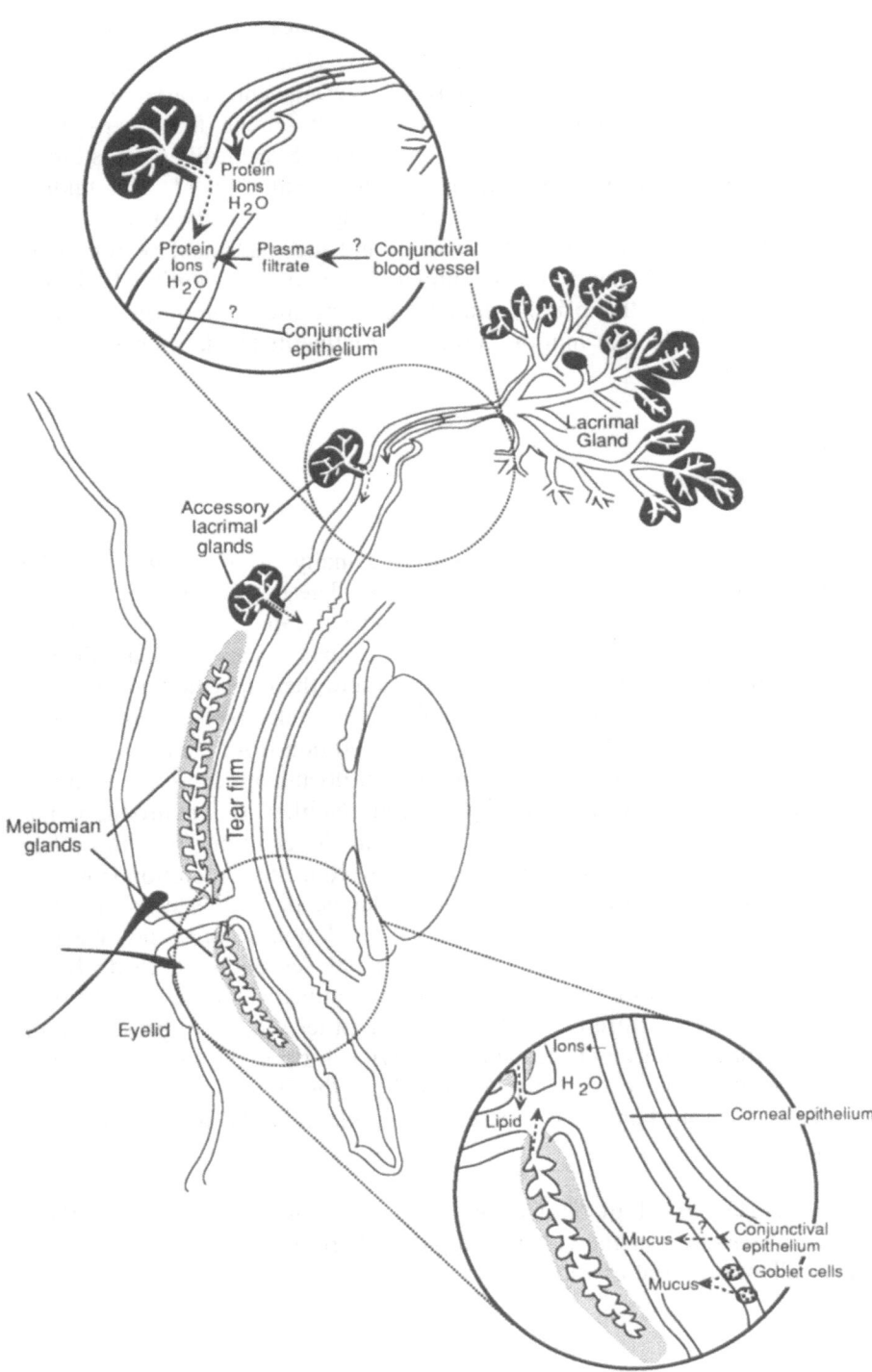

Second, Sullivan and Ariga used their findings that testosterone increases secretory IgA secretion from lacrimal glands to develop another treatment [51]. They found that androgen therapy ameliorated the autoimmune sequelae in lacrimal glands from adult female MRL/Mp-*lpr/lpr* mice, an animal model for Sjögren's syndrome. Specifically, testosterone decreased the lymphocytic infiltration into the lacrimal gland. This finding could also provide a basis for new systemic drugs to treat dry eye.

Continued investigation of the stimuli and mechanism of secretion by each of the orbital glands could similarly provide a scientific basis for treatment of dry eye that arises from deficiency or alteration of the lipid and mucous layers of the tear film or additional treatments for deficiencies of the aqueous layer.

5 Conclusions

Tears are the sum of the secretions of the many orbital glands and the epithelia that line the ocular surface (Fig. 13). The net secretion is a three-layer structure that is remarkably stable and yet can respond to the challenges of the environment to protect the ocular surface. To maintain the tear film, the orbital glands and epithelia secrete their specific, and in some cases unique, secretory products including lipids, electrolytes, water, protein, and mucus. That electrolyte and water secretion from the main lacrimal gland is under neuroendocrine control is well documented, as are many of the details of the mechanism of secretion. Neither the neuroendocrine regulation nor the specifics of the mechanism of secretion from the other orbital glands is well studied. There is some evidence that secretion from the accessory lacrimal glands, the meibomian glands, the goblet cells, and the corneal epithelium is under neuroendocrine regulation. There is no evidence about the regulation of conjunctival epithelial secretion of electrolytes, water, or mucus or of the contribution of conjunctival blood vessel permeability to tears. Future research using modern techniques of tissue culture and molecular biology is necessary to describe further the neuroendocrine regulation of all the orbital glands as well as the individual processes involved in the mechanism of secretion, providing a basis for improved therapy for dry eye.

Acknowledgements. I thank Deanna Dicker and Robin Hodges for their technical assistance in the research reported here and Leona Greenhill for her excellent editorial assistance.

References

1. Jones LT (1966) The lacrimal tear system and its treatment. Am J Ophthalmol 62:47–60
2. Jordan A, Baum J (1980) Basic tear flow: does it exist? Ophthalmology 87:920–930
3. Botelho SY, Hisada M, Fuenmayor N (1966) Functional innervation of the lacrimal gland in the cat. Arch Ophthalmol 76:581–588
4. Brown SI, Dervichian DG (1969) The oils of the meibomian glands. Arch Ophthalmol 82:537–540
5. Gilbard JP, Rossi SR, Heyda KG, Dartt DA (1990) Stimulation of tear secretion by topical agents that increase cyclic nucleotide levels. Invest Ophthalmol Vis Sci 31:1381–1388
6. Aragona P, Candela V, Caputi AP, Micali A, Puzzolo D, Quintieri M (1987) Effects of a stable analogue of PGE$_2$ (11-deoxy-13, 14-didehydro-16(S)-methylester PGE$_2$: FCE 20700) on the secretory processes of conjunctival goblet cells of rabbit. Exp Eye Res 45:647–654
7. Dartt DA (1989) Signal transduction and control of lacrimal gland protein secretion: a review. Curr Eye Res 8:619–636
8. Kelly RB (1985) Pathways of protein secretion in eukaryotes. Science 230:25–32
9. Nikkinen A, Lehtosalo JI, Uusital H, Palkama A, Panula P (1984) The lacrimal glands of the rat and guinea pig are innervated by nerve fibers containing immunoreactivities for substance P and vasoactive intestinal peptide. Histochemistry 81:23–27
10. Lehtosalo J, Uusitalo H, Mahrberg T, Panula P, Palkama A (1989) Nerve fibers showing immunoreactivities for proenkephalin A-derived peptides in the lacrimal glands of the guinea pig. Graefes Arch Clin Exp Ophthalmol 227:455–458
11. Jahn R, Padel U, Porsch P-H, Soling H-D (1982) Adrenocorticotropic hormone and α-melanocyte-stimulating hormone induce secretion and protein phosphorylation in the rat lacrimal gland by activation of a cAMP-dependent pathway. Eur J Biochem 126:623–629
12. Sullivan DA (1987) Endocrine control of the ocular secretory immune system. In: Berczi I, Kovacs K (eds) Hormones and immunity. MTP Press, Lancaster, England, pp 54–92
13. Berridge MJ, Irvine RF (1984) Inositol trisphosphate, a novel second messenger in cellular signal transduction. Nature 312:315–321
14. Smith WL (1989) The eicosanoids and their biochemical mechanisms of action. Biochem J 259:315–324
15. Berridge MJ (1985) The molecular basis of communication within the cell. Sci Am 253:142–152
16. Dartt DA, Møller M, Poulsen JH (1981) Lacrimal gland electrolyte and water secretion in the rabbit: localization and role of (Na$^+$ + K$^+$)-activated ATPase. J Physiol 321:557–569
17. Lechleiter JD, Dartt DA, Brehm P (1988) Vasoactive intestinal peptide activates Ca^{2+}-dependent K$^+$ channels through a cAMP pathway in mouse lacrimal cells. Neuron 1:227–235
18. Mircheff AK (1989) Lacrimal fluid and electrolyte secretion: a review. Curr Eye Res 8:607–617
19. Dawidowicz EA (1987) Dynamics of membrane lipid metabolism and turnover. Annu Rev Biochem 56:43–61
20. Alexander JH, van Lennep EW, Young JA (1972) Water and electrolyte secretion by the exorbital lacrimal gland of the rat studied by micropuncture and catheterization techniques. Pflugers Arch 337:299–309
21. Botelho SY, Martinez EV, Pholpramool C, van Prooyen HC, Janssen JT, De Palau A (1976) Modification of stimulated lacrimal gland flow by sympathetic nerve impulses in rabbit. Am J Physiol 230:80–84

22. Ichikawa A, Nakajima Y (1962) Electron microscope study on the lacrimal gland of the rat. Tohoku J Exp Med 77:136–149
23. Gilbard JP, Dartt DA, Rood RP, Rossi SR, Gray KL, Donowitz M (1988) Increased tear secretion in pancreatic cholera: a newly recognized symptom in an experiment of nature. Am J Med 85:552–554
24. Tangkrisanavinont V (1984) Adrenergic control of lacrimal secretion in rabbits. Life Sci 34:2373–2378
25. Pholpramool C (1979) Secretory effect of prostaglandins on the rabbit lacrimal gland in vivo. Prostaglandins in Medicine 3:185–192
26. Cripps MM, Bennett DJ (1990) Peptidergic stimulation and inhibition of lacrimal gland adenylate cyclase. Invest Ophthalmol Vis Sci 31:2145–2150
27. Gilbard JP, Dartt DA (1982) Changes in rabbit lacrimal gland fluid osmolarity with flow rate. Invest Ophthalmol Vis Sci 23:804–806
28. Dartt DA, Shulman M, Gray KL, Rossi SR, Matkin C, Gilbard JP (1988) Stimulation of rabbit lacrimal gland secretion with biologically active peptides. Am J Physiol 254:G300–G306
29. Kelleher RS, Hann LE, Edwards JE, Sullivan DA (1991) Endocrine, neural and immune control of secretory component output by lacrimal acinar cells. J Immunol 146:3405–3412
30. Allansmith MR, Kajiyama G, Abelson MB, Simon MA (1976) Plasma cell content of main and accessory lacrimal glands and conjunctiva. Am J Ophthalmol 82:819–826
31. Vigneswaran N, Wilk CM, Heese A, Hornstein OP, Naumann GOH (1990) Immunohistochemical characterization of epithelial cells. I. Normal major and accessory lacrimal glands. Graefes Arch Clin Exp Ophthalmol 228:58–64
32. Gillette TE, Allansmith MR, Greiner JV, Janusz M (1980) Histologic and immuno-histologic comparison of main and accessory lacrimal tissue. Am J Ophthalmol 89:724–730
33. Ruskell GL (1985) Innervation of the conjunctiva. Trans Ophthalmol Soc UK 104:390–395
34. Tseng SCG, Hirst LW, Farazdaghi M, Green WR (1984) Goblet cell density and vascularization during conjunctival transdifferentiation. Invest Ophthalmol Vis Sci 25:1168–1176
35. Neutra MR, Phillips TL, Phillips TE (1984) Regulation of intestinal globet cells in situ, in mucosal explants and in the isolated epithelium. Ciba Found Symp 109:20–39
36. Seidler U, Sewing K-Fr (1989) Ca^{2+}-dependent and -independent secretagogue action on gastric mucus secretion in rabbit mucosal explants. Am J Physiol 256:G739–G746
37. Boat TE, Cheng PW, Klinger JD, Liedtke CM, Tandler B (1984) Proteinases release mucin from airways goblet cells. Ciba Found Symp 109:72–88
38. Woodward DF, Hawley SB, Williams LS, Ralston TR, Protzman CE, Spada CS, Nieves AL (1990) Studies on the ocular pharmacology of prostaglandin D2. Invest Ophthalmol Vis Sci 31:138–146
39. Tiffany JM (1985) The role of meibomian secretion in the tears. Trans Ophthalmol Soc UK 104:396–401
40. Baron C, Blough HA (1976) Composition of the neutral lipids of bovine meibomian secretions. J Lipid Res 17:373–376
41. Tiffany JM (1978) Individual variations in human meibomian lipid composition. Exp Eye Res 27:289–300
42. Parakkal PF, Matoltsy AG (1964) The fine structure of the lipid droplets in the meibomian gland of the mouse. J Ultrastruct Res 10:417–421
43. Linton RG, Curnow DH, Riley WJ (1961) The meibomian glands: an investigation into the secretion and some aspects of the physiology. Br J Ophthalmol 45:718–723
44. Miraglia T, Gomes NF (1969) The meibomian glands of the marmoset (*Callithrix jachus*). Acta Anat 74:104–113
45. Montagna W, Ellis RA (1959) Cholinergic innervation of the meibomian gland. Anat Rec 135:121–128

46. Klyce SD, Crosson CE (1985) Transport processes across the rabbit corneal epithelium: a review. Curr Eye Res 4:323–331
47. Maurice DM (1973) Electrical potential and ion transport across the conjunctiva. Exp Eye Res 15:527–532
48. Abelson MB, Smith LM (1991) Mediators of ocular inflammation. In: Duane TD, Jaeger EA (eds) Biomedical foundations of ophthalmology. Harper and Row, Philadelphia, chap 27
49. Greiner JV, Weidman TA, Korb DR, Allansmith MR (1985) Histochemical analysis of secretory vesicles in non-goblet conjunctival epithelial cells. Acta Ophthalmol 63:89–92
50. Gilbard JP, Rossi SR, Heyda KG, Dartt DA (1991) Stimulation of tear secretion and treatment of dry eye with 3-isobutyl-1-methylxanthine. Arch Ophthalmol 109: 672–676
51. Ariga H, Edwards J, Sullivan DA (1989) Androgen control of autoimmune expression in lacrimal glands of MRL/Mp-*lpr/lpr* mice. Clin Immunol Immunopathol 53:499–508

Chapter 4

Basic Principles and Classification
of Dry Eye Disorders

M.A. Lemp

1 Introduction

The term "dry eye" is a rubric to describe a variety of ocular disorders of
diverse pathogenesis but sharing signs of ocular surface abnormalities with
symptoms of discomfort, a feeling of dryness, grittiness, and/or foreign body
sensation. The origins of these manifestations include decreased tear secretion, abnormalities of conjunctival mucin secretion, meibomian gland dysfunction, lid surfacing abnormalities, and primary ocular surface disease.
This chapter focuses on the physicochemical mechanisms of the tear film
formation, maintenance, and rupture, biochemical characteristics of tears,
the morphology of the ocular surface, tear-epithelial interactions, and the
renewal cycle of the corneal epithelium. A classification of these disorders is
presented based on major pathogenetic mechanisms. A presentation of the
various theories on the pathogenesis of ocular surface disease follows with
the final discussion of the implications of recent discoveries for the future of
the diagnosis and management of these disease states.

2 Structure, Formation, Rupture, and Maintenance
of the Tear Film

Tears support the normal structure and function of the corneal and conjunctival surfaces. The tear film acts to smooth out irregularities in the
corneal epithelium and actually serves as the anterior refracting surface of
the eye, presenting the first interface between air and an aqueous medium
[1]. There is evidence that tears also play a role in regulating hydration of
the cornea by way of tonicity changes secondary to evaporation of the tear
film. Mishima has demonstrated that an osmotic gradient develops across
the cornea because of tear film evaporation resulting in movement of water
from the aqueous to the cornea into the tear film; he has estimated that this
flow approximates $3\,\mu l\,cm^{-1}\,h^{-1}$ in rabbit studies. When hypertonic solu-

M.A. Lemp/R. Marquardt (Eds.) The Dry Eye
© Springer-Verlag Berlin Heidelberg 1992

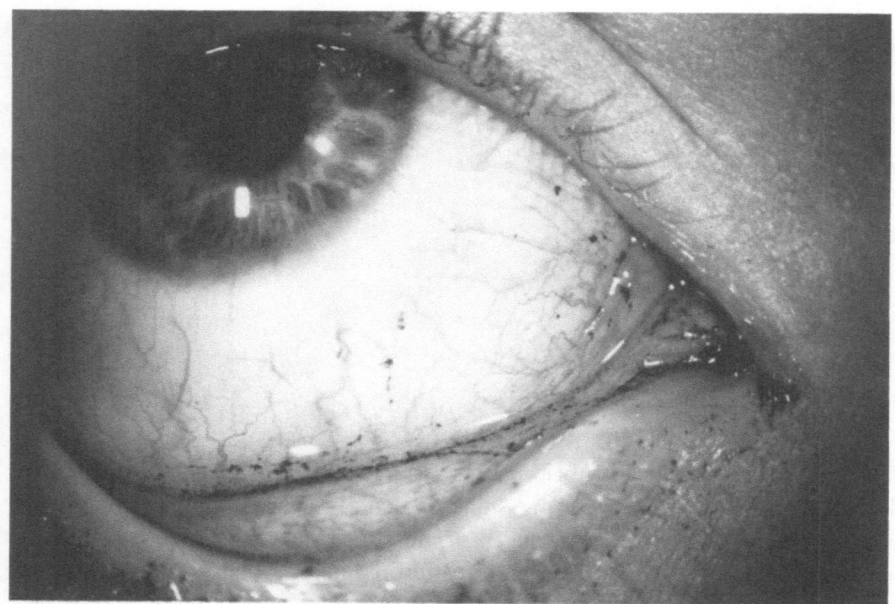

Fig. 1. Black microspheres engulfed by mucin network on the ocular surface

tions are introduced into the tear film this movement can be exaggerated both across the corneal and conjunctival surfaces, as suggested by Mishima and Maurice and as noted clinically in the reduction of corneal epithelial edema after instillation of hypertonic drops.

Tears also provide the corneal epithelium its primary source of oxygen obtained from the atmosphere and dissolved within tears; the cornea is avascular and not supplied with another ready source of oxygen. Tears represent, in effect, the only oxygen source; they are important in providing for the aerobic metabolism of the corneal epithelium. The relative contribution of oxygen dissolved in the tears versus oxygen supplied by the circulation in the conjunctiva is not known. Tears play a role in the healing of central corneal wounds by providing a pathway by which blood cells make their way from the conjunctival and limbal circulation to the tear film into central corneal openings. Tears also contain a number of substances with antibacterial properties, including lysozyme, beta-lysin, and lactoferrin. Tears flush the surface of the eye removing exfoliated cells from the ocular surface plus debris and extraneous foreign bodies by way of entrapment in a mucin network on the surface (Fig. 1).

There is an intimate relationship between the ocular surface and the tear film. The entire tear film is about 7 μm in thickness. Wolf initially described the three-layer structure of tears consisting of an innermost mucin layer coating the epithelial surface, an intermediate much thicker aqueous layer,

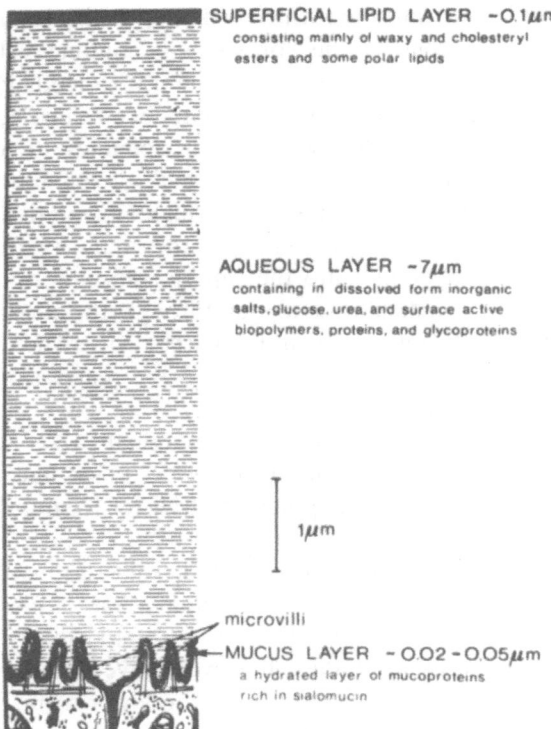

SUPERFICIAL LIPID LAYER ~0.1μm
consisting mainly of waxy and cholesteryl
esters and some polar lipids

AQUEOUS LAYER ~7μm
containing in dissolved form inorganic
salts, glucose, urea, and surface active
biopolymers, proteins, and glycoproteins

1μm

microvilli

MUCUS LAYER ~0.02-0.05μm
a hydrated layer of mucoproteins
rich in sialomucin

Fig. 2. Structure of the tear film

and a thinner outermost lipid layer (Fig. 2). The structure first postulated by Wolf has been subsequently confirmed by other investigators who demonstrated the presence of the lipid layer both by noting the interference patterns and by direct testing of the surface of the tear film for lipid activity.

2.1 The Aqueous Component of the Tear Film

The aqueous component of the tears which provides over 90% of the thickness of the tear film is produced by the main and accessory lacrimal glands [2]. It is thought that 95% of tears arise from the orbital and palpebral portions of the main lacrimal gland; the rest is thought to come from the accessory glands of Krause and Wolfring. Anatomical dissection of cadaver specimens has demonstrated that there is considerable variability in the number and mass of accessory lacrimal gland tissue in normal subjects. This considerable variability may well account for the relative importance of the main lacrimal gland in providing adequate aqueous tear production in given individuals. The aqueous portion of the tears is secreted as an isotonic or slightly hypotonic solution (see the chapter by Dartt, this volume, for a thorough discussion of aqueous secretion). The flow of aqueous tears originates in the ductule openings of the main and accessory lacrimal glands in the superior fornix. This fluid flows into the fornicial spaces, the lacrimal "rivers" and over the exposed portions of the corneal and conjunctival surface. The direction of flow of aqueous fluid is from temporal to medial; this directional flow is driven by the action of the orbicularis oculi muscle, the fluid being drawn immediately into the two punctal openings in a relaxation phase immediately subsequent to a blink. The bulk of this flow occurs to the lacrimal rivers. Some aqueous fluid is lost through evaporation and reabsorption through the conjunctival surface, but the majority of fluid flows out through the punctal openings into the superior and inferior canaliculi, then into the common canaliculus, and out through the nasal lacrimal duct emptying out by the inferior meatus in the nasal cavity. There is, however, a considerable reabsorption of this fluid across the mucosa of the nasolacrimal duct during its passage.

There is almost no exchange of tears between the marginal "rivers" and the preocular surface tear film except during a blink. A "black line" described by Maurice is a narrow strip of thinning limiting transfer from the marginal "river" to the preocular film.

When small samples of tears $(0.1-0.4 \mu l)$ are collected from the marginal tear film, and osmolarity is measured using freezing point of depression, normal subjects showed a value of $302 \pm 6 \, mosmol/l$; this is approximately isotonic with saline. Earlier studies, however, have found a slightly lower osmolarity from tear samples obtained from the lower fornix. The aqueous tear volume can be studied using fluorimetry measuring the decay rates of concentration of fluorescein instilled in the tear film as a measure of tear film dilution by newly secreted tears. Employing this methodology, tear volume values of $6-8 \mu l$ have been reported. The marginal strips have been reported to contain approximately $3.0 \mu l$, the preocular tear film $1 \mu l$, and the forniceal spaces approximately $3 \mu l$. The flow of aqueous tears has been reported to be about $1.2 \mu l/min$ (range $0.5-2.2$). This so-called "basal" rate of tear secretion occurs in the eye without any evidence of stimulation. Stimulated tear flow can increase 100-fold. Significant decrease in tear volume in patient with moderate to severe keratoconjunctivitis sicca (KCS) has been reported. The thickness of the tear film has been estimated by a variety of methods and is reported to be between 6 and $7 \mu m$.

It has been proposed by Jones that aqueous tear secretion driven from both the main and accessory lacrimal glands can be divided into "basic" or "basal" secretion and "reflex" secretion. He further proposed that "basal" secretion can be measured by performing a Schirmer test following a drop of topical anesthetic. Subsequent studies have demonstrated a 300% increase in tear turnover rate following lid margin stimulation in the anesthetized human eyes. In addition, tear flow rate in such eyes is found to be greater than that in unanesthetized eyes after the testing stimulus was reduced. These data therefore suggest that tear secretion is driven reflexly, and that a

Schirmer test performed after topical anesthesia is not a measure of "basal" tear flow. In fact, the existence of "basal" tear secretion has been called into question [3]. It is probable that aqueous tear secretion is stimulus driven at all times. Further supporting evidence for this contention lies in the fact that under conditions of considerable decrease in external stimuli, for example, general anesthesia or nightly sleep, aqueous tear secretion diminishes. A similar reduction in salivation occurs during sleep. The reduction in aqueous tear secretion during sleep is thought to be related to a high prevalence of recurrent corneal erosions and contact lens problems occurring during sleep.

It has also been suggested that, while tearing is decreased during sleep, there has been an inadequate explanation for the destination of tears during sleep in the absence of a blinking mechanism to drive tear exit. It has been suggested that there may be a mass movement of fluid from the tear film accross the conjunctiva to blood resulting from sodium ion transport during sleep. It is thought that tears are lost in the eye by way of three roots: (a) via bulk flow into the canalicular system; (b) via evaporation from the exposed surface of the eye, which has been measured to be about $0.085\,\mu l/min$; (c) via absorption of water across the conjunctival surface as a result of a sodium pump across the conjunctival epithelium. There is evidence of considerable absorption of tears across the mucous membranes of the superior inferior and common canaliculi and the nasolacrimal sac.

2.2 The Lipids of the Tear Film

The lipids of the tear film are thought to be excreted by the meibomian glands of the lids. There are approximately 20 meibomian glands in each upper and lower lid. It is possible that some lipid reaching the tear film is excreted by the lid glands of Zeis and Moll. The meibomian glands are deep in the lid structure and can be visualized by transilluminating the lid (Fig. 3); their gross morphology can be outlined by transillumination photography employing infrared film. The factors controlling excretion rates in meibomian glands are poorly understood. If one can extrapolate, however, from what is known concerning the oil glands of the skin, it is probable that excretion of meibum from these glands is at least somewhat influenced by hormonal changes. It is thought that in infections of the meibomian glands and/or dysfunctional conditions, there is a qualitative change in the excretion (see Dartt, this volume, for a complete discussion of meibomian gland secretion). In fact there is a qualitative increase in free fatty acids (see below).

The lipid secreted by the meibomian glands is made up of a variety of lipid entities, including nonpolar sterol and waxy esters (around 58%) plus other esters, free sterols, triglycerides, and free fatty acids. Polar lipids are reported to account for about 15% of meibomian gland secretion. The meibomian lipid is secreted as a fluid. The lipid flows onto the aqueous preocular tear film; this can sometimes be seen as visible streams com-

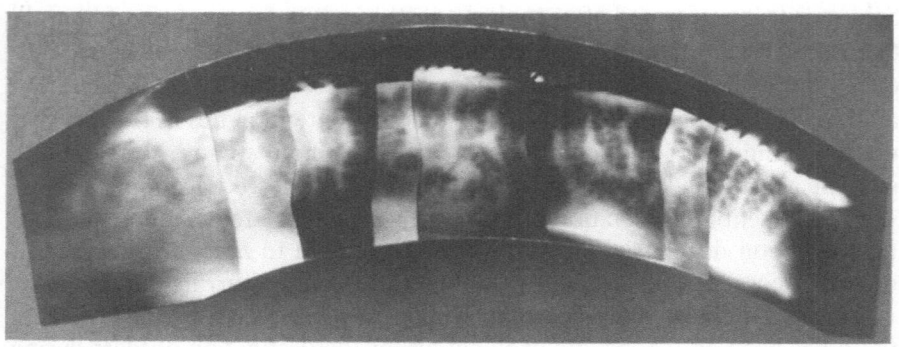

Fig. 3. Transillumination infrared photography (montage) of the lid (meibography). The structure of the meibomian glands. (Courtesy of W. Shields)

ing from the meibomian orifices. The orientation of the lipid forming the outermost layer of the preocular tear film is thought to be such that the polar components spread fastest with their charged polar groups oriented toward the aqueous phase. The more slowly spreading nonpolar lipids quickly cover this polar layer to form a thicker "duplex" film.

The existence of anterior lipid layer of the preocular tear film has been inferred from biomicroscopic observation of interference patterns seen from the surface of the tear film. Such patterns have been observed by Koby et al. A method for estimating thickness of the lipid portion of the tear film relating to the color bands observed has been reported by McDonald and Norn. More recently a uniform field biodifferential interference microscope has been developed by Hamano and associates; they described three patterns reflective in the lipid layer, i.e., an amorphous pattern, a marmoreal pattern, and a flow pattern. Other methods to study these lipid patterns include the use of a modified slit lamp, specular microscopy, keratometry, and a noninvasive low-illuminence grid pattern reflection instrument which attaches to a Zeiss slit lamp and is known as a toposcope.

During blinking it is thought that the lipid layer undergoes considerable compression and decompression. This layer is characterized by a high degree of stability, which accounts for its resistance to deformation when subjected to high mechanical demands. In vitro studies indicate that the meibomian gland secretion can form stable layers 80–100 Å in thickness; other studies have indicated values of 200–2000 Å.

It is thought that the lipid layer of the tear film serves at least three important functions to enhance the stability of the tear film. (a) It tends to retard evaporation from the tear film. In rabbits this has been measured to be a 4- to 20-fold diminution in evaporation. (b) It has been suggested that meibomian gland secretion prevents contamination of the tear film by the more polar lipids secreted by the sebaceous glands of the eye lids. The application of a drop of this sebum to the tear film causes an immediate

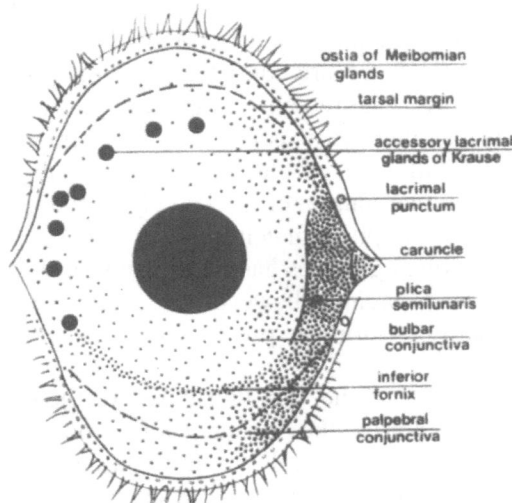

ostia of Meibomian glands

tarsal margin

accessory lacrimal glands of Krause

lacrimal punctum

caruncle

plica semilunaris

bulbar conjunctiva

inferior fornix

palpebral conjunctiva

Fig. 4. The topographical distribution of goblet cells in the conjunctiva

breakup with the formation of a dry spot. (c) As the eye lids open subsequent to a blink, the spreading lipid lowers the surface tension of the tears, which in turns draws water into the tear film and thickens the aqueous phase. This so-called Marangoni effect appears to occupy an important role in maintaining tear film thickness.

2.3 The Mucin Component

As noted above, the innermost layer of the tear film consists of a coating immediately overlying the epithelial surface of the cornea and conjunctiva. This layer is complex but consists mostly of mucous (hydrated) glycoproteins associated with a mixture of protein electrolytes and cellular material. The thickness of this layer has been variously reported as only a few hundredths of a micrometer to over one micrometer. The source of the mucin layer has been reported to include: (a) 1. the conjunctival goblet cells, (b) 2. the lacrimal glands, and (c) 3. the corneal and conjunctival epithelial cells.

The goblet cells are unicellular, mucus-secreting glands scattered throughout the bulbar and palpebral conjunctiva. The topographical distribution of these cells (Fig. 4) is highly varied and has been described in numerous early works. Kessing, studying whole-mount dissections of cadaver conjunctiva, described the greatest density of these cells to be in the inferior palpebral conjunctiva. Ralph, studying biopsy specimens, found between 8.8 and 10 goblet cells per millimeter in this area. Subsequent studies by Marquardt demonstrated between 25 and 40 cells per millimeter. The goblet cell density is found to be quite similar in different age groups; however, there is a slight decrease in goblet cell density in subjects in the seventh decade of life or older. Histochemical studies have demonstrated that human goblet cells stain with periodic acid–Schiff (PAS) and alcian blue; these staining characteristics at pH 1–2.5 are consistent with the presence of sulfated and sialoglycoproteins. Fluorescein-conjugated antibody studies against fractions of human tear mucous glycoprotein have demonstrated the presence of this material within the goblet cells. Such findings have not been reported from other putative sources of tearlike glycoprotein, for instance, lacrimal gland and nongoblet epithelial cells.

PAS and alcian blue staining of protein granules has been demonstrated within human lacrimal acinar cells. Such findings, however, are nonspecific for glycoproteins and do not necessarily confirm the presence of substances that contribute to the tear film.

A third putative source of the mucin of the tear film is the epithelial cells themselves. Investigators have reported the existence of a mucous secretory system within the nongoblet epithelial cells of the conjunctiva. This system involves subsurface secretory vesicules with histochemical staining properties consistent with the presence of sialomucins. As mentioned above, these histochemical stains are not specific for the glycoproteins of the mucin layer of the tear film.

Histopathological studies of the surface of the eye reporting different thicknesses in the mucus layer and different morphological characteristics may be due to differences in processing. Recently a two-layered structure of the mucin layer has been described, i.e., an innermost component tightly bound to the epithelial cell surface and thought to constitute a glycocalyx secreted via the subsurface epithelial vesicles. Above this is a much thicker, looser "mucus blanket" thought to be the product of goblet cells of the conjunctiva. The differences in the physical chemical properties of these two components of the mucus layer have not been well studied.

Holly and Lemp have demonstrated that tear mucus glycoproteins lower the tear surface tension from a level of about 70 dyne/cm to 40 dyne/cm. This is thought to be effected by an interaction between mucin and the surface lipid layer. They propose that the corneal surface epithelium is hydrophobic due to the lipid content of the cell wall, and that the mucin forms a loose adsorptive coating which temporarily forms a new surface that is wettable by the overlying aqueous tear layer. This theory is based on a series of experiments in which the mucin layer was carefully wiped from the surface, presumably exposing the underlying epithelial cells. This exposed surface was found to be nonwettable by saline and artificial tear preparations containing proteins. When the surface was wiped by mucus plug, however, aqueous solutions then spread spontaneously on the surface. Subsequent investigators have criticized these experiments suggesting that this method produced damage to the corneal surface, and that the hydrophobicity noted was caused by this trauma. The wettability of the corneal surface is discussed in greater detail below.

2.4 Wettability of the Corneal Surface

The cell walls of the superficial corneal epithelial cells are composed of proteins and lipids. There is evidence that a glycoprotein is secreted by the corneal surface cells forming an outer glycocalyx. The chemical composition of both the epithelial cell wall and the glycocalyx are poorly defined. Mishima reported that wiping of the corneal surface rendered it unwettable by tears. The mechanism by which tears actually wet the corneal surface has been a subject of speculation and investigation for some years. It has been suggested that proteins dissolved within the aqueous phase of the tear film lower its surface tension, thus contributing to its stability. Alternatively, the lipids of the meibomian gland secretions were thought to be selectively rubbed into the epithelial surface, increasing its surface activity.

The wettability of solid surfaces can be defined by studying the spreading characteristics of fluids. Lemp et al. measured the contact angle of solutions containing various constituents of tears on the rubbed corneal surface of rabbits. They determined that both mucin and simple proteins are capable of lowering the surface tension of tears. Conjunctival mucin, however, spread by the action of the lids adsorbs onto the corneal surface and is thought to be a critical factor in establishing a new adsorbed layer over the corneal surface which is wet by aqueous tears. Further studies by Holly and Lemp of excised rabbit corneal surface and also that of epithelial monolayers cultured from the corneal epithelium were studied with pure hydrophobic liquids. Their results indicated that the corneal epithelium free of adsorbed mucin shows a low-energy surface. While the epithelial surface has an affinity toward aqueous phases, this is insufficient to account for complete wetting. Using bovine submaxillary mucin, they demonstrated that mucin adsorbed on such a low-energy surface yields a new surface with a higher critical surface tension with considerably higher affinity toward water. They suggested that the primary role of conjunctival glycoproteins (mucin) is to transform a low-energy corneal surface into a higher energy surface via adsorption. This action of mucin, in combination with its effect increasing the affinity of tears for water and lowering the surface tension of tears, is thought to be sufficient to achieve complete wetting of the corneal surface. Other investigators, however, hold to the view that the cell membranes of corneal surface cells are entirely wettable by virtue of the charged groups on the glycoproteins, proteins, and glycocalyx creating a strong interaction between the strong dipole of water and the polar cell surface.

2.5 Tear Film Formation, Stability, and Rupture

As the upper lid moves down over the corneal and conjunctival surface, it compresses the outer lipid layer of the tear film between the two lid edges;

the aqueous layer remains in place beneath. Presumably at the same time the lids act to spread conjunctival mucin which is newly absorbed onto the corneal surface. The outer lipid strip is compressed greatly and probably reaches a thickness of 0.1 mm; this is such that no spillover of lipid onto the skin would be expected. The moving lid controls the speed of spreading liquid, and there is never an aqueous tear layer surface exposed to the atmosphere. The corneal surface should be wetted if its surface tension is greater than the sum of the surface tension and interfacial tension of the tear film. It is thought that the interfacial tension between the aqueous tear-mucin interface is quite low. The role of mucin in lowering both the surface tension of the tears and the interfacial tension facilitates rewetting of poss-ible discontinuities (dry spots) of the tear film.

2.6 Tear Film Rupture

If after the upper lid has completed its upward excursion, a further blinking is prevented, the preocular tear film thins and eventually ruptures, creating "dry spots." The time between the last complete blink and the appearance of the first randomly distributed dry spot is referred to as the breakup time. This is a measure of the stability of the tear film. The tear film is a tenuous structure tending toward disruption. To explain the mechanisms by which tear film rupture occurs (if a new film is not reestablished with a blink) several hypotheses have been advanced. Holly has suggested that the mucin layer becomes contaminated with lipids to such an extent that this layer becomes hydrophobic. Aqueous layers over hydrophobic surfaces are known to rupture when thickness decreases below a critical value, i.e., 10^{-2} cm (a value which is much higher than the thickness of the tear film). The tear film therefore could not be expected to remain continuous over such a hydrophobic location. Holly further thinks the most likely source of contamination is the superficial lipid layer. Evaporation, the presence of debris in the tear film, or local fluid forces driven by surface tension gradient (Marangoni flow) all tend to make the tear film thinner. It is thought that there is a diffusion of lipid molecules from the superficial lipid layer across this very thin aqueous phase to the mucin layer. Once the mucin layer is saturated with lipid to such an extent that it becomes hydrophobic in certain locations, the tear film spontaneously ruptures. Such lipid-contaminated mucin is thought to work its way out of the tear film by way of the formation of a mucin network, comprised of fibrils, threads, and clots. This network is driven downward by the force of the lid and eventually becomes a recogniz-able mucus thread in the inferior fornix ultimately exiting via the medial canthus.

In contrast to this, Ruckenstein and Sharma believe that the key step in tear film rupture is instability and eventual rupture of the mucin layer caused by van der Waals expulsion forces acting on the mucin layer. The aqueous layer is then thought to rupture when it comes in contact with the underlying hydrophilic epithelium. Lin and Brenner have suggested yet another possibility causing tear film rupture. They have demonstrated that the break-up may be caused by long-range intermolecular forces, known as dispersion forces, associated with coherent dipole-dipole interactions among neutral molecules.

Each of these hypotheses may reflect events operative in the rupture of the tear film. All are consistent with the observation that the tear film established by the blinking mechanism is somewhat tenuous and tends toward disruption. Periodic reformation by way of blinking is necessary to maintain a continuous tear film over the preocular surface.

3 Renewal of the Ocular Surface

There is an intimate relationship between the ocular surface and the overlying tear film. The cornea and conjunctival surfaces are in a continual state of replenishment, with older cells being sloughed off (exfoliation) and newer, deeper cells coming to the surface. The renewal of the corneal epithelium has been a subject of intense study; less is known about conjunctival cell replacement. The corneal epithelium is regularly arranged, with a uniform thickness of five cell layers. The innermost basal cells are columnar to cuboidal in shape and are attached to the underlying basement membrane by hemidemisomal junctions. Basal cells are thought to provide for the generative activities of the epithelium. Overlying the basal cells is a layer of wing-shaped cells with broad shape and processes extending to the apical areas of the basal cell layers. More superficially are several layers of flattened cells. The surface of the cornea, when seen under high magnification of the scanning electron microscope, shows many microvillous projections from the cells, greatly increasing their surface area; these probably facilitate attachment of the tear film. The biochemistry of the corneal epithelium has been studied and found to differ from that of the conjunctiva. Corneal epithelial biochemistry is characterized by high levels of intracellular glycogen and by both anaerobic and aerobic metabolism, primarily via the hexose monophosphate shunt. It is thought that these energy sources, fueled by oxygen obtained from the tears and conjunctival capillaries of the lid, provide the respiration necessary for continuous cellular turnover and repair.

Epithelial cells are continually renewed, with cellular division occurring in the basal cell layer. A gradual upward and outward movement of new cells reaching the surface culminates in the eventual exfoliation of dead cells in the surface. Using tritiated thymidine and autoradiography in the rabbit model, Hanna and O'Brien found that one in every 75 basal cells is in a premitotic synthetic state over a 2-h period; they have calculated an average life cycle for a new epithelial cell of 3.5–7 days in the rabbit.

It has been reckoned, however, that a mitotic rate based on the above data is insufficient to account for replenishment of epithelial cells from the surface. In the search for a possible source of dividing cells interest has centered on the limbus. It has been known for many years that if the corneal epithelium is removed in its entirety, the conjunctival epithelium becomes a source for a centripetal movement of epithelial cells to recover the cornea. The role of the conjunctiva in the regeneration of normal uninjured corneal epithelium has not been elucidated.

Davanger and Evensen have focused attention on the limbus, an area of distinctive histological architecture, as a probable source of major epithelial regeneration. This annular band of tissue is approximately 1 mm in width and surrounds the cornea proper. It is characterized by the presence of Vogt's palisades, deep subepithelial outpouchings of richly vascularized papillae. These papillae are more discrete in younger and heavily pigmented individuals. They are more prominent inferiorly and show considerable variation among individuals. Between the papillae are numerous invaginations of goblet cell free epithelial cells. The area covered by the basal cells is larger due to the increased interfacial area caused by the invagination; the basal cells are adjacent to a well-developed capillary net. This is a region of considerable pigmentation in pigmented species of animals and in humans who are deeply pigmented.

Davanger and Evensen further buttressed their hypothesis by noting the frequent occurrence of peripheral corneal pigment lines suggesting a direction of movement of cells centripetally. Melanocytes have been observed to reside in the neighborhood of blood cells that are usually absent from the cornea. Further evidence of centripetal movement of cells lies in the recent observation that there is a radial arrangement of hemidesmisomal alignment along the basement membrane in normal murine eyes. It is a common clinical observation that in heavily pigmented individuals there are often radial pigment lines extending variable distances from the corneal periphery into the cornea and suggesting a possible streaming of pigment-laden epithelial cells from the limbus. This can be more accentuated after injury.

Based on these observations and on other indirect evidence, Thoft and Friend have proposed the "x,y,z hypothesis" which states that corneal epithelial cell maintenance depends upon a continual, centripetal migration as well as proliferation and declamation. In an attempt to better define the question of possible migration of the epithelial sheets in the normal uninjured cornea, Buck marked the peripheral cornea with a rotating needle containing a mixture of India ink and thorium dioxide. After 7 days the marker was visible in the underlying corneal stroma; the marker-containing epithelium had moved away from the stromal marks a mean distance of 94 ± 17 µm or about 17 µm per day. This migration was seen in the superficial and wing cells but was not present in basal cells. Recent experimental evidence involving tissue culture of human corneal epithelial cells has further supported the notion of the greater regenerative capacity in the peripheral cornea. Ebato, Friend, and Thoft found that explants from the peripheral cornea show greater outgrowth and a higher mitotic rate than those of the central cornea. Furthermore, in contrast to central explants, those from the periphery demonstrate confluence with small presumably new cells.

That corneal epithelial cells are capable of significant movement is evident from studies of epithelial healing following experimental wounds. The rapid sliding of epithelium after corneal injury was first noted by Peters in 1885. Subsequent studies have demonstrated that shortly after injury there is a sliding of adjacent epithelial cells with a pseudopodal extension of their processes into the defect in an attempt to cover it. Coincident with this movement is a lag period of approximately 1 day in which there is a cessation of DNA synthesis and a basal cell mitosis in the area surrounding the wound. Approximately 24 h after injury, DNA synthesis begins in the underlying stromal cells, and a wave of epithelial cell mitosis moves towards the wound crater, finally involving the basal cells which cover the wound. This activity eventually results in normal thickness of the epithelium covering the wound. Epithelial sliding is thought to be a wound repair mechanism unique to the cornea and is dependent upon intracellular glycogen. It can be retarded by glycogen depletion with certain metabolic poisons. Therefore epithelial healing in the cornea appears to consist of at least two stages: an initial sliding process which covers the defect rapidly and a second phase of mitotic activity resulting in the thickening of the epithelium. It has been observed that reepithelialization proceeds first downward, subsequently horizontally, and finally from below.

In a study of corneal abrasions in 21 patients Dua and Forrester followed closure patterns using fluorescein stain and planimetry. They noted that all abrasions involving the central cornea in which the limbus was intact healed in a similar manner; there was a nonuniform advancement of two, three, or more foci of epithelial sheets producing multiple convex fronts which meet, giving rise to Y- or double-Y-shaped patterns from which epithelial cells form a whirl pattern.

Following injury to the corneal epithelium the conjunctiva can be a source of cellular renewal to recover the cornea. Danjo et al. studied the mitotic rate and goblet cell density of conjunctival epithelium following total or central corneal epithelial removal. On day 1 following total removal of the corneal or limbal epithelium the mitotic rate of the surrounding perilimbal conjunctiva was ten times normal; following a central 5- or 10-mm epithelial removal, the perilimbal mitotic rate increased at three to four times normal. In addition, goblet cell density decreased. This is strong evidence that the conjunctival epithelium plays a major role in the resurfacing of large and limited corneal injuries, and that there is a substantial movement of cells from the periphery to the center of the cornea. Recent electron microscopic studies have demonstrated that conjunctivally derived "corneal epithelium" remains morphologically abnormal for as long as 7 months.

All epithelial cells contain keratin. There are over 20 kinds of keratin within cells, and these can be used as markers for specific types of epithelium. The introduction of monoclonally produced keratin-specific antibodies has provided investigators with a powerful tool in the study of epithelial cell behavior. Employing this technology researchers have become interested in the role of a specific subset of epithelial cells known as stem cells. These long-lived cells are present in all renewing tissues and are thought to be responsible for cellular regeneration. Stem cells are slow cycling and take up tritiated thymidine to an insignificant degree. They are believed to represent a stable population of primitive cells undergoing regular cell division, in turn giving rise to a population of intermediately differentiated cells called transient amplifying cells. These cells divide several times, amplifying the number of stem cell derived cells before subsequent terminal differentiation.

The dermatological literature contains studies of similar cells. Investigators have differentiated a primitive, slow-cycling, basal keratinocyte population from a highly proliferative and more differentiated group of keratinocytes located both basally and suprabasally. Cellular differences have been noted in the corneal limbus indicating the limbus as a site of corneal stem cells. Earlier sex chromatin studies, in addition to the previously cited India ink studies of Buck, provide further support for the migration of cells from the limbus to the center (Fig. 5). Very recent data from anti-keratin antibody research have demonstrated that corneal basal cells are more differentiated in their keratin expression than are limbal basal cells. The schema of stem cells giving rise to transient amplifying cells which then become fully differentiated corneal cells has been established as a working hypothesis buttressed by a substantial body of experimental data. The exact location and density of transient amplifying cells is as yet not clearly delineated.

In an in vitro system of cultured epithelial cells Soong used double labeling simultaneously for vinculin and actin. He demonstrated an intimate relationship between cytoplasmic filamentous actin stress fibers and focal extracellular vinculin (110–130 kDa), which act as cell and substrate adhesion foci. Soong has postulated that epithelial sheets of cells advanced by a "front-wheel drive" mechanism whereby focal attachments (vinculin) to substrate develop, becoming contiguous with oriented actin fibers which pull the cells ahead. Further support for vinculin as a putative agent in cell adhesion to substrate was presented Zieske and Gibson, who studied scraped keratectomized and thermally burned corneas in the rat. They found a 110-kDa protein synthesized at focal points at the leading edge of migrating epithelium and probably playing an important role in effecting

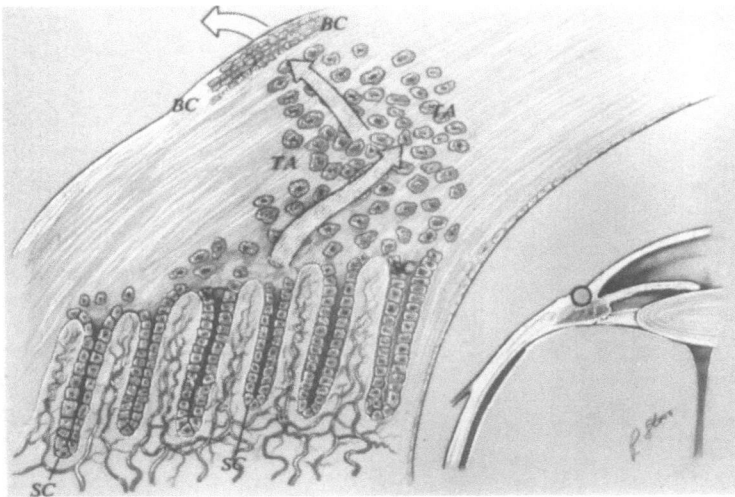

Fig. 5. Schematic drawing showing movement of cells from the corneal limbus with Vogt's palisades, stem cells (*SC*), transient amplifying cells (*TA*), and differentiated corneal basal cells (*BC*)

epithelial cell movement and wound healing. This protein size, location, and presumed functions are consistent with the characteristics of vinculin.

In an extensive clinical descriptive study, Bron categorized a variety of clinical conditions in which swirled, radiating lines (vortex patterns) in the corneal epithelium are a common feature. These include Fabry's disease, toxic keratopathy such as chloroquine and amiodarone, striate melanocytosis, healing corneal abrasions in association with iron lines in the cornea, band keratopathy, corneal edema, and in the periphery of the penetrating keratoplasty. Bron has advanced the thesis that the resemblance in patterns seen in these diverse clinical entities depends upon growth properties of the epithelium rather than on any specific stimuli. A centripetal "pigment slide" is observed in the corneas of highly pigmented individuals. It is assumed that this pigment lies within epithelial cells. The pigment is presumably derived from branching melanocytes located with fingerlike projections in the limbus. Such an epithelial marker would therefore delineate sliding of peripheral cells centrally. In lightly pigmented individuals alternative markers might be accumulated intracellular metabolic products such as those seen in Fabry's disease of chloroquine and amiodarone keratopathy (Fig. 6). The inferiorly decentered apex of the vortical pattern is consistent with a predominant cell movement downward. The constant feature is a radial centripetal slide from the limbus to the corneal center.

It seems likely that there is more than a single focus for the regeneration of corneal epithelium. While basal epithelial cells are clearly capable of

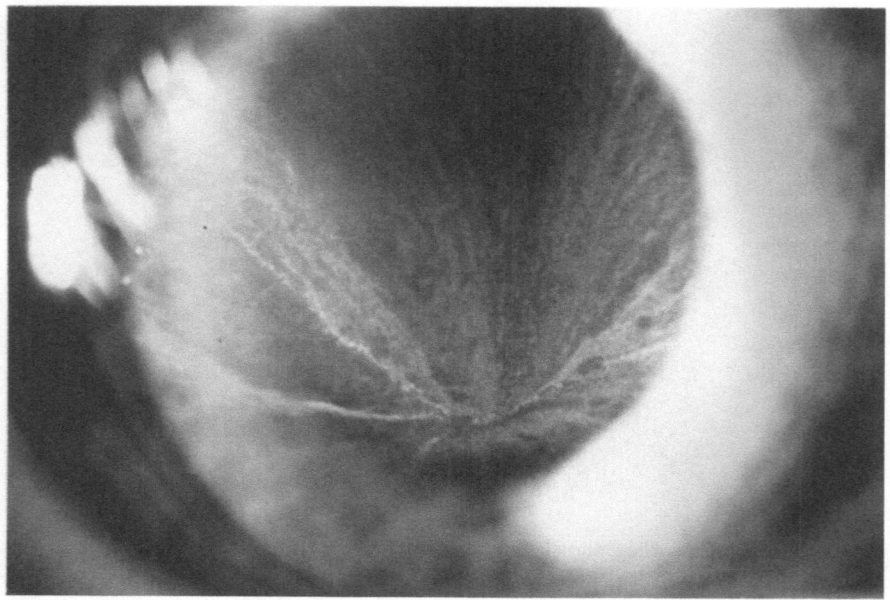

Fig. 6. Vortex keratopathy displaying radiating pathways of epithelial slide in a patient taking amiodarone

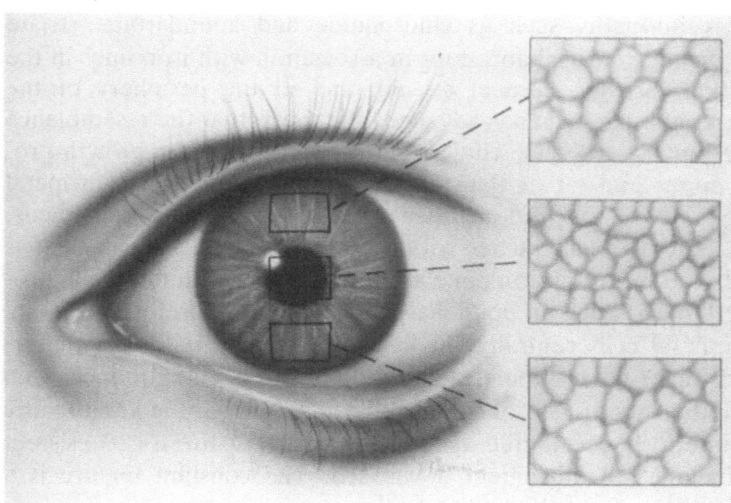

Fig. 7. Schematic drawing demonstrating differences in epithelial cell size by topographical distribution. Small cells predominating at the corneal center are newer cells

mitosis throughout the cornea (particularly in response to injury), the major contributors to regeneration appear to be located in or near the limbus. With normal exfoliation there is a centripetal movement of cells probably at the wing cell layer and immediately superjacent squamous cell layer although lateral movement of basal cells cannot be excluded. These mobile cells undergo division, replenishing epithelial cells lost from the corneal surface via the exfoliative process.

Recent studies employing specular microscopy of the corneal surface in the human by Lemp and Mathers [4] suggest that at least one of the driving forces in the centripetal movement of epithelial cells is a preferential exfoliative loss of cells from the central cornea driven by the shearing force from the upper lid. The evidence presented includes a statistically significant shift to small, presumably new cells in the central cornea as opposed to the limbus (Fig. 7). The upper lid is capable of considerable posterior force on the corneal surface; presumably this is greatest near the corneal apex, giving rise to a preferential loss of cells in the central cornea. In keratoconjunctivitis sicca this process appears to be accentuated (see below).

4 Classification of Tear Deficiency States

Based on the physiological considerations discussed above, it is possible to construct a classification system of tear film abnormalities in which specific pathogenetic mechanisms are identified. While each of the following abnormalities may exist in isolation, there is sometimes an overlap between these entities in which multiple abnormalities occur (Table 1).

4.1 Aqueous Tear Deficiency

The aqueous tears the products of the main and accessory lacrimal glands constitute the bulk of the preocular tear film. In certain situations there is an absolute or partial deficiency in aqueous tear production. This can occur as a rare congenital abnormality such as alacrima. This can be unilateral or bilateral; it may be due to hypoplasia of the lacrimal and/or a congenital paresis of the VII cranial nerve.

Another relatively rare cause of aqueous tear deficiency is familial dysautonomia (Riley-Day syndrome). This is a condition occurring in Jews of Eastern European origin and affects both sexes equally. It occurs as part of generalized dysfunction of the autonomic nervous system and includes the following characteristics: blood pressure lability, cyclic vomiting, motor incoordination, emotional difficulties, increased sweatin, dermal discoloration, and a tendency to frequent respiratory infection. There is an exaggerated response to sympathomimetic and parasympathomimetic drugs.

Table 1. Classification of tear deficiency states

Aqueous tear deficiency
  Keratoconjunctivitis sicca
  Keratoconjunctivitis sicca associated with Sjögren's syndrome
  Congenital alacrima
  Familial dysautonomia (Riley-Day syndrome)
  VII nerve paresis
  Postdacryoadenitis
  Posttrauma
  Postirradiation
  Chemical burns
  Pharmacologically induced
Mucin deficiency
  Hypovitaminosis A
  Cicatricial ocular pemphigoid (late aqueous deficiency, AD)
  Erythema multiforme (Stevens-Jonhson syndrome) (late AD)
  Chemical burns (late AD)
  Trachoma (late AD)
Lipid abnormalities
  Congenital anhydrotic ectodermal dysplasia
  Meibomian gland dysfunction (blepharitis)
  Isoretinin treatment
Lid surfacing abnormalities
  Exposure keratitis
  VII nerve paresis
  Symblepharon
  Lid-corneal surface incongruities
  Incomplete blinking
  Three and nine o'clock staining with contact lens wear
Epitheliopathy
  Anesthetic cornea (V nerve lesions)
  Corneal scars

In addition to decreased aqueous tear secretion, there is a decrease in corneal sensation; corneal ulceration occurs. Riley-Day syndrome is associated with a short life span, as most of those afflicted succumb to infection.

Much more common, however, is the development of an aqueous deficient tear state in adults. Aqueous tear secretion decreases with aging but in most individuals is not severe enough to cause problems. In some individuals, however, particularly women, tear production decreases to the extent that there is the development of ocular surface disease and irritative symptoms. This condition occurs most commonly in the fifth decade and later in life. In relatively mild cases the main symptom is a foreign body sensation or "scratchiness." These symptoms can progress to become constant with intense burning or irritation which can prove debilitating to the patient. The most commonly observed clinical signs include increased debris in the tear film (due to an increased rate of epithelial cell desquamation) and a relative stagnation of normal tear flow, a scanty marginal tear strip, increased mucous threads within the tear film particularly in the inferior fornix, decreased wetting of Schirmer test strips, and staining of the exposed

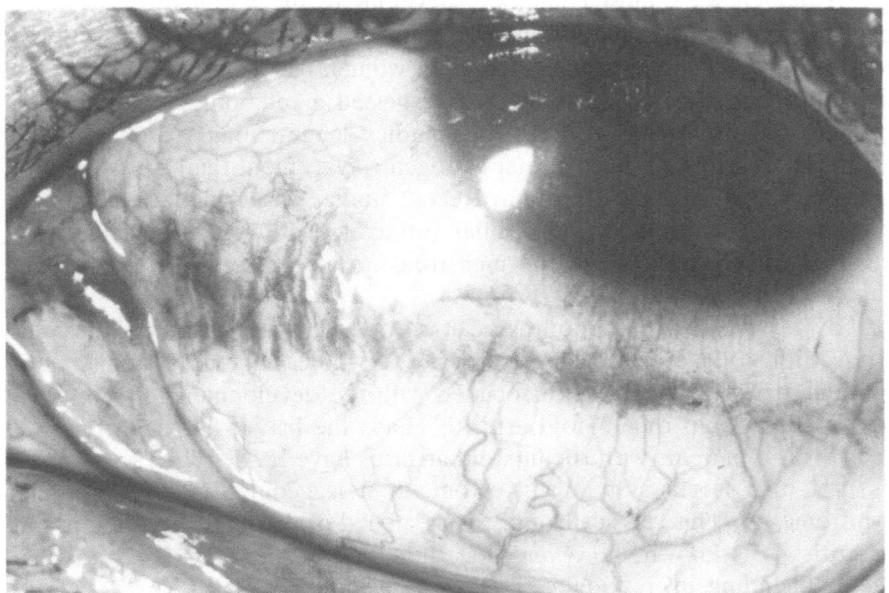

Fig. 8. Rose bengal staining of the ocular surface in KCS

portions of the corneal and conjunctival surfaces with rose bengal stain (Fig. 8). The severity of this condition fluctuates. More severe cases, however, progress to develop filamentary keratitis, which is a painful condition characterized by the appearance of numerous strands or filaments attached to the corneal surface. There is evidence to suggest that these filaments represent breaks in the continuity of the normal epithelial cell sheets, probably secondary to desiccation and/or excessive shear forces from the upper lid. The filaments contain partially desquamated sheets of epithelial cells mixed with mucin; a variant is the stationary mucus plaque.

A characteristic finding in KCS is the presence of variable amounts of stagnant mucin within the tear film and on the ocular surface. It is thought that this is due to the increased precipitation of lipid-contaminated mucin resulting from reduced aqueous tear production.

Eyes with KCS are more susceptible to infection. There is a breakdown in several aspects of the ocular surface defense mechanisms. At least three components of the tear film with antibacterial activity have been identified, i.e., lysozyme, beta-lysin, and lactoferrin. Both lysozyme and lactoferrin have been reported to be reduced in the tears of patients with KCS. In addition, with the reduction of aqueous tear flow, the normal flushing action of the tears is impaired. There is a high prevalence of concomitant lid infections in patients with KCS. This can lead to more serious infections of the ocular surface, including conjunctivitis and keratitis.

Although KCS most commonly develops in the absence of any other overt systemic abnormality, there is a frequent association of KCS with systemic disease. The prevalence of KCS in women particularly in menopausal and postmenopausal age groups has suggested a relationship to hormonal changes. There are no well-controlled studies documenting this relationship, but anecdotal reports suggest that estrogen replacement therapy can exert a beneficial effect on this condition. Recent studies on hormonal receptors in the lacrimal glands and on the ocular surface and studies on ocular cellular changes in association with the menstrual cycle have further strengthened this association (see below).

By far the most common association of KCS with systemic illness has been with collagen vascular disorders. A whole host of systemic autoimmune diseases have been associated with the development of a dry eye. Within this group rheumatoid arthritis heads the list. It has been reported that 14% of patients with rheumatoid arthritis have KCS. When KCS occurs as part of a larger systemic involvement, it is generally called Sjögren's syndrome [5]. This classically consists of a triad of dry eyes, dry mouth, and arthritis. It is known, however, that there can be multiple organ involvement, including liver, kidney, spleen, gastrointestinal tract, lung, thyroid, and the adrenal glands. Because of the frequent involvement of the labial glands of the mouth, biopsies of these glands have been used as a diagnostic test for Sjögren's syndrome.

The histological changes in KCS are those of generalized atrophy of the acinar and interstitial tissue of the lacrimal glands. Particularly in those patients with Sjögren's syndrome there can be intense lymphocytic and plasma cell infiltration. These changes resemble those seen in autoimmune disease, reinforcing the impression that KCS has an autoimmune basis.

There is increasing evidence that the dry eyes associated with Sjögren's syndrome represent a distinct subset of patients with aqueous tear deficiencies. These patients are prone to more severe complications of the disease process including the association of scleritis (including necrotizing scleritis; Fig. 9), rheumatoid nodules of the sclera (Fig. 10), and corneal ulceration leading sometimes to performation (Fig. 11).

KCS is usually a bilateral disease and seldom occurs unilaterally. It can be seen in one eye after VII nerve paresis, viral dacryoadenitis, mechanical trauma to or surgical removal of the lacrimal glands, irradiation of the eye, and chemical burns.

4.2 Mucin Deficiency

In contrast to the aqueous-deficient dry eyes, there exists a group of conditions which are characterized primarily by morphological changes in the conjunctiva which in turn lead to instability of the tear film. In the previous section the critical role of mucin produced by the goblet cells of the con-

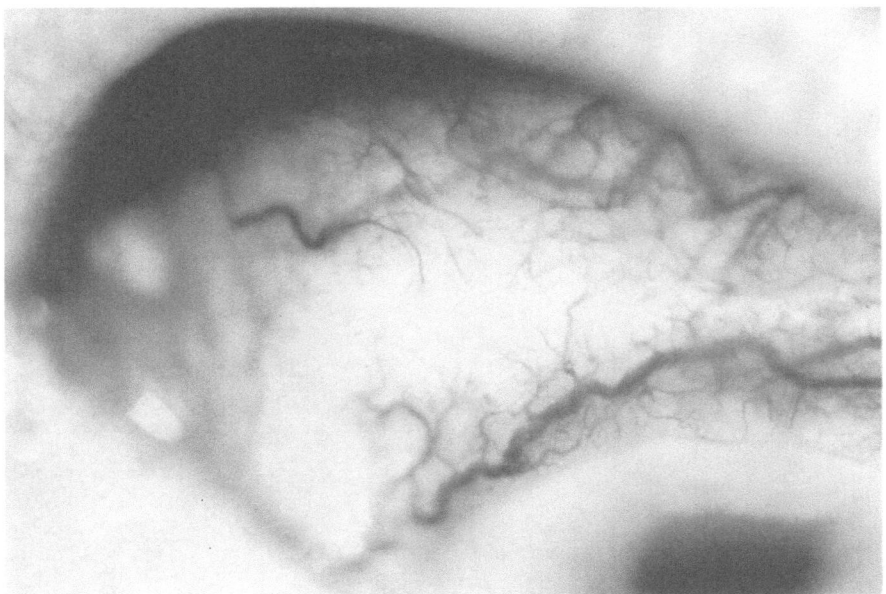

Fig. 9. Necrotizing scleritis (scleromalacia perforans)

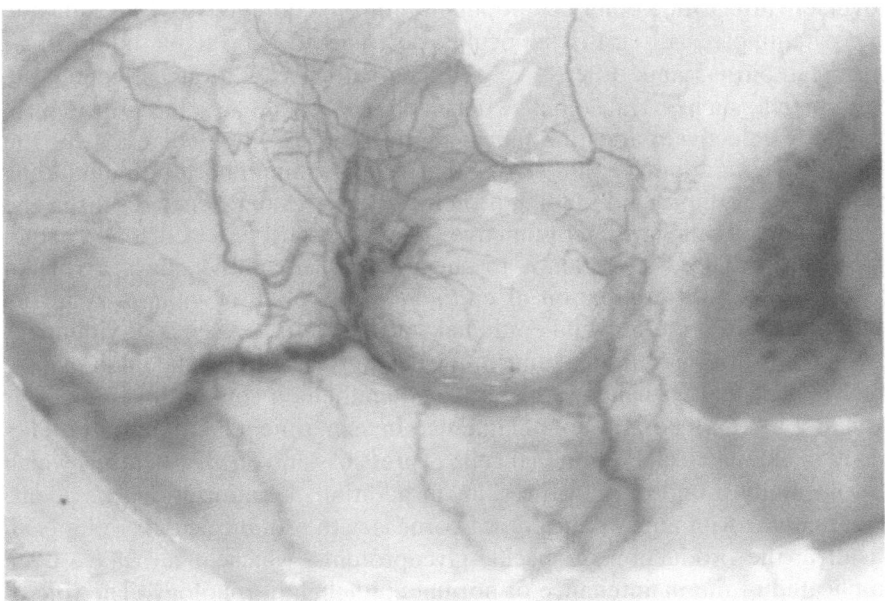

Fig. 10. Rheumatoid nodule of the sclera in a patient with Sjögren's syndrome

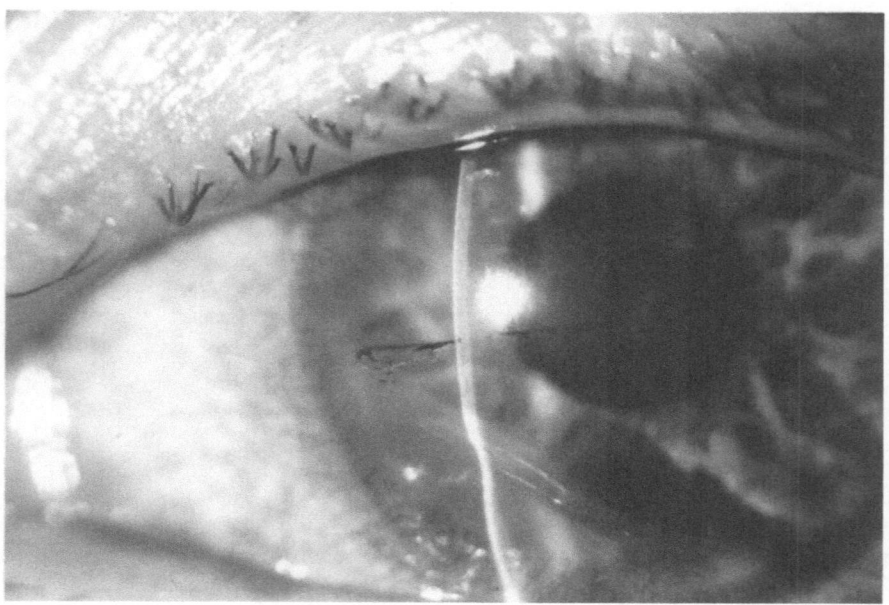

Fig. 11. Peripheral corneal ulceration in Sjögren's-associated KCS

junctiva has been discussed. There are a number of conditions known to adversely affect the goblet cell population of the conjunctiva. These include hypovitaminosis A, cicatricial ocular pemphigoid, erythema multiforme, chemical burns, and other severe inflammatory conditions affecting the conjunctiva, such as trachoma. A deficiency of vitamin A is the prototypical condition selectively affecting mucin production. The epithelial cells of the conjunctiva, and indeed all layers of the cornea, contain both retinol binding protein and retinoic acid-binding protein. Vitamin A deficiency results in the loss of goblet cells in the conjunctiva; this is an early effect of this vitamin deprivation. There is evidence to suggest that vitamin A plays a role in controlling the differentiation of epithelial cells. Lack of vitamin A favors the production of keratinized epithelial cells while the presence of vitamin A favors the differentiation of mucin-producing cells. It has been shown by Tseng et al. that corneal and conjunctival epithelium contain low molecular weight (40-kDa) keratin tonofilaments. In experimental vitamin A deficiency in animal models epithelial cells express 65- and 56 kDa keratins which are normally found only in the skin; in addition, keratinization is evident. Treatment of vitamin A deficient rat corneas with retinoic acid or retinol can result in the production of specific glycoproteins, which in turn have been implicated in the maintenance of normal epithelial morphology. The role of vitamin A in the maintenance of a normal conjunctival and corneal surface is as yet unclear.

The initial histological change observed in vitamin A deficiency appears to be the disappearance of conjunctival goblet cells; the initial clinical change seen is the appearance of areas of nonwettability on the conjunctival and corneal surface. Further development of this condition is associated with keratinization of both cornea and conjunctiva epithelia. It has been demonstrated that in the presence of loss of goblet cells there is an instability of the tear film, giving rise to rapid breakup. It is probable that, in addition to the adverse affects on the tear film itself, keratinization of the surface also affects wetting. Topical treatment with vitamin A analogs have been shown to reverse the phenomenon.

While vitamin A deficiency selectively affects conjunctival goblet cells, other conditions that indiscriminately destroy normal conjunctival architecture also affect goblet cells. These conditions include chronic cicatricial ocular pemphigoid, erythema multiforme, chemical burns, trachoma, and certain forms of drug-induced disease. When these inflammatory changes are marked, it is common for the openings of the main and accessory lacrimal glands also to be affected giving rise to an aqueous tear deficiency. The hallmark, however, of the primary mucin deficient condition is an unstable tear film manifest as an abnormally rapid tear film breakup time.

4.3 Lipid Abnormalities

In general, problems associated with lipid abnormality are those of glandular dysfunction rather than glandular absence. Congenital anhidrotic ectodermal dysplasia has, however, been reported to be associated with an absence of obvious meibomian gland openings. Since the lipids produced by the meibomian glands are important in the stabilization of the tear film, abnormalities in their production have an adverse affect on tear film stability. Recent work by Mathers et al. has elucidated some of the mechanisms associated with these dysfunctional states. Meibomian gland dysfunction is associated with abnormalities of the excreta thickness and volume of the meibomian glands (meibum; Fig. 12). The secretion responding to digital expression is normally clear and flows freely. In contrast, in meibomian gland dysfunction there is probably a qualitative shift in the constituents of the meibum with a change in melting point and obstruction of the meibomian orificies. These alterations in meibum viscosity range from turbidity of the meibum seen in seborrheic meibomian dysfunction to a more coagulated type of expression in obstructive meibomian dysfunction, resulting in a formed column of meibum similar to that in a toothpaste tube. It has been shown that this obstructive meibomian gland dysfunction is associated with a decreased volume of excreta and results in an increase in tear film osmolarity, which is presumably due to accelerated evaporation from the surface. This in turn can lead to a type of "pseudo-dry eye state."

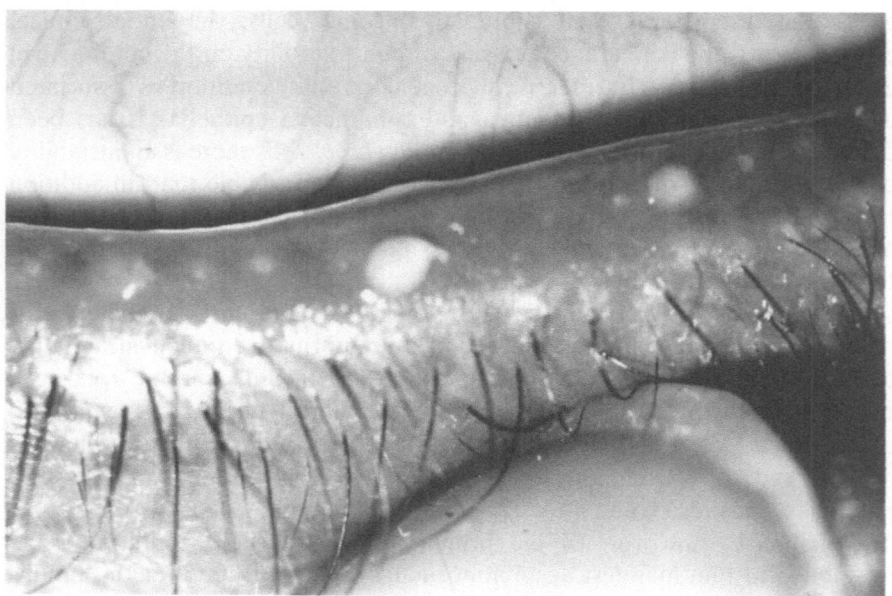

Fig. 12. Thickened excreta (meibum) from meibomian glans in obstructive meibomian gland dysfunction. (Courtesy of W.D. Mathers)

Obstructive meibomian dysfunction has been correlated with morphological changes in glandular structure showing drop-out of glands and involution and atresia of ductules by transillumination infrared photography of the lids (meibography). Similar temporary involutional changes are associated with systemic treatment with isoretinin (Accutane).

4.4 Lid Surfacing Abnormalities

As discussed earlier, the precorneal tear film is inherently unstable, i.e., after formation of a continuous film subsequent to a blink, the tear film thins and develops areas of discontinuity unless there is resurfacing by way of a new blink. The shear force produced by moving lids drives the removal of lipid-contaminated mucous strands and thus plays a vital role in rejuvenation of the mucus layer of the tear film. It is necessary for periodic resurfacing of the tear film by way of the blinking action of the lids to maintain a normal continuous precorneal tear film. (The action of the lid also drives a preferential exfoliation of corneal epithelial cells in the central area of the cornea, as discussed above.)

When normal lid movement is compromised, the area of the cornea and conjunctiva not covered by a blink represents a well-defined area of non-wetting resulting in localized desiccation. Eventually secondary changes

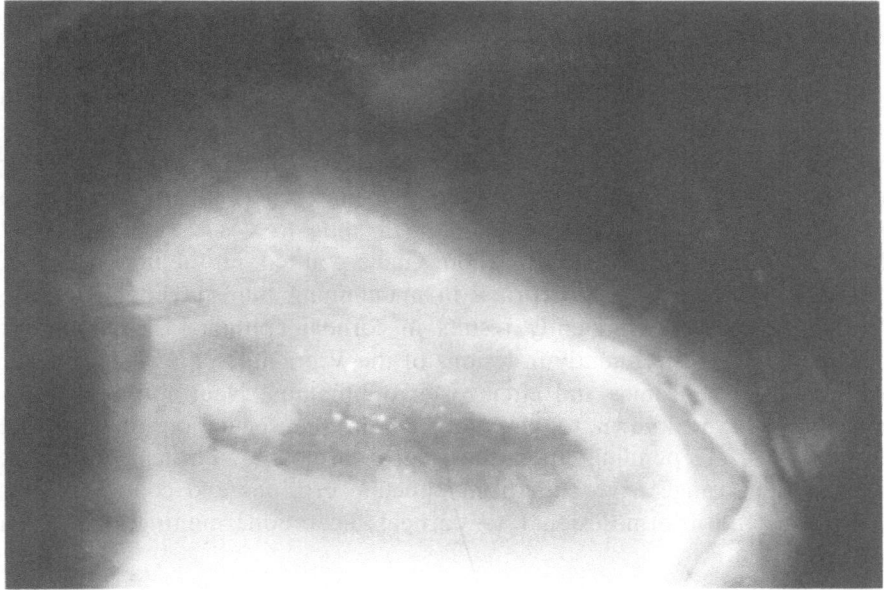

Fig. 13. Localized nonwetting of cornea in exposure keratitis

(keratinization) occur in the desiccated epithelium making the area even less wettable.

Localized drying is seen in exposure keratitis, most commonly in connection with VII cranial nerve paresis. There is some surfacing of the tear film in patients with a VII nerve paresis with an intact Bell's phenomenon by upward rotation of the globe. This mechanism, however, is usually insufficient to maintain an adequate tear film, particularly over the inferior one-third of the cornea. The localized desiccation causes forms of exposure keratitis which can range from mild superficial punctate erosions to well-demarcated areas of severe desiccation (Fig. 13). Secondary keratinization in the area further complicates the wetting problem, and prolonged hydration is often necessary to restore the integrity of the cornea.

Lid movement can also be restricted by the development of symblepharon. Symblepharon is particularly prominent in cicatrizing ocular pemphigoid and erythema multiforme and chemical burns. Successful maintenance of a tear film also requires a reasonable congruity between the lids and the ocular surface in order to produce sufficient and uniform shear. In the absence of proper apposition of the lid and the ocular surface the shear diminishes, and the tear layer is not resurfaced adequately. Such localized nonwetting can also occur in contact lens wearers with incomplete blinking giving rise to so-called three and nine o'clock peripheral staining.

4.5 Epitheliopathy

Because there is an intimate relationship between the corneal surface and
the tear film, alterations in the normal morphology of the corneal epithelium
can affect the stability of the tear film. The corneal epithelium is thrown into
multiple microvillous projections. These villi or plicae increase the surface
area of the corneal epithelium allowing for more adsorptive sites for tear
mucin. Abnormalities in the morphology of the corneal surface give rise to
problems in tear surfacing in that area leading to desiccation, epithelial
breakdown, and even frank ulceration. Gaule pointed out the importance of
nervous innervation to the cornea in maintaining the epithelial integrity.
Corneal anesthesia frequently results in corneal epithelial abnormalities.
This is seen most frequently in lesions of the V cranial nerve such as occur
with acoustic neuromas and after zoster ophthalmia. Neurohumoral transmitters are now known to be important in the regulation of epithelial
turnover [6]. Depending upon the degree of loss of corneal sensation,
clinical signs range from superficial punctate erosions and coarse mucous
plaques (dendritiform lesions) to corneal ulceration, melting, and even
performation.

5 Pathogenesis of Ocular Surface Disease

The causative factors in the production of ocular surface disease in dry eye
states constitute a subject of extensive investigation and speculation (Table
2). Since the morbidity in dry eyes is related in great measure to changes
that occur on the ocular surface, an understanding of the multiple factors
which can be operative in the production of ocular surface disease is critical.
The following theories have been advanced relating to the production of
ocular surface disease in dry eye states.

5.1 Desiccation

It has classically been thought that ocular surface disease in dry eye is
related to decreased aqueous tear production. It is now known that a variety
of neurohumoral transmitters play a role in the production of aqueous tears.
These include adrenocorticotropic hormone, α-melanocyte stimulating
hormone, corticotropin-like intermediate lobe peptide, enkephalins, and
prolactin (see Dartt, this volume). In patients with Sjögren's disease and
possibly those with non-Sjögren's aqueous-deficient tear disease there is
evidence of a chronic inflammatory process in the main and accessory

Table 2. Factors causing dry eye symptoms

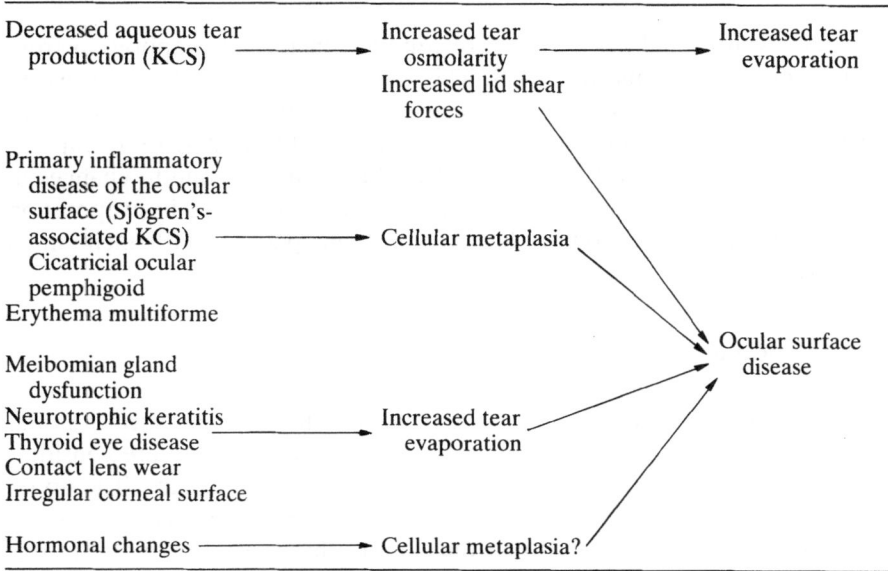

lacrimal glands. This leads to dysfunction of the acinar tissue of the lacrimal glands and ultimately to atrophy. This is thought to be an autoimmune process. Recently, the possibility that a chronic viral infection could play a role in the induction of these inflammatory changes in the lacrimal glands has been suggested; the Epstein-Barr virus has been implicated.

The role of desiccation secondary to decreased aqueous tear secretion as the major pathogenetic mechanism in the production of ocular surface disease has been supported by the work of Gilbard, Farris and associates studying osmolarity of the tear film [7]. They have reported that in KCS there is a statistically significant rise in tear film osmolarity. They believe that there is a movement of fluid out from the epithelial cells in response to this osmotic shift. Similar rises in tear film osmolarity have been reported in contact lens wearers, patients with thyroid disease with increased inter-palpebral area, in neurotrophic keratitis, and in patients with meibomian gland dysfunction (see above).

Animal models have been created inducing a dry eye state by closing off the openings of the aqueous tear producing glands and removing accessory lid tissue. There is a rise in tear film osmolarity in these models. In addition, in vitro studies of epithelial cell cultures have demonstrated changes suggestive of desiccation when exposed to hyperosmolar bathing solutions. Similar changes have been reported in a small series of human subjects. The efficacy of hypotonic artificial tear solutions remains a subject of some controversy.

5.2 Evaporation

Rolando, Refojo and associates have reported increased evaporation from the tear film in patients with KCS. This theory is not mutually exclusive to the preceding one and in some respects could be interpreted as being supportive of the desiccation theory. Why there should be increased evaporation in KCS is not entirely clear, but it could possibly be due to changes in the superficial lipid layer of the tear film. Similar increases in evaporation have been reported in contact lens wearers and patients with meibomian gland dysfunction.

5.3 Lubrication

It is known that the lids move in close contact with the ocular surface in the course of a blink. There is also evidence to suggest that there are considerable posterior forces from the upper lid onto the corneal surface. The upper lid creates substantial shearing forces which would be minimized by lubricity provided by the tear film between the lid and the corneal surface. As this lubricity is decreased, an increase in shearing force would be expected with a substantial abrasive effect from the upper lid on the surface of the cornea. Recent studies employing specular microscopy of the human cornea have suggested that there is a preferential shearing force from the lid to the central area of the cornea resulting in a decrease in average cell area in central cornea (these smaller cells being newer cells with a preferentially higher epithelial cell turnover rate in the central area of the cornea.) In similar studies of patients with KCS there was a statistically significant shift to small cells in the central cornea, suggesting an accelerated turnover of cells in this area. This could be accounted for by a substantially increased shearing force secondary to decreased lubricity in KCS.

5.4 Cellular Metaplasia

It has been shown using cellulose acetate filter paper applied to the conjunctival surface that one is able to lift off a sampling of surface cells which can then be stained and analyzed for morphological characteristics. Employing this technology, Nelson described morphologic changes in patients with ocular pemphigoid and demonstrated a decrease in goblet cell density. Tseng et al. further developed this technique and related goblet cell density decreases to chronic inflammation. They further studied changes in the conjunctiva in dry eye states and found evidence of conjunctival squamous cell metaplasia. Although most of the specimens demonstrated in this study were patients other than those with KCS, i.e., chronic conjunctival inflammation with scarring such as cicatricial ocular pemphigoid and erythema multiforme. There were only mild changes in patients with KCS. These studies have led to the development of a strategy for the use of topical retinoid treatment for these conditions. A recent multicenter clinical trial has not demonstrated a statistically significant improvement in patients receiving topical retinoids. Recent studies have demonstrated that some patients with Sjögren's syndrome, however, show surface morphological changes which include the presence of inflammatory cells, suggesting a more severe inflammatory process in KCS related to Sjögren's syndrome.

5.5 Hormonal Changes

The high prevalence of KCS in women in the menopausal and post-menopausal age groups has led to speculation about a possible relationship between systemic hormonal changes and the development of ocular surface disease. No definitive study has yet linked hormonal deficiencies, for example, in estrogen, with decreased tear production. Laboratory work, however, has shown that prolactin can decrease aqueous tear production and establishes for the first time a hormonal link. Attempts to establish the presence of estrogen receptors in the conjunctival surface have not proved rewarding; however, the development of more sensitive tests for the identification of these receptors may yet establish their presence. Cellular changes of the conjunctival surface in association with the menstrual cycle, however, have strengthened the case for systemic hormonal influence on the ocular surface.

5.6 Primary Inflammatory Disease of the Ocular Surface

The disparity between tear production (as measured by Schirmer test) and the degree of ocular surface disease seen in some dry eye patients has raised the possibility that there might be a form of primary ocular surface disease unrelated to the volume of tears. There are several animal models of severe ocular surface disease which appear to be similar to that seen associated with dry eyes in humans; these include the canine and murine models. These models appear to be immunogenically mediated. They are characterized by severe ocular surface disease which is out of proportion to the decrease in aqueous tear production. The recent evidence cited above employing impression cytology has indicated that in KCS there may be a substantial difference in the ocular surface disease occurring between patients with Sjögren's and those with non-Sjögren's KCS. Impression cytologic studies have demonstrated inflammatory cell infiltrate on the ocular surface in Sjögren's patients. These findings could have substantial implications in the development of new treatment strategies.

5.7 Associated Conditions

As previously discussed, the lipid excreta from meibomian glands of the lids (meibum) is important in the maintenance of a normal tear film. There is a frequent association between meibomian gland dysfunction and decreased aqueous tear production in patients. Indeed, an association between dry eyes and rosacea lid disease has been reported. More recently experimental studies in rabbits with closure of the meibomian gland orifices has shown that there is an increase in tear film osmolarity, decrease in conjunctival goblet cell density, and decrease in corneal epithelial glycogen levels.

It is probable that the origin of ocular surface disease differs in different dry eye states and is in many of them multifactorial. To successfully manage these potentially serious problems, an understanding of the pathogenetic mechanisms operative in these conditions is necessary.

6 Implications for Future Diagnosis and Management of Dry Eye

Recognition that the term dry eye does not refer to one disease state but to a variety of related conditions united by a common expression in the development of ocular surface disease is crucial to improvements in both the diagnosis and management of these problems. New studies reported by Dartt (this volume) which detail the discovery of many new substances that influence aqueous tear production may well lead the way to the development of new stimulating agents to improve tear production in patients with remaining functional acinar tissue. On the other hand, in patients in whom ocular surface disease predominates, particularly those with immunologic disease, the development of topical or systemic agents which would inhibit or modulate autoimmune inflammatory processes appears to be a promising avenue for exploration. Additional studies to further elucidate the mechanisms in the production of meibomian gland dysfunction are also crucial in developing new ways of managing this aspect of the disease. The past decade has witnessed a remarkable increase in our knowledge about this fascinating and complex field which afflicts so many patients. The prospects for further substantive advances in our ability to diagnose and manage these disease states appears promising indeed.

References

1. Holly FJ, Lemp MA (1989) Tear physiology and dry eyes. Surv Ophthalmol 22:69–87
2. Bron AJ (1985) Prospects for the dry eye. Trans Ophthalmol Soc UK 104:801–826

3. Jordan A, Baum JL (1980) Basic tear flow, does it exist? Ophthalmology 87:920–930
4. Lemp MA, Mathers WD (1981) Corneal epithelial cell movement in humans. Eye 3:438–445
5. Shearn MA (1971) Sjögren's syndrome. In: Smith CH Jr (ed) Major problems in internal medicine, vol 2. Saunders, Philadelphia
6. Cavanagh HD, Colley AM (1989) The molecular basis of neurotrophic keratitis. Acta Ophthalmol (Copenh) 67:115–134
7. Farris RL (1986) The dry eye: its mechanism and therapy with evidence that contact lens is a cause. CLAOJ 12:234–246

Chapter 5

Diagnosis of Dry Eye

M.S. Norn

1 Introduction

Dry eye is a sign that is characteristic of various morbid states having different causes. It is therefore reasonable to choose the diagnostic method that seems best suited to the disease expected and then to supplement this, if need be, by other methods.

Lemp (this volume) classifies dry eye conditions into five principal categories:

- Aqueous deficiency. When this is suspected, tear production (Schirmer's test) should be measured, and possibly also the tear flow and the elements produced by the lacrimal gland (lactoferrin, lysozyme). Other parameters should also be included, such as breakup time (BUT) and staining.
- Mucin deficiency. The mucous apparatus is examined. The number of goblet cells can be determined (by biopsy or, preferably, imprinting technique), or the size of the mucous thread can be assessed after staining with alcian blue.
- Lipid problems. The lipid phase is analyzed superficially in the pre-corneal film (tear film preocular film) by the interference method in the slit lamp.
- Lid surfacing problems. These are disclosed by careful slit lamp examination, in some instances supplemented by vital staining of Marx' line and the meibomian glands.
- Epitheliopathy. The cornea is examined carefully by sclerotic scatter and staining, among other methods.

The choice of method should take into account the accuracy of possible methods. Reproducibility can be assessed by the coefficient of variability (standard deviation as percentage of the mean). The clinical value of the method depends on its sensitivity, specificity, and overall agreement between results of diagnostic test and presence/absence of disease. The emphasis in this chapter is on diagnostic methods that are of particular value

M.A. Lemp/R. Marquardt (Eds.) The Dry Eye
© Springer-Verlag Berlin Heidelberg 1992

in general ophthalmological practice. A method must yield a prompt result and require only very simple facilities. The result depends on the modification employed. Achieving comparable results by different workers calls for standardization of the methods down to the last detail. I have therefore given a detailed description of various methods. This is followed by a brief report of other modifications. Finally, I present the methods of investigation requiring more elaborate laboratory facilities.

1.1 Subjective Complaints

A patient with dry eye does not necessarily complain of such. A large proportion of patients report pain, itching, a sandy sensation, stickiness, or other irritative symptoms, but not specifically dry eyes.

Can a person with no subjective complaints have a tendency to dry eye? Experience shows that he can indeed. The problem arises in relation to a person's desire to wear contact lenses. Patients with low tear parameters are poor candidates for contact lenses. McMonnies [1] has formulated a questionnaire for tracing such problematic patients prior to the fitting of contact lenses. This includes dry eye symptoms such as those "after having been in dry, smoky environs, after alcohol consumption, after swimming in fresh chlorinated water, associated with corneal exposure during sleep, associated with the side effects of certain medications, and perhaps associated with rheumatoid arthritis or lupus or thyroid abnormality, perhaps associated with mucous membranes in other parts of the body, perhaps with a report of previous treatment of a dry eye condition".

To this we may raise the objection that most normal persons complain of irritative symptoms when exposed to tobacco smoke and excessively chlorinated bathing water. Appropriately, however, the list includes dryness of other mucous membranes (e.g., the oral mucosa), to which may be added pronounced dental problems in Sjögren's syndrome type I and rheumatoid arthritis (Sjögren II). Previously instituted medication may point to Stevens-Johnson syndrome. Finally, the list may be supplemented by aggravation in certain environments, for example, "sick" buildings [2], with an abundance of fleecy materials (carpets, fleecy walls and ceilings), sites with inadequate dust exhausts, turpentine vapors, work with rock wool [3], and prolonged work with data processing machines. In such situations the great majority of those present complain of irritative symptoms suggesting environmentally induced dry eye. The symptoms subside on holidays and weekends.

Affective tearing (epiphora in response to psychogenic weeping) may be absent in patients with dry eye. Some patients may even state that previously when weeping they had secreted tears but are now unable to do so. Provoked tear secretion may fail (peeling of onions).

May a subject with epiphora suffer from dry eye? Certainly – this is a phenomenon called paradoxical epiphora. It is seem most often in elderly persons whose tear secretion has been impaired due to age-related atrophy of the lacrimal gland combined with a reduced outflow of tears (from impaired strength of the muscular fibers of the tear pump round the lacrimal sac or an abnormal nasolacrimal duct). When out-of-doors, the patient has epiphora (reflex-stimulated tear secretion exceeds the reduced outflow of tears); indoors, the nonstimulated tear secretion is so minimal that the condition must be characterized as that of dry eye.

These observations show that subjective complaints are of limited value in the diagnosis of dry eye. Diagnostic tests therefore play an important role. I must stress, however, the great value of questioning. This allows one to establish the necessary rapport to render a probable diagnosis, to make a reasonable differential diagnosis (against infectious conjunctivitis and other eye diseases), to point out the proper cause of the suspected dry eye, and to suggest the correct physical examination.

1.2 Ordinary Method: Slit Lamp Examination

It should be pointed out, first, that an ordinary slit lamp examination without any aids cannot disclose keratoconjunctivities sicca (KCS). The eye affected by KCS appears surprisingly normal, even without hyperemia. It is no wonder, therefore, that KCS is underdiagnosed. Many cases are mistakenly regarded as nervous complaints or simple chronic conjunctivitis. Patients exposed to such mistaken diagnoses are deprived of appropriate treatment.

1.2.1 Cornea

The KCS-affected eye may look dull as a result of inadequately covering precorneal film. In my view this cannot be settled on the basis of ordinary slit lamp examination. However, Edmund [4], as early as 1951, demonstrated a reduced corneal gloss in cases of KCS when undertaking photoelectric measurements of the light reflex from the cornea (normal value 155.83 ± 1.12 units in men and 155.42 ± 1.30 in women; nonsignificant difference).

The cornea should be closely examined in the slit lamp for disclosure of all signs of dry eye in its widest sense. It is therefore important to employ different techniques and adjustments during the examination. We use diffuse lighting (frosted glass, a wide slit width, subdued light in the room) and direct light with a wide and with a narrow slit. The cornea is best seen with the dark pupil as background. A narrow slit width with a wide angle should be used for examination of the illuminated optical section of the cornea. We often vary the slit width to assess details, for example, corneal edema or epithelial bullae (dry eye due to epitheliopathy). Such a varied technique is necessary for disclosure of dots and map-corneal dystrophy [5], for instance. I have found it advantageous to include an oblique or a horizontal slit.

1.2.2 Different Methods of Lighting

Indirect lighting is necessary for studying details. The light of the slit lamp is focused on a point just outside the area to be examined. We often perform the two examinations concurrently, studying the corneal area exposed to direct light and the neighboring area. The finding of epithelial bullae serves to ascertain whether the refractive index of the bulla is higher or lower than that of the surrounding corneal bulla (shadow effect contralateral to light direction = positive refraction = cell debris = microcyst; ipsilateral shadow = regular shadow corresponding to a low index = cyst, vacuole).

Retrograde lighting (regredient, retroillumination) is that reflected from a structure (iris, opaque lens) behind the region to be examined. This technique discloses filiform mucous coatings (KCS), opacities, epithelial vacuoles, edema, and fingerprint degeneration [5,6].

Specular reflection is suitable for examination of the corneal epithelium, endothelium, and the lipid layer of the precorneal film. The rays of the slit lamp enter obliquely, and the microscope is placed in the opposite direction, thus rendering the angle of incidence equal to that of reflexion. The technique discloses irregularities of the reflecting surface (see Sects. 7, 9.4).

The sclerotic scatter technique uses the cornea as light conductor. The method is especially well suited for disclosing incipient corneal edema, for example, at the initial stage of epitheliopathy. The method was described by Graves [7,8] as early as 1923. An intense, broad pencil of rays from the slit lamp is focused on the sclera and the limbal cornea. The microscope is focused on the central area of the cornea, which has a milky appearance in cases of incipient edema. The slit-lamp light causes a total inner reflection of the whole cornea. This is broken in the form of a light scatter at the site of a possible edema. The phenomenon is best observed at the lowest magnification, or even better at no magnification [9]. Accordingly, I undertake the sclerotic scatter analysis at the lowest magnification, supplemented by naked-eye inspection.

Polarized light, under normal conditions, shows thin, parallel lines in one direction across the cornea and corresponding lines at right angles to these. This latticework covers almost the entire cornea, the periphery being indistinct. The lattice shows defects over the area of a superjacent mucous thread (filiform formations in KCS), and in the presence of vacuoles, micro-bullae, excoriation edema, or corneal opacity. I have used a Haag Streit 900 slit lamp and provided this with a polarizer (below the lamp component, above the mirror in a holder) and an analyzer, which can revolve before the microscope, the polarizing plate replacing the clear protective plate in front of the microscope. The examination is performed in subdued light. The two polarizing plates are rotated until the ordinary light becomes extinct. Polarizing elements are then luminous on a dark background. The pupil is the best background for examination, possibly best when dilated.

1.2.3 Debris Precorneally and in the Inferior Fornix

We often find small fragments, air bubbles, and structures resembling flakes of mucus, pus, or epithelial cell nests floating in the precorneal film, in the tear meniscus (lacrimal river), and in the conjunctival sac of the inferior fornix. Debris in the tear film is a constant finding in patients with KCS. Unfortunately, debris is in no way pathognomonic; such phenomena may be seen in normal subjects and in fairly large numbers in cases of bacterial conjunctivitis. In my experience a diagnosis of dry eye cannot be established on the basis of these findings. However, they stress the fact that the differential diagnosis against bacterial conjunctivitis is often of immediate importance. In this connection particularly a leukocyte esterase stix test may be of interest (see Sect. 9.6).

1.2.4 Leukoplakia, Symblepharon

Pemphigoid and Steven-Johnson syndrome are examples of dry eye. In the acute phase one examines for conjunctival vesicles; in the brief acute disease, differential diagnosis is against the frequent conjunctival cysts (mass of goblet cell secretion or lymphocytic vessel dilatation). In the chronic phase one inspects for leukoplakia and symblepharon.

Leucoplakia manifests itself by well-defined conjunctival areas. These are white, slightly elevated, and impossible to rub off with a cotton swab. They never, or only very rarely, show staining with rose bengal, alcian blue, or tetrazolium. Leukoplakia consists of keratinized epithelial cells. Among 29 patients with benign mucosal pemphigoid leukoplakia was found in 13 (two with two patches in one eye); 14 patches were located on the inferior tarsus and one on the superior [10]. The patches of leukoplakia were oval, with the longest diameter parallel with the lid margin, irregularly scattered over the tarsus, in two cases even extending over the inferior lacrimal point. These averaged 4.1×2.3 mm in size (range 1–10 mm). Leukoplakia is not seen in KCS.

Symblephara indicate shrinkage of the conjunctival sac and are an important sign of benign mucosal pemphigoid and Stevens-Johnson syndrome. The patient is requested to look straight up, and the inferior tarsus is pulled forcefully down and temporally, directly down (Fig. 1), and finally down and nasally. Pulling from side to side is required to disclose all the strands in the inferior fornix. Similarly, strands are sought medially, laterally, and superiorly. In 29 eyes with benign mucosal pemphigoid a total of 59 symblephara were counted, the majority passing vertically or obliquely from the inferior tarsus to the bulbar conjunctiva. Only 5% occurred superiorly, 15% centrally in the inferior fornix, and the remainder evenly

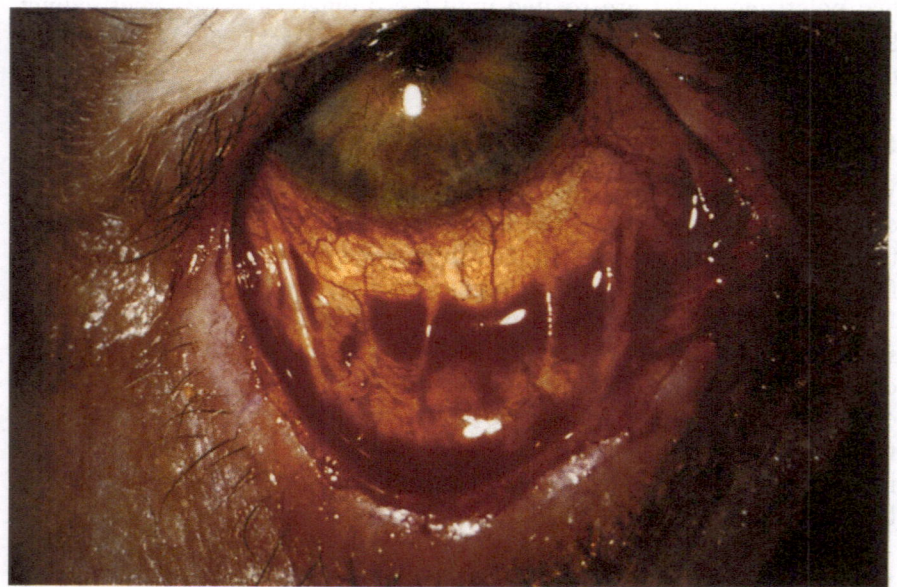

Fig. 1. Symblepharon strands in the inferior conjunctival fornix in a case of benign mucous membrane pemphigoid. (Rose bengal)

distributed medially and laterally. The strands were not specially stainable. Symblephara are not seen in cases of KCS but may occur following fairly deep cauterization or operation for strabismus.

1.2.5 Conjunctival Hyperemia

As noted above, KCS is usually not marked by hyperemia. Congestion is present only in association with secondary bacterial infection. Environmentally induced dry eye, on the other hand, may show hyperemia, especially on the bulbar conjunctiva. This can be objectified by a photo, particularly if a standardized gray scale is used in the photo.

1.2.6 Eyelids

Lagophthalmos, or incomplete closure of the eye, may be a cause of dry eye. In the slit lamp or on gentle closing (uniformly on both sides) one can see clearly whether the lids meet tightly. Is there inadequate blinking, floppy eye, perhaps exophthalmos? The muscular strength of the eyeball is studied by binocular forced blink of the lids under resistance. Possible signs of ectropion or entropion (is the lacrimal point connected correctly with the lacrimal lake?) can be disclosed in the slit lamp.

  Tear pump activity is assessed in the slit lamp. Does the lacrimal point move medially in response to blinking, with uniform eyeball muscle action and corresponding wrinkling of the skin under the inner canthus? Does one lacrimal point meet the other correctly when blinking (kissing points)? Reduced outflow of tears produces compensatory reduction in the tear secretion. Are the lacrimal points normal? Does Marx' line (see Sect. 8.6) run normally?

The lid margin is inspected with a view to hyperemia, scales, and crusts because chronic blepharitis is often complicated by (or is the cause of?) dry eye. One often finds an irregular row of meibomian glands, some possibly emptying into the aqueous phase behind the normal row. One also sees many blocked orifices, some with a plug. Such irregularities are frequent in elderly subjects but are not especially characteristic of dry eye [11].

The tear meniscus (lacrimal river, streaming lacrimation) may be reduced in height in KCS. This is measured with the measuring instrument of the slit lamp. However, a primitive technique (measurement <0.2 mm) has been of no aid to me as a guide (however, see Sect. 9.1). An irregular tear meniscus seems to be merely an age-related phenomenon and is not a characteristic sign of dry eye.

2 Tear Quantity

Measurement of tear production per unit of time is, of course, an essential factor in the diagnosis of dry eye. The measurement is usually performed by absorption on filter paper placed folded round the lower lid with its short end situated within the conjunctival sac as a wick.

2.1 Schirmer's Tear Test

In 1903 Otto Schirmer introduced his three tear production tests with filter paper absorbing tears from the conjunctival sac (lacrimal basin). The length of the moistened paper outside the conjunctiva is measured in millimeters [12]. Schirmer preferred measurement on an open eye, but we generally prefer a closed eye, this being more convenient for the patient and independent of blinking. This modification was introduced by Henderson and Prough [13] in 1950, and the test should therefore perhaps be given their names (see [14]); Schirmer's name, however, is traditionally attached to tear secretion tests based on filter paper.

2.1.1 Method

Standardized filter paper (Whatman's no. 41) is used. The paper strips are delivered ready-cut in closed polythene envelopes, with two strips in each individually closed envelope (Halberg et al.; 589 black ribbon filter paper). The packet contains a millimeter scale and instructions (Clement Clarke).

Each filter paper has an indentation. The proximal part is rounded and 5 mm long, prepared for insertion into the conjunctival sac. The distal part, below the indentation, is 35 mm long. Of the two strips one has a straight end and the other an oblique, to make them distinguishable from each other after removal (right against left eye).

The polythene envelope is to be cut (torn) open in a manner to ensure that the part the nearest to the long ends of the two filter paper strips is the closest to the opening. The short end remains sterile in the deepest section of the remaining envelope. The two strips are then folded at the sites of the indentations while still lying protected inside the envelope. One can take the strips out of the envelope by grasping the long distal part (with the fingers or tweezers). The patient is informed about the purpose of the examination and is told that the test will take 5 min (which may be considered a long time), and that the paper may irritate, but that the examination is harmless. The patient is then instructed to look upward, the observer pulls the lower lid down a little and inserts the short rounded end of the filter paper inside the lateral one-third of the lower lid with as little manipulation as possible. The rounded part touches the bottom of the inferior fornix and the indentation the lid margin. The 5-mm-long proximal section of the filter paper is thus contained in the conjunctival sac while the 35-mm-long section distal to the indentation hangs down before the cheek.

Generally both eyes are subjected to the test simultaneously. A filter paper strip is inserted successively into each eye at the shortest possible interval. It is important to note which strip is inserted into which eye (the one cut straight into the right eye and the oblique into the left). A clock with a second hand is started immediately after insertion of the first paper. The filter paper must sit correctly and not touch the cornea (in the diagram of the written instruction the strip has been placed incorrectly in the middle of the lower lid).

The patient must sit with both eyes closed and remain quiet. After exactly 5 min the first strip to be inserted is removed and after the same interval after insertion the second strip. These are both read after having been placed on the enclosed millimeter scale. We measure the exact distance from the fold (indentation) to the site of transition from moist to non-tear-stained paper, thus excluding the wick of 5 mm. If the transitional zone is difficult to see (a good light is required), transillumination may disclose it. If the transitional zone is oblique or irregular, the mean value is taken. If the strip is moistened throughout, the result is over 35 mm. One may repeat the test with a shorter examination period and then calculate for a 5-min period or insert another filter paper at the moment when the first one is at the point of spilling over.

The filter paper should be read immediately after its removal from the eye, before the fluid extends farther over the paper. Waiting until maximum absorption occurs outside the eye increases the value by 0.5–1.5 mm. The paper may dry and thus render reading difficult or impossible.

The test is performed without anesthesia prior to any other tests to avoid their possible influence on the result. The interference-lipid test, however, may be carried out safely prior to Schirmer's test (see Sect. 7). It is difficult to decide on the optimal order of tests for dry eye because one test interferes with the next. Schirmer's test, for instance, interferes with BUT and staining. Pronounced rose bengal staining occurs at the site where the paper touches the palpebral and the bulbar conjunctiva. (We may perhaps ignore staining within the involved region.)

2.1.2 Sources of Error

If Schirmer's test is performed in a carefully standardized manner, as described above, various sources of error can be ruled out. If the paper used is not standardized, the length of absorption depends on the quality and absorbent capacity of the paper and of the direction of its fibers. However, the standardized paper can absorb only a fairly small quantity of fluid. In experiments in vitro I have found Halberg paper to absorb less fluid than glass capillary tubes, and in vivo fluorescein-stained tear fluid has been seen in nasal secretion but only in small amounts in simultaneously inserted filter paper [6].

The extent of moistening (in millimeters) of the standardized paper correlates closely with the quantity of absorbed fluid (in micrograms) [15]. The site at which the filter paper is inserted is essential. In 220 experiments two strips of Schirmer's filter paper were inserted simultaneously into one eye: one into the lateral one-third and one into the medial one-third of the lid. The result was a significantly higher value laterally than medially (however, see [16]). This is probably because the medially located lacrimal point and lacrimal duct act as a capillary tube effectively sucking tear fluid away from the region in competition with the filter paper strip inserted close by [17].

Contact with the sensitive cornea intensifies tear secretion; the sensitivity of the cornea is substantially greater than that of the conjunctiva or lid margin [18]. Touching of the cilia or cheek as well as other forms of irritation should be avoided because of the reflex action of such on tear production. Both eyes should remain closed; if one eye is kept open during testing of the opposite eye the latter becomes irritated (due to eye movements). The feeling of discomfort is least if both eyes remain closed throughout the test period.

Occlusion of the lacrimal punctum reduces the value of Schirmer's test. In 32 cases the nasolacrimal duct was occluded by pressing a finger against the lacrimal sac. The mean Schirmer test value on compression was 3.96 ± 0.43 mm versus 7.88 ± 0.86 mm before and 8.29 ± 0.55 mm 2 min after compression (statistically significant); this presumably reflects reflex inhibition of tear secretion [19].

The absorbing part of the paper should not be exposed to fat when being inserted (the proximal part must not be touched by the observer). However, an unknown amount of meibomian secretion cannot be prevented from greasing the paper, which touches the margin.

In ten experiments I have noticed a tendency to lowered tear secretion on simultaneous insertion of two filter paper strips laterally, one of which had been greased by sebum from about ten nasal skin glands (12.0 ± 2.18 versus 17.7 ± 2.66 mm (unpublished observation).

2.1.3 Normal and Pathological Values

The cutoff value for Schirmer's test is 10 mm for a test period of 5 min, provided the test has been made by the standardized procedure described above. The result is regarded as pathological if the value is 10 mm or below (Copenhagen criteria for Sjögren's syndrome). Schirmer himself took 15 mm as the cutoff, but he tested with an open eye [12]. Sjögren chose 5 mm, Boyer 6 mm, and Jones 10 mm [6]). Bijsterveld [20] tested 550 normal subjects and 43 patients with KCS and found 5.5 mm to be the best cutoff point. Tear production depends on the patient's age, as secretion decreases with age. Zappia [21] suggests the following age-related values (in 5 min): 11–20 years, 19 mm; 21–30 years, 20 mm; 31–40 years, 18 mm; 41–50 years, 13 mm; 51–59 years, 13 mm; and 60 years or above, 9 mm. There is no difference in sex incidence and no dependence on oral contraception [22].

Regarding sensitivity and specificity Bijsterveld found 83% and 85%, respectively, on the basis of his cutoff value of 5.5 mm in 5 min. Farris [23] found a sensitivity of no more than 10%, against a specificity of 100%. In 24- and 25-year-old normal subjects Hansen et al. [17] observed 13% false-positive reactions at a cutoff value of 5.5 mm and of 35% at a value of 15 mm in 5 min. The coefficient of variation is surprisingly high; Shapiro [24] noted 100% (33.1 ± 33.2; $n = 880$) and Hansen et al. [17] 60.5%.

Pathological cases include more than those dry eye (Sjögren's syndrome, KCS, pemphigoid). Tear production also may be reduced in cases of occlusion of the nasolacrimal duct (reflex action).

Schirmer's test is a coarse test, and it is therefore tempting to express the result in relation to a "gray zone" of 5–15 mm in 5 min. A test result above 15 mm is regarded as normal and one below 5 mm as pathological. A result falling in the gray zone is inconclusive. On the other hand, this is a reasonably reliable test for determining fluctuations in the condition of patients with KCS. We should therefore continue to present test results in terms of millimeters per 5 min and employ the best standardization possible and an internationally approved cutoff value (10 mm per 5 min) until a better method becomes available for evaluating tear secretion under practical clinical circumstances.

2.1.4 Modifications of Schirmer's Test

Historically Schirmer's test I is made on an open eye. Schirmer's test II measures reflex-stimulated tear secretion (homolateral nostril irritated by a hair pencil). Schirmer's test III measures reflex-stimulated tear secretion provoked by letting the patient look in the direction of the sun (one should beware of retinal photocoagulation). Chemical stimulation is used today in the diagnosis of facial palsy (NH_3, formaldehyde, onion). Schirmer test I with open eye gives a higher value with an anesthetized open eye than with an anesthetized closed eye [25]. Schirmer's test with local anesthesia gives a lower value than a test without anesthesia – so-called basal tear secretion, i.e., in the absence of functioning main gland. To confirm this Jones [26] dried the inferior fornix with cotton for 1–2 min after local anesthesia prior to insertion of filter paper. Lambert found the Schirmer test value with topical anesthesia to be 60% of the normal value (27). Comparison with fluorophotometric measurement, however, disclosed that even Schirmer's test on an anesthetized eye includes a certain reflex-stimulated tear secretion [28], also detectable in the initial rapid phase of this type of Schirmer's test [29]. We may conclude that anesthesia should not be used in Schirmer's test, a certain tear reflex being unavoidable in any case. Furthermore, the anesthesia contributes to a greater coefficient of variation.

Regarding the use of filter paper medially, Henderson, among others, inserted paper strips nasally close to the inferior lacrimal point (see Sect. 2.1.2).

Litmus (lacmus) paper has been used for Schirmer's test by Sjögren [6], among others, to make the demarcation line more readily visible on the filter paper; tear-moistened paper changes to blue while the dry paper remains red. The paper may be retained as documentation material. The absorptive properties of the paper have not been standardized, however.

In cases of total absence of tears in the filter paper after 2 min Mackie replaces the paper by another and removes this after 5 min [30]. Jonasdottir, on the other hand, could not verify the need for this modification [31]. Due to such sources of error as greasy filter paper and evaporation from the paper Holly [32] introduced lipid-extracted paper in an envelope. Jonasdottir has used methanol-chloroform-extracted Halberg paper without having found this modification necessary in practice [31], presumably because lipid from the lid margin plays an essential role. Holly's modification, on the other hand, is suitable for kinetic studies [32]. If Schirmer's test is performed over only a fairly short period, one cannot directly compute the production over 5 min, the secretion being greatest during the initial period. Jones reckoned that a test result for a 1-min period is to be multiplied by 3 to correspond to 5 min [33]. The moisture content of the filter paper is measured electrically by measuring resistance (Periotron, Harco Electronics).

Kurihashi [34] inserted a cotton thread instead of a filter paper strip in Schirmer's test. The proximal part of the thread has either been stained in advance by fluorescein (10%) to render the moistened part visible, or the thread is read without staining, or the thread is impressed on fluorescein paper after its removal from the eye (method III). The thread is 0.20 mm in diameter and just over 6 cm long (of American prima cotton 82/3, Yokota, Osaka, Japan). The cotton thread irritates the eye less than filter paper, the test period being limited to 5 s (3 or 7 s). The test is performed without anesthesia on closed eye. The cutoff value 10 mm per 5 s. The coefficient of variation can be calculated at 15%–31%, though on the basis of the mean of three measurements. Lacrimal passage occlusion seems to give a higher value than Schirmer's test. This may be due to the cotton thread absorbing mainly the tear meniscus during the few seconds that the test lasts, whereas filter paper used in Schirmer's test absorbs tears secreted over 5 min.

3 Tear Flow

Normal tear flow presupposes a proper relationship between tear production and tear outflow. In dry eye this relationship may be disturbed as a result of reduced tear production; however, it may remain normal if the outflow has been relatively increased. Tear flow can be assessed by introducing a dye or radioactive substance into the conjunctival sac (tear basin) and measuring its concentration after a certain period. Grudzdew [6] introduced such a method in 1938: a starch solution is instilled, and the tear dilution is measured by inserting into the conjunctival sac a cotton swab dipped in Lugol's solution. Staining methods with collargol or argyrol (complex silver compounds) have since been used, and more recently most often fluorescein [6].

3.1 Tear Meniscus Dilution Test

A method is easy to employ in practice in the slit lamp is the tear meniscus dilution test, using a mixture of 1% rose bengal and 1% fluorescein. The dye dilution after 5 min is determined in the inferior tear meniscus (lacrimal river, tear streak). The advantages of the dye mixture are an intense color scale in relation to tear dilution and applicability in subsequent studies of conjunctiva and cornea (KCS, Bijsterveld score; Sect. 8.2) and Marx' line (Sect. 8.6). One instills 10 μl dye mixture (fluorescein sodium 50 mg, rose bengal 50 mg, sodium chloride 45 mg, phenylmercuric nitrate as preservative 0.0025 mg, distilled water to 5 g), perhaps simply from a bottle mounted with a disposable cannula (steristar red needle gauge 25, 0.5 × 16 mm). The

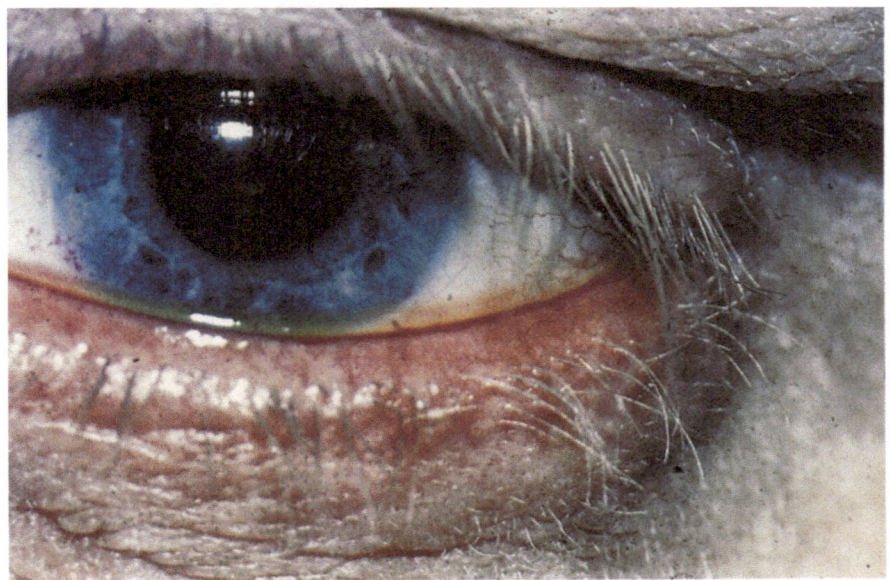

Fig. 2. Tear meniscus dilution test. After 5 min. The meniscus along the lower eye lid is pale orange in this case, corresponding to a dilution grade of 1:256

patient must not close or squeeze his eyes but sit with them open and with normal, gentle blinking.

After exactly 5 min the tint is assessed in the tear meniscus along the lower lid, corresponding with a scale of six dilution grades (figures in parentheses indicate the dilution grade in proportion to the original color of the dye mixture): red (1:4), pale red (1:16), orange (1:64), pale orange (1:256), yellow (1:1024), and pale yellow (1:4096), only visible as fluorescence in blue-filtered light in the slit lamp (Fig. 2). The color is estimated roughly or is compared with a color scale constructed on the basis of the fourfold dilutions, stored in six sealed glass capillary tubes of tear meniscus dimension (Fig. 3). On comparison with a capillary tube scale a white background should be employed if examination of the tear meniscus uses the sclera as background, and a black background if the pupil is the background in the slit lamp.

Error may be introduced by the tear meniscus being regular in thickness or height, as is often the case; in addition, the color may vary, being generally the palest laterally. The whole lacrimal river is examined, with reading over a representative area, which most often covers the middle. Dye may be lost initially by sqeezing and overflow down the cheek. An appreciable loss necessitates a renewed test, possibly with local anesthesia a few minutes before this [6].

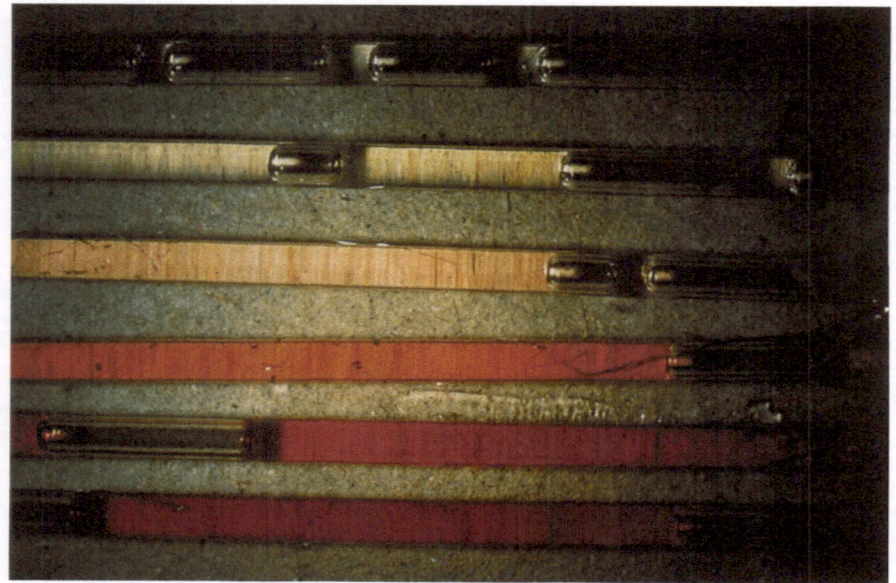

Fig. 3. Capillary tube color dilution scale for the tear meniscus test. (Rose bengal–fluorescein mixture)

The tear meniscus becomes yellow in the great majority of normal subjects. In KCS it remains red or assumes a bright orange color. The latter is regarded as pathological and a pale orange color as normal [35]. On examination of 186 eyes (93 normal subjects) a yellow or pale yellow color was seen in 65%, pale orange in 29%, intense orange in 10%, and pale red in 0.5% – in other words, 10.5% false positives. In KCS 78% (27 eyes) were found to have pathological values. In stenosis of the nasolacrimal duct (functional or mechanical, dacryocystectomy, ectropion) pathological test results were found in 100% (a total of 111 eyes). The test is, in other words, more sensitive in nasolacrimal duct occlusion than in KCS [36].

3.2 Jones' Test

Jones has described a test similar to that outlined above but using fluorescein alone [6,37]. In addition, outflow of tears to the nose can be measured by a cotton swab test (I), possibly combined with rinsing of the conjunctival sac of dye and subsequent lavage of the nasolacrimal duct (Jones' test II).

Modifications. Brandt has modified Norn's tear meniscus dilution test by reading after only 3 min and employing a greater number of grades on the color scale [38]. Brandt's method is best suited for measuring hypersecretion.

Port [39] photographs the tear meniscus at 1-min intervals after instillation of 2% fluorescein. The result has been compared with a dye dilution scale in nine capillary tubes.

3.3 Scintigraphy

Rosamondo introduced lacrimal scintigraphy in 1972, instilling 10 µl normal saline solution containing 200 µCi technetium into the conjunctival sac [40]. This is controlled on gamma-camera oscilloscope display. The normal value is 0.083 µl/min ($n = 35$; SEM 0.003) as turnover rate in the basal phase (after a more pronounced elimination during the first 7.5 min). Sørensen found no correlation between scintigraphy and Schirmer's test [40].

Pathological values occur primarily in association with nasolacrimal duct occlusion. However, individual cases of dry eye are also mentioned. The method is suitable for solution of many theoretical problems, for example, the grade of the reflex-stimulated tear secretion provoked by Schirmer's test.

3.4 Fluorophotometry

Mishima et al. in 1966 introduced dynamic, refined fluorophotometry for the investigation of tear flow [41]. There is no difference in sex incidence. Occhipint et al. [42] found no correlation to Schirmer's test except at values above 35 mm, corresponding to a higher turn-over rate of fluorescein-stained tears. In normal eyes a tear elimination coefficient of 15.4% ± 11.9% per minute ($n = 52$) has been found in the precorneal film, measured at the site of the corneal center [43].

4 Tear Quality

4.1 Crystallization

Tears left on a glass slide dry, forming fern-like crystals. Crystallization is less pronounced if tear quality is poor (dry eye from different causes). The phenomenon is related to ferning of mucus in a vaginal smear, as described by Papanicolaou in 1946 [44]. The crystallization of tears was described by Sole in 1955 [45], Tabara et al. in 1982 [46] and Rolando in 1983 and 1984 [47,48]. It was named tear mucus ferning, presumably because the sample is drawn from mucus-containing conjunctival fluid. Ferning is, however, hardly a direct indication of mucus deficiency but rather of altered tear protein composition, osmolarity etc. [49].

4.1.1 Qualitative Ferning

The rounded end of a glass rod (5 mm in diameter) is pressed against the bottom in the middle of the inferior conjunctival fornix. The adhering conjunctival fluid is transferred to a glass slide. The end of the glass rod touches, or nearly touches, the slide and is then removed leaving a well-defined circular drop on the slide. The rod must not be passed across the slide but must only just leave the drop. The drop dries up on the slide about 10 min later at room temperature. The specimen can be subjected to microscopy directly after desiccation or within few hours. Ordinary microscopy is employed with 40–100 × magnification.

Grading of the specimen is performed according to Rolando [47,48,50]. Grade I indicates ferning evenly distributed over the entire desiccated drop; grade II, crystallization with minor gaps (defects); and grade III, ferning with large defects. Finally, grade IV is a desiccated drop with scattered grains but no ferning or with only a suggestion of ferning at most. In this semiquantitative grading the size of the desiccated drop is of no importance. The essential thing to notice is whether the drop has formed a coherent crystallizing sheet. Ferning decreases after constitution in vivo (particles) [49], expression of meibomian glands, or instillation of oil in vivo, or if ointment is applied to the glass slide [50].

Grade I or II is present in the great majority of normals (83%). There is no difference in sex incidence, but a tendency towards less ferning (a higher

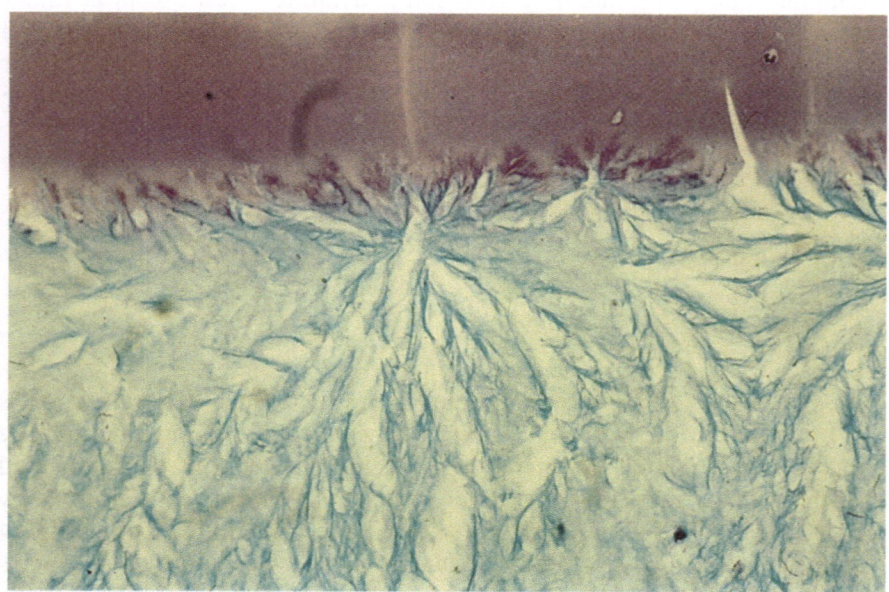

Fig. 4. Crystalization of dryed-up tears: acute angle ferning

grade) in persons aged over 40 years [49,51]. Of KCS-affected patients 92% show grade III or IV [49,51]. The quality of ferning is also reduced in pemphigoid and Steven-Johnson's syndrome [46]. Other states with signs of dry eye may show deficient ferning, for example, chemotherapy of pronounced colon cancer [52] and cystic fibrosis [53]. On the other hand, ferning improves in persons exposed to intense draft, presumably due to increased tear flow [54].

Modifications. For sampling the glass rod has been replaced by a spatula, a platinum wire, smears scraped with a knife, or tear fluid aspirated in a Pasteur pipette, capillary tube. A few microliters (no exact quantity stated) is transferred, giving a drop of 2–3 mm in diameter on the slide [49]. The type of instrument is presumably of minor importance where qualitative analysis is concerned. Liotet et al. [49] suggest a slightly different grading. They attach importance to right-angle branches of the fern pattern in grade I (see Sect. 4.1.2). Phase-contrast microscopy is performed. Microscopy should preferably be performed within a few hours. In my experience the specimen can keep at most for 36 h in a refrigerator (4°C); according to others, it can keep for some weeks [49].

4.1.2 Quantitative Ferning

I have quantified the ferning method by using exactly 2.5 µl tear fluid absorbed from the lateral part of the tear meniscus in a thin capillary tube (1 mm = 0.5 µl). The tear fluid sample is dropped onto a glass slide to be dried. The area showing crystallization is calculated by counting with an ocular micrometer lattice, correction being made for the relationship between the two ferning types, acute-angle ferning (Fig. 4) and right-angle ferning (Fig. 5). The former has only 0.11 times the value of the latter (demonstrated by in vitro experiments [44]). The method has a coefficient of variation of 6% and is of use for experimental studies [50]. Results of clinical examinations are not yet available.

A quantitative conjunctivocytologic pipette sample may disclose ferning, much of which vanishes, however, during the preparation (staining, rinsing, mounting). In such samples the ferning value depends on the amount of mucus, presumably because the mucus contained in the sample preserves the fern pattern during the preparation. In KCS cases no ferning has been detected despite an abundant amount of mucus in the sample [44].

5 Tear Film Stability Breakup Time

If a blink is occasionally omitted, gaps gradually occur in the precorneal film. This liquid layer (precocular tear film, lacrimal film) covers the exposed

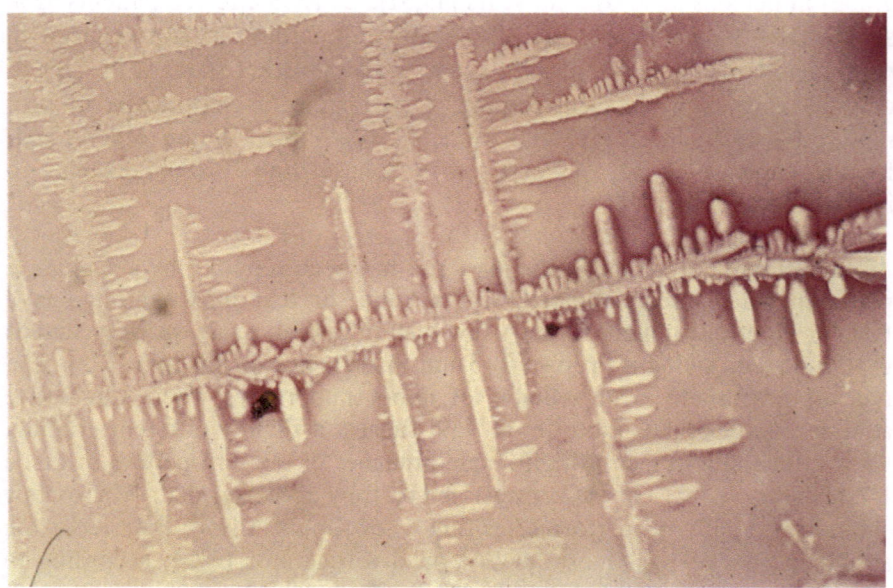

Fig. 5. Ferning; right-angle ferning. (Alcian blue in a quantitative pipette sample)

part of cornea and conjunctiva. The conjunctiva being irregularly folded, gap formations cannot be recorded here. The time elapsing from a blink to occurrence of gaps in the precorneal film constitutes a measure of the stability of the tear film, an important parameter in the diagnosis of dry eye. The gap phenomenon was described by Decker as early as 1876. The interval to detection of a gap was first measured by Go Ing Haen and Marx in 1926 by moving a lamp before the eye and examining gaps seen in the reflection of light in a magnifying glass [6]. Not until 1969, when the slit lamp and fluorescein came into use, could the BUT test be employed clinically [55,56,57]. The gap is hardly a complete hole in the precorneal film. The cornea is covered by a thin moisture film at the bottom of the hole.

BUT depends on many factors, including the viscosity of the tear film itself and the surface tension (contact angle). These depend on the composition of the film layer; the film consists superficially of a lipid layer and, the boundary layer between this and the aqueous layer consists of intensely active lipid breakdown products. Further, they depend on the thickness of the intermediary layer, on the deep mucous layer, on the epithelial layer itself with its villi, and possibly also on edema and other irregularities. It is thus evident that all types of dry eye may reduce the BUT value: environmental dry eye (diminished lipid layer), KCS (diminished aqueous phase), pemphigoid (reduced mucus), and epitheliopathy.

5.1 Method

The patient is informed about the investigation and is placed at the slit
lamp. The light in the room is turned down. Then 10 µl of 0.125% fluorescein is instilled into the eye (possibly as Fenton's solution: 0.125% fluorescein, 0.3% oxibuprocain, 0.025% phenylmercuric nitrate, sodium chloride to
isotonicity [58], dropped from the bottle through a red steristar disposable
cannula 25G 0.5 × 16 mm [6]).

The patient blinks normally a few times while placing his head in the
slit lamp support (cheek and forehead supports). The patient is thereafter
instructed not to blink. The observer then studies the precorneal film in
10–20 × magnification with a high, fairly wide (1–2 mm) light slit, light
inclination about 30°, mounted blue filter (cobolt), and microscope at right
angles to the cornea. If the color is satisfactory, the patient is requested to
blink once more with normal intensity. The moment that the blink is over
the observer starts his stop watch. Now the patient is no longer allowed to
blink, the observer must not touch the patient's lid, and the patient is
requested to force his eyes to be kept normally open. If the patient does
blink, or if the stained tear film is uneven, the test must be repeated. With
the patient's eye still kept open the observer now studies the fluorescein-
stained precorneal film by moving the slit lamp horizontally at a slow rate
from side to side with unaltered angle between light and microscope. The
observer scans the cornea from one limbus to the other until a black gap
(dry spot) is seen in the precorneal film. The stop watch is stopped the
moment that the gap begins to increase in size. Such a gap may turn up
anywhere in the precorneal film, although perhaps most commonly in the
lower temporal region close to the tear meniscus, where the film is thin
because the tear meniscus absorbs fluid. However, careful successive screening of the whole corneal area is required because the initial gap may occur
anywhere in the film.

The vertical light slit should be so high that the total cornea can be
included successively in the examination. The stop watch is not to be
stopped as long as a dark spot represents only a doubtful gap. After a true
dry spot has been demonstrated, this very soon expands to a slit or even
presents dry twigs radiating from the gap. The observer should not await
further enlargement of the gap before stopping the watch (Fig. 6). The test
is usually performed two or three times on either eye. The mean is calculated for each eye separately (difference?). In the short-term BUT test it
is necessary to notice where the first gap turns up to ascertain whether the
gap appears in the same place on repeated test (sign of epithelial bulla,
erosion, or other local epithelial disorder). If the BUT is particularly long,
one test is sufficient; this is interrupted after 1 min, for instance, when
normal values are found. If the first BUT period is short (10 s), the test
should be repeated two or more times to determine, on the basis of the
mean value, whether it really has disclosed a pathological state.

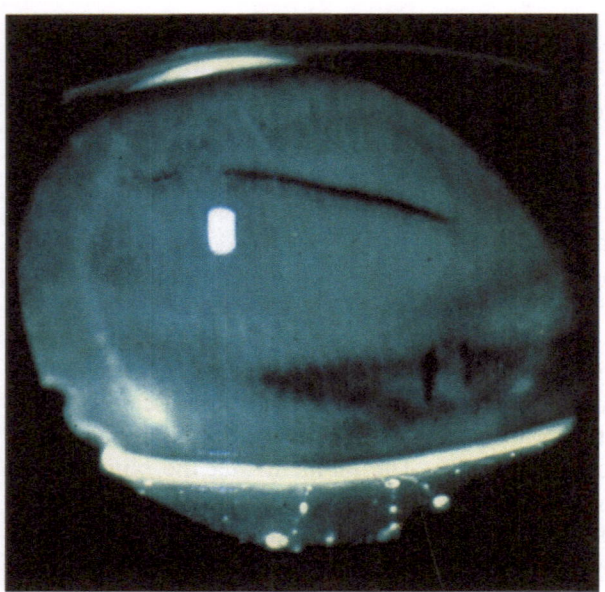

Fig. 6. Break up time. Two small dry spots are seen in the lower part, a long slit in the upper part. (Fluorescein-stained precorneal film)

5.2 Sources of Error

Palpebral fissure may be a source of error. The patient must not be prevented from blinking by keeping the lids wide apart with the observer's (or the patient's) fingers. After a few tests the patient can be instructed verbally to keep his eyes open naturally. Artificially wide opening produces an uncontrollably short BUT because the lids (margo palpebrae) may lose contact with the precorneal film. The patient's palpebral fissure should be of normal size during the test.

The initial gaps in the fluorescein-stained precorneal film may be due to air bubbles (foam) of small foreign bodies. If such formations disturb the reading, the observer asks the patient to resume gentle blinking, after which the test is repeated.

Because of the dye concentration used the test proceeds promptly. If repetitions are required, reinstillation may be necessary and the test procedure repeated. The relatively pale fluorescein staining requires subdued light of environs and well-adjusted slit-lamp light.

Retarded discovery may also be a source of error. The gap may occur in an area past search at the moment and thus not be detected until the next search from one limbus to the opposite one. Hence, the horizontal search in the slit lamp should not be delayed.

Previous instillation alter the BUT test appreciably. The BUT is reduced by oil, ointment, silicone emulsion, anti-foam, benzalkonium chloride

(0.01%), cocaine (2%), and bad indoor climate (sick building syndrome). It is increased by mucomimetics (methyl cellulose, polyvinyl alcohol, polyvinyl pyrrolidine, carbowax, dextran 10% [59]). The BUT test is influenced by anesthesia [60], but not by the mild anesthetic in Fenton's mixture [55].

Preceding Schirmer's test reduces the BUT very considerably because the filter paper absorbs the tear film. A small piece of paper 5 × 5mm in size in the inferior fornix has no influence [19].

The coefficient of variation of double BUT test is 31% ($n = 646$ [59]). The intraindividual variation is great [61]. This is probably because each BUT test is actually a new test with altered conditions after blinking (new debris, perhaps new admixture of meibomian secretion, altered lipid decomposition, altered cover of mucus over the cornea, etc.). Nevertheless the BUT is a unique parameter for dry eye and cannot be replaced by other parameters. The BUT is thus independent of tear flow [19].

5.3 Normal and Pathological Values

A BUT value over 10s is normal [62]. The BUT is independent of age, sex, size of palpebral fissure, ethnic origin, environmental temperature, and moisture [6,22], although uncertain tendencies have been demonstrated. In 15% of 64 normal subjects I have noted a BUT of 10s or less (mean of three measurements). A BUT of 10s or less is a pathological value indicating dry eye, independently of the cause. Pathological values are recorded in KCS, Sjögren's syndrome, pemphigoid (in 84% of 29 eyes, even in cases with a normal tear flow [10]), draft in the eye in a motorcar [54], the sick building syndrome (presumably due to a reduced lipid layer in the precorneal film [63]), in vapor of lipid-soluble substances (e.g., turpentine), and cigarette smoking [6]. A BUT of zero is found in dry eye due to epitheliopathy [56]. On the other hand, one finds a normal BUT in such disorders as simple chronic conjunctivitis, infectious conjunctivitis, allergic conjunctivitis, and in clinical states with reduced corneal sensitivity [55].

5.4 Modifications of the BUT Test

Fluorescein concentration and application differ greatly in the investigations of the various workers. Insertion of fluorescein-imbibed filter paper must be a considerable source of error if the paper is placed direct against the conjunctiva. The tear film concentration and dilution also become unpredictable if the strip is applied with saline on the paper. I have chosen a low concentration (0.125% in 10 µl drop) to obtain standardized conditions. In practice, I use Fenton's mixture to be able to let the BUT test be succeeded by applanation tonometry without further instillation. Others prefer a higher fluorescein concentration (0.5%), this being easier for beginners to read. A high concentration tends to give a lower BUT value. Use of the large fluorescein molecule fluorexon likewise gives a lower value. At the higher concentration the test cannot be carried out until after a series of blinks. The waiting time alters the concentration unpredictably. A smaller quantity of fluid is obtainable with a special dosing pipette, and the fluorescein concentration must then be increased correspondingly. An amount of $1-2\,\mu l$ 5% fluorescein [61] is recommended on the assumption that the smaller the quantity of fluid, the less pronounced is the source of error.

Different excitation filters have been used (Scott OG 530, combined with BG 12 or with Zeiss 485) to render the gap formation in the precorneal film plainly visible. I use the ordinary cobalt-blue filter in Haag Streit's slit lamp.

Other modifications include closing of the nontested eye to avoid blinking reflex (which affects both eyes, however), wiping away of fluid in the inferior fornix, widening the palpebral fissure, etc. This modification explains the greatly differing BUT results.

Self-reported BUT has been used by Wyon and Wyon. They have shown that after one or two tests with usual BUT measurement (without anesthesia), where the patient is asked if he can acknowledge a feeling of dryness on indicated precorneal gap formation, it is possible (in new tests) to have the patient state the interval from blink to self-reported gap formation. The time is measured with a stop watch [54]. This self-reported BUT (termed BUTS) without fluorescein is significantly correlated to the ordinary BUT ($r = 0.41$; 24 pairs), but BUTS is three times longer than BUT (mean 46.7 s versus 13.6 s).

Noninvasive BUT uses a large half-bowl as a globular perimeter with lit-up grid and observation of the corneal reflex (grid pattern). This allows reading the BUT without instillation of fluorescein or other manipulation [64]. Comparison with the usual BUT technique has shown that fluorescein reduces the BUT value.

6 Mucus Tests

Mucus is produced in the conjunctiva by goblet cells and, in addition, by epithelial cells throughout the lacrimal basin. It constitutes an important lubricating mechanism and removes foreign bodies (Fig. 7). The number of goblet cells is reduced in KCS, pemphigoid, and vitamin A deficiency. In the cases of the latter disorder goblet cells regenerate soon after even a single vitamin A capsule.

6.1 Alcian Blue Staining

Alcian blue stains mucus specifically (chondroitin and mucoitin sulfate complexes). Alcian blue, introduced as a vital stain in 1962 [65], is a

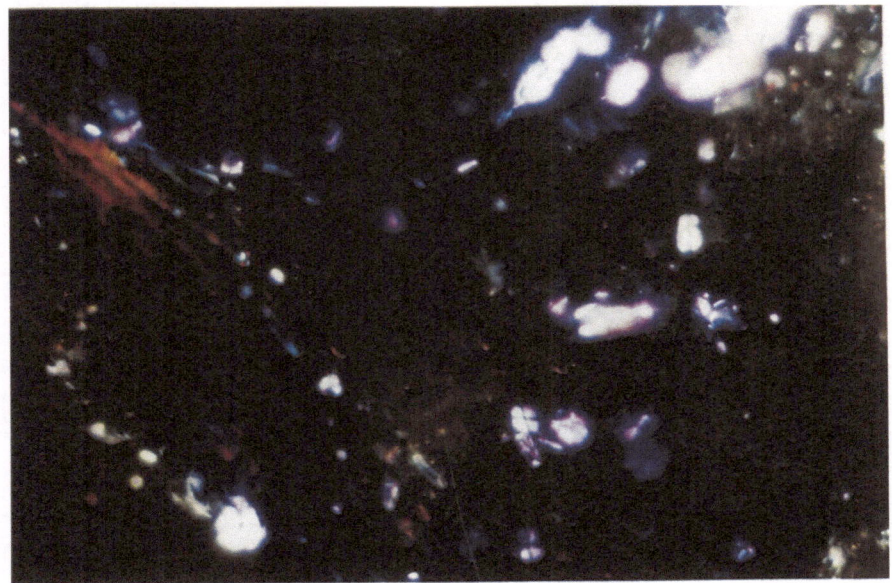

Fig. 7. Powder in mucous thread from the inferior conjunctival fornix. (Polarized light, toluidine blue, ×100)

complex cyclic compound conbtaining copper and is used as a wool dye (alcian blue 8GX; Michrome 24, Edward Gurr, London). It is used in a 1% aqueous solution, preserved with 0.3% phenylethyl alcohol. A drop of 10 µl is instilled into the eye, and the staining is recorded after excess stain has run off (normal blinking for a few minutes).

Staining with alcian blue discloses dots on the epithelium representing mucous coatings, sometimes shaped as threads. Normals show only few scattered dots, especially in the lower nasal part of the bulbar conjunctiva, the caruncle, and on Marx' line on the lid margin. In KCS pronounced punctate staining is seen all over the exposed parts of cornea and conjunctiva, possibly with filaments and flakes. The color is as intense as after staining with rose bengal [65]. In pemphigoid there is only a minimal tendency toward staining of the cornea [10].

6.2 Staining with Mixture of Tetrazolium and Alcian Blue

This dye mixture differentiates between mucus (stained blue) and neutrophilic leukocytes plus mildly degenerate epithelial cells stained red by tetrazolium. The mixture is composed as follows: iodonitrotetrazolium 100 mg, alcian blue 25 mg, phenylmercuric nitrate 0.1 mg, and distilled water to 10 g. Iodonitrotetrazolium is colorless. Enzymatic reduction of this in live cells with increased cell membrane permeability transforms it to the

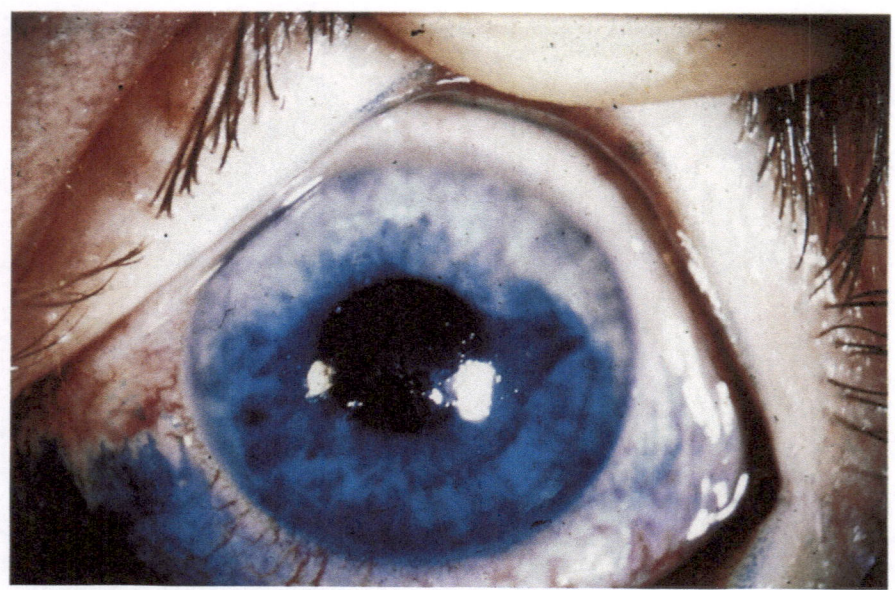

Fig. 8. Alcian blue stained lime-burnt cornea, 30 min after an accident (Franguolis, Thessaloniki, Greece)

red substance formazan. Its chemical formula is: 2-(p-iodophenyl)-3-(p-nitrophenyl)-5-(phenyltetrazolium chloride (pure AR 1-8377, Sigma). Tetrazolium was introduced as a stain on conjunctiva and cornea in 1971 [66].

Normal subjects only occasionally show a few stained dots on the lower nasal part of the bulbar conjunctiva. In KCS we find pronounced blue and red punctate staining on exposed areas of cornea and bulbar conjunctiva. The red color seen in KCS confirms that the exposed area contains many live though affected epithelial cells. (Rose bengal also stains dead epithelial cells.) In pemphigoid red punctate staining is rarely seen on exposed areas, more often red staining on both tarsi [10].

Alcian blue staining is contraindicated in cases showing totally bared connective tissue without epithelium. The ground substance of connective tissue is stained by alcian blue. The discoloration may become permanent in pronounced cases (tattooing; Fig. 8). In cases of dry eye or a suspicion of such the connective tissue is not bared. The contraindication concerns exclusively very deep erosions. Frank epithelial defects, and cauterizations.

6.3 Mucous Thread Measurement

The mucous thread in the inferior fornix exists in all normal eyes as a stainable continuous thread produced by pasting together of detached bits of

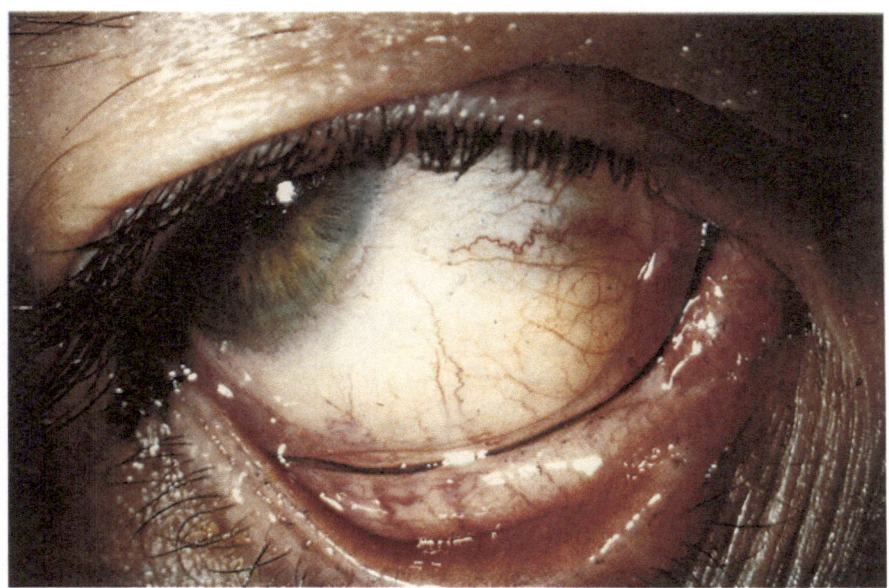

Fig. 9. Mucous thread in the inferior conjunctival fornix. (Alcian blue 1%)

mucus from the tears during blinking (Fig. 9). A corresponding, though smaller, thread is collected in the superior fornix. Continued blinking makes the threads move medially toward the inner canthus, where they are pressed onto the skin to end as "sleep". The mucous thread can be assessed in the slit lamp after staining with rose bengal or alcian blue. After staining the mucous thread can be taken out and transferred to a glass slide (Fig. 10), for example, by touching it by wooden pegs and thus making both ends adhere to these [6].

In normal subjects the mucous thread measures $3.1 \pm 0.7\,mm^2$ covered by mucus (alcian blue stain) with vacuoles admixed (extra $1.3 \pm 0.3\,mm^2$). There are very few tetrazolium-stained leukocytes (0.02 ± 0.16; $n = 19$) [66]. In pemphigoid the mucous thread is totally absent in 63% of cases [10]. Only few and small mucous flakes are seen in the inferior fornix between symblephara; a normal mucous thread is seen in no more than 8%. The average extent of the mucous thread has been measured at $1.5\,mm^2$ mucus ($0.70\,mm^2$ vacuoles and $0.2\,mm^2$ leukocytes; $n = 55$) [10]. Examination in the slit lamp can disclose the reduced mucus production in two-thirds of patients with benign mucous membrane pemphigoid by staining alone (absent mucous thread). This affords a possibility of differentiation from conjunctival shrinkage from other causes (Fig. 11). In KCS the dimensions of the mucous thread are increased, if anything [66]. On staining with rose bengal it seems to be thicker than normal (see following section).

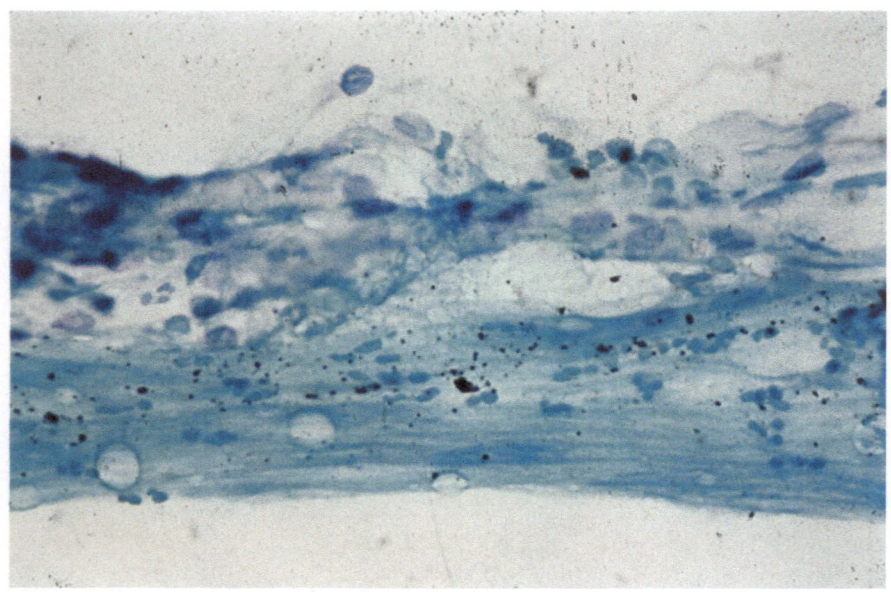

Fig. 10. Mucous thread from the inferior conjunctival fornix, transferred to a glass slide. Mucous fibrils are stained *blue*, nuclei of epithelial cells *violet*. (Formolfuchsin–alcian blue, ×100)

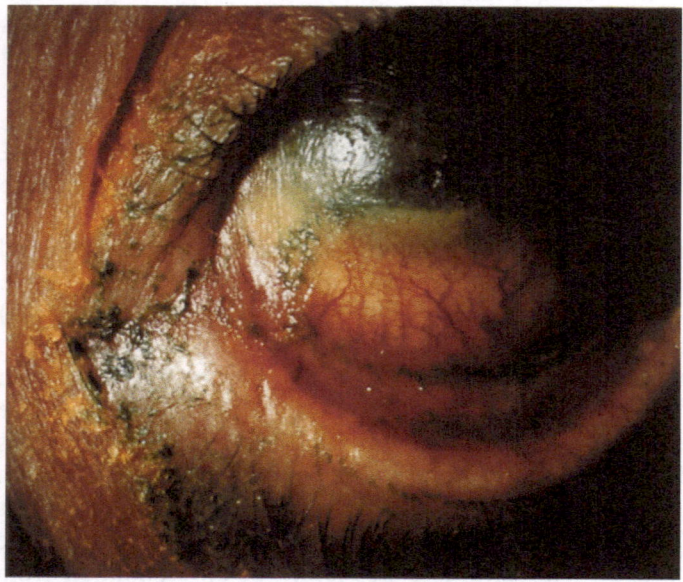

Fig. 11. Benign mucous menbrane pemphigoid. Only few mucous flakes are seen (cf. Fig. 9). (Alcian blue 1%)

6.4 Mucous Flow

The movement of the mucous thread in the medial direction can be measured by staining the medial half and measuring the movement of the transitional zone in relation to the lower lacrimal point after a certain time interval. Staining is performed with ¼% alcian blue. A drop of 10 µl is instilled into the medial half of the conjunctival sac, the medial lower lid being everted by the observer's finger on the outside of the lid. At the same time the lateral half is pressed against the bulbar conjunctiva. After 15 s the finger is removed, and the distance between the inferior lacrimal point and the transitional zone between stained and unstained mucous thread is measured through a measuring ocular in the slit lamp. The patient is instruced to blink normally. The measuring is repeated after exactly 10 min. The difference between the two measurements indicates the movement of the mucous thread in 10 min [67].

In normal subjects the average mucous flow in 103 eyes was 1.13 mm/min, independent of age, sex, environmental temperature, or moisture. The flow ceases during sleep and in general anesthesia and is accelerated by intense blinking [67]. The mucous flow is abated in the dry eye: KCS (0.42 mm/min), facial nerve palsy (0.42 versus 1.5 mm/min in the contralateral normal eye), entropion (0.20 mm/min), and pemphigoid, if a mucous thread exists at all. The mucous flow is normal in infectious conjunctivitis, chronic simple conjunctivitis, blepharoconjunctivitis, exophthalmos, etc. In KCS the rose bengal stained mucous thread is extraordinarily broad. This is due partly to an increased epithelial desquamation in KCS, which produces an intensified staining of dead epithelial cells (not mucus but rose bengal stained), and partly to the abated mucous flow, which perhaps causes the amount of mucus in this place to accumulate despite a reduced production.

6.5 Quality of Mucus

Conjunctival mucus is produced partly by goblet cells and partly by epithelial cells. The type of mucus depends on the site of production; it is of a different kind in patients with KCS. Analysis of the quality may therefore lead to interesting results of enzyme studies: neuraminidase, hyaluronidase. Glucoseoxidase, etc. [6] (see Sect. 10.8).

6.6 Biopsy, Imprint Technique

In pemphigoid biopsy is relatively contraindicated because it gives rise to further shrinking, and the biopsy specimen must be large to be representative of the goblet cell density. The problem is elegantly solved by the imprint technique (see Sect. 10.7).

7 Lipid Tests: Tear Film Interference

The preocular tear film (lacrimal film, precorneal film) is covered superficially by a thin lipid layer which prevents evaporation even on blinking
[68]. The thickness of this lipid layer can be measured by means of its
interference pattern in the slit lamp with an adjustable lamp (goose neck
lamp), as first demonstrated by McDonald in 1969 [69]. The examination
can, however, easily be carried out with no other aid than the slit lamp [70].
The test is of importance on suspicion of dry eye. This is so because in some
conditions (KCS) the lipid layer is increased in thickness (possibly due to
slower elimination of the tear film owing to a diminished aqueous phase).
Certain cases of environmentally induced dry eye, on the other hand, have a
thinner lipid layer (perhaps evaporated in the atmosphere).

7.1 Method

The patient is placed in front of the slit lamp in a room with subdued light.
The slit lamp mirror (in Haag Streit's slit lamp) is replaced by the back of
the mirror which reflects diffusely (ground glass). Another possibility is to
use a ground glass plate, polaroid filter, or simply a piece of parchment
paper (tracing paper) in front of the mirror in the pencil of rays of the slit
lamp. The slit lamp is adjusted so that the angle of incidence is equal to the
angle of reflexion (mirror reflex test). The patient is placed with his chin on
the chin support and forehead against the forehead support. The intensity of
light in the slit lamp is raised to maximum (with a broad pencil of rays). The
light is focused on the precorneal film, while the patient looks fixedly at a
point just above the source of light and continues to do so throughout the
test period. The slit is now opened for passage of a maximum pencil of rays,
exposing the cornea to a diffuse white light. The light is then focused on the
mirror reflex image of the lipid layer centrally on the cornea with the dark
pupil as background. Magnification is $\times 15-20$.

We may notice small particles in the aqueous phase, which facilitate the
focusing. The lipid layer is superficial, situated anterior to the corneal
epithelium. The aqueous phase is about $7\,\mu m$ thick. The observer must
draw the slit lamp a little toward himself with the joystick to make the interference image of the lipid layer stand out more sharply than that obtained
by the ordinary examination of the anterior surface of the cornea.

If the lipid layer is just over $134\,nm$ thick, the reflected light from its
anterior surface (lipid-air boundary layer) interferes with the reflected pencil
of rays from its posterior surface (lipid-aqueous phase boundary layer). The
blue light (wavelength $4000\,\text{Å} = 400\,nm$) is in the opposite phase and is thus
eliminated, while the red light ($800\,nm$) is in the cophase and is therefore
visible. The blue light forms an opposite phase when the lipid layer represents one-half of a blue wavelength ($= 200\,nm$). By correction for the

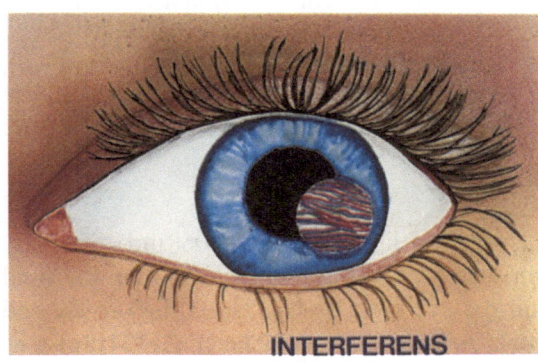

Fig. 12. Examination of the lipid layer of the lacrimal film, interference pattern

refractive index of the lipid layer (1.50) the critical lipid layer thickness becomes $200 \times 0.67 = 134$ nm.

If the slit lamp discloses a lipid layer resembling a petrol puddle on a pool of water, in other words, distinct, red, curved, radiant lines in and beyond the illuminated corneal field (Fig. 12), the lipid layer must be not less than 134 nm thick. In this situation we actually see all the colors of the rainbow distributed irregularly in patterns, all in motion.

If, on the other hand, we see only a grayish plane, possibly with a small number of pale, bluish lines, the lipid layer is thinner. The patient may then be requested to close the eye gradually, or the observer may carefully support the patient's lower eyelid with a finger on the outside of the lid and close it gradually, for instance, by one-sixth palpebral fissure height each time. The lipid layer gradually becomes thicker in response to gradual narrowing of the palpebral fissure. The observer records the palpebral fissure height at which the lipid pattern appears, i.e., when the reflecting lines become visible. This constitutes the semiquantitative measure of the thickness of the lipid layer. If, for instance, the lipid pattern appears when the eye is half closed, the thickness is estimated at $134 \times 0.5 = 67$ nm. If the eye is closed to a fissure height of one-sixth, the lipid layer thickness is only $134 \times 1/6 = 22$ nm. If further closing leaves no lipid pattern, this is due either to a wrong slit lamp adjustment or to a thick lipid layer. If the lipid layer is more than 134 nm thick, it is too thick to provoke interference. The layer resembles silk with a rough surface in an open eye. The observer can verify this by distending the patient's lids with his/her fingers until the lipid pattern with its red color comes out, the lipid layer being now artificially widened. In this situation the result is clearly above 134 nm.

In ptosis the eyelid must be raised to an about 12 mm palpebral fissure, after which the thickness of the lipid layer is to be measured as described above.

The test should not be carried out directly after sleep because the lipid layer is not removed during sleep, when transportation of tears and mucus has ceased.

The lids should not be exposed to such manipulation that the meibomian glands are emptied. This increases the amount of lipid in the precorneal film [71]. The eye should also not be treated with ointment, oil, silicone emulsion, nor with the preservative benzalkonium chloride.

7.2 Normal and Pathological Values

Testing 206 normal subjects, I found a lipid layer of $0.068\,\mu m$ ($68\,nm$ ± $2\,nm$; average ±SEM [70]), corrected for the refractive index of the lipid layer. This indicates that the normal eye must be half closed before the red interference phenomenon occurs. A maximum lipid layer ($>134\,nm$) was noticed in no more than 5% of cases. There was no difference in sex and age incidence. The lipid layer is possibly somewhat thinner in Eskimos (62 ± $3\,nm$) compared with Caucasians (69 ± $4\,nm$; $n = 74$ in both groups) [72]. The thickness of the lipid layer is independent of BUT and the presence of foam [73]. The coefficient of variation was 12.7% in 20 duplicated tests [73].

In KCS the lipid layer has been found to be increased in thickness (109 ± $6\,nm$, $p < 0.001$; $n = 20$), having reached maximum in 40% [70]. The lipid layer may, however, also be increased in other morbid conditions (chronic blepharoconjunctivitis, infectious conjunctivitis, in contact lens wearers, and in persons with increased expressibility of meibomian glands [71]. The layer is normal in chronic simple conjunctivitis and allergy.

A reduced lipid layer is seen in a climatological dry eye: in turpentine vapors (painters) and in the sick building syndrome, where the thin lipid layer may be the cause of the complaints of dry eye. (The lipid layer is dissolved in the climatological fat-soluble aerosol. This causes evaporation from the tear film to increase, the BUT to be reduced, and the corneal epithelium to be damaged [2]).

7.3 Modifications

Josephson [74] warns against the use of too intense light to avoid tear reflex and disruption of the lipid layer. He has studied the thickness of the lipid layer not only on the cornea but also on the bulbar conjunctiva close to the temporal border of the limbus. He has undertaken both static and dynamic examinations on a video recorder. The examination can be quantified more thoroughly by photographing the palpebral fissure initially and again on the appearance of the interference phenomenon.

Olsen [75] introduced an objective, photometric reflectometry – slit lamp examination at wavelengths of 500 and 700 nm. In ten normal subjects he found a lipid layer thickness of 40 nm.

The function of the meibomian glands can be assessed by triple staining with lipid-specific Sudan III, lissamine green, and fluorescein (Fig. 13). The orifice is sometimes blocked (in an average of 55% of the glands in

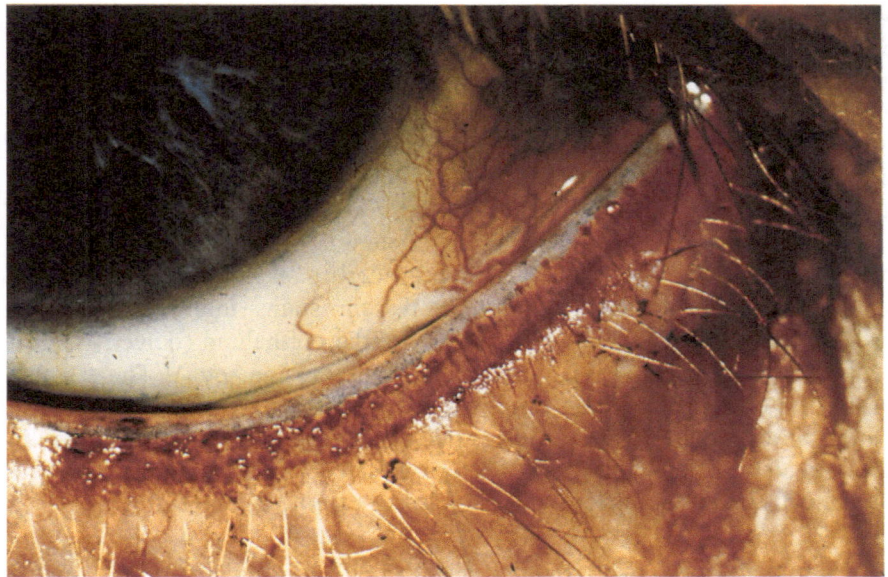

Fig. 13. Vital staining of the orifices of the meimbomian glands. A few active glands are visible (*red*) in the lateral part of the margin. (Sudan III and lissamine green)

normals), in some cases by epithelial plugs. Several orifices are irregularly placed, especially in elderly normals and in cases of conjunctivitis, including KCS [11].

7.4 Discussion

The semiquantitative interference method described above is easy to employ with no aids (beyond a slit lamp). Its theoretical background is, however, subject to criticism, there being no inevitable correlation between the thickness of the lipid layer and the height of the palpebral fissure. In addition, the composition (quality) of the lipid layer may be equally as important as its quantity, or even more so (proportion of lipid invaded from the skin to secretion of meibomian glands, melting point of the lipid, cholesterol content, free fatty acid [76]).

8   Staining

Dry eye can be diagnosed by demonstrating dessication in an exposed region of the epithelium by staining. Henrik Sjögren (the Swedish eponym of

Sjögren's syndrome) in 1933 introduced rose bengal for detection of KCS. Marx used the stain as an ocular vital stain as early as the 1920s [6]. Rose bengal stains dead, degenerate, and dessicated epithelial cells as well as mucus and is thus not specific to dry epithelial cells. In dry eye dessicated epithelial cells are often covered by mucus. Hence, a differentiation between dessicated epithelial cells and mucus is not strictly necessary in practice. Differentiation is, however, obtainable by double staining (rose bengal and alcian blue, Fig. 14; see below).

Other stains have also been used. Lissamine green causes no smarting pain. Since it has the same staining properties as rose bengal, it may sometimes be preferred to this. Fluorescein stains intercellular spaces provided there are breaches of continuity in the epithelium (defective intercellular seam, dropping out of epithelial cell, erosion, etc.). The staining properties of fluorescein thus differ essentially from those of rose bengal [6]. One stain cannot replace the other, but the two supplement each other. In cases of dry eye rose bengal is preferred, since this stains dessicated epithelial cells (staining nucleus and, to a lesser extent, cytoplasm).

8.1 Specificity of Stains

Figure 14 gives a survey of the specific properties of stains in staining cornea and conjunctiva [6]. Dessicated epithelial cells are stained in vivo by 1% rose bengal. When 10% rose bengal is used, cells only just beginning to be affected by dessication likewise become stained. In normal subjects this staining is localized as in those with KCS (Fig. 15). Rose bengal also stains dead cells. We can distinguish between dead and dessicated epithelial cells in vivo by staining with 1% trypan blue as well (dead cells stained blue, dry cells red) or avoid concurrent staining of mucus by using 1% alcian blue (mucus stained blue and cells red). Iodonitrotetrazolium stains dry, live cells red. This can be combined with lissamine green (stains dry and dead cells blue). Thus, vital stains of different specificities can be combined if assessment of special conditions is desired (see also Sects. 6.3, 7).

8.2 Rose Bengal Staining

Rose bengal (4,5,6,7-tetrachloro-2′,4′,5′,7′-tetraiodofluorescein sodium) is used. I use 1% rose bengal (extra CI 45440 from the British Drug House no. 20103) alone or possibly mixed with fluorescein for differential diagnosis (fluorescein sodium 50 mg, rose bengal 50 mg, sodium chloride 45 mg, phenylmercuric nitrate 0.05 mg, distilled water to 5.0 g). The patient is warned that the drops may cause a smarting pain. A drop of 10 μl is instilled through a cannula mounted on the bottle (red steristar gauge 25; 0.5 × 16 mm). The patient thereafter blinks naturally and is placed in front of the slit lamp. The staining can be studied as soon as excess stain in the precorneal film has disappeared, i.e., after 1–2 min. The reading may be post-

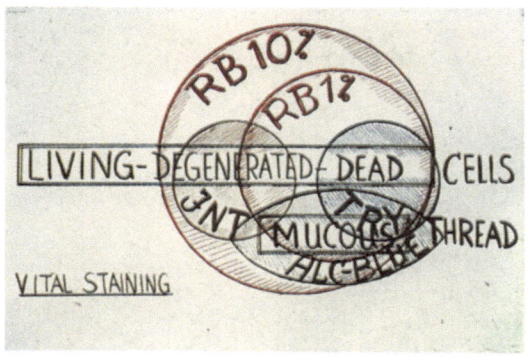

Fig. 14. Diagram of specificity of vital stains. *RB*, Rose bengal; *JNT*, iodonitrotetrazolium; *TRY*, trypan blue; *ALC*, alcian blue

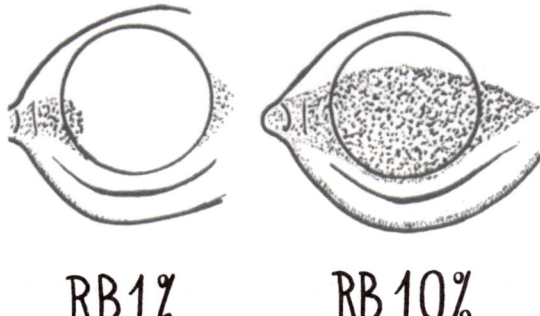

Fig. 15. Rose bengal staining of normals with 1% (*left*) and 10% (*right*)

poned maximally 5 min in association with lacrimal river dilution test (see Sect. 3.1). After 5 min the red color begins to fade [6].

The quantity of dye is a moot point. An amount of 2.5 µl 1% rose bengal can be used, instilled from an automatic precision pipette with sterile tips. Reading in the green light of the slit lamp may be carried out after few blinks. Other workers employ transfer with a glass rod or use rose-bengal-imbibed filter paper moistened by a drop of sterile saline and then inserted into the upper or the lower conjunctiva. Filter paper direct on the conjunctiva causes too much irritation. A glass rod or filter paper gives inaccurate, and often too small quantities of dye. Rose bengal is delivered in single-dose containers (Smith and Nephew). An Italian firm delivers nearly all clinically useful stains in such single-dose containers. If the patient fears smarting pain, local anesthesia may be given prior to staining (0.2% oxibuprocain 5 min before), or lissamine green may be chosen instead. Smarting is more intense the greater the stainability (KCS).

Rose bengal staining is seen even in normal subjects, though usually only as a few dots. These generally occur in the lower nasal part of the bulbar conjunctiva, particularly in elderly individuals, as well as on caruncle and Marx' line (see Sect. 8.6). On observation for dry eye it is therefore important to be familiar with the normal staining picture, and grading is

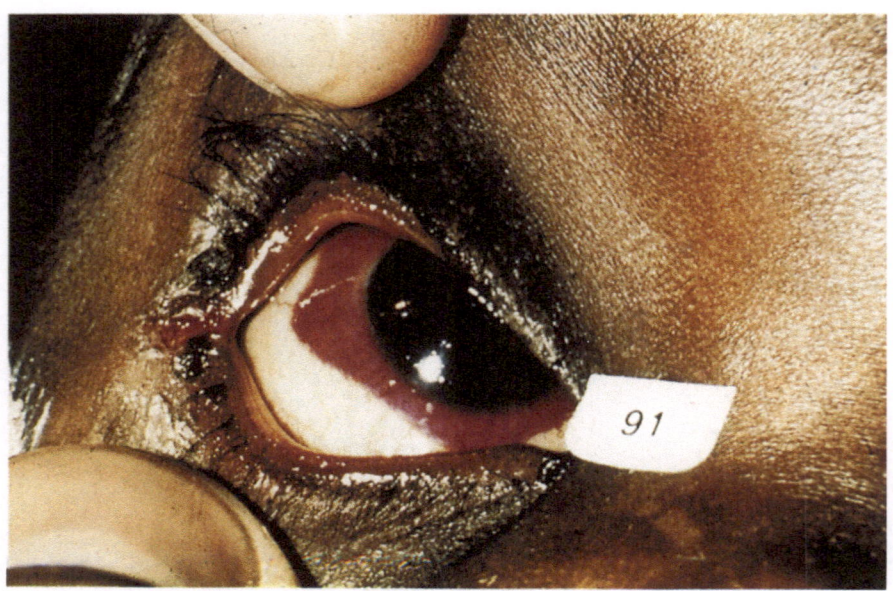

Fig. 16. Staining with rose bengal in a case of vitamin A deficiency (Jim Sauter, Kenya)

useful. This grading depends, however, on the type of dry eye for which the patient is examined. In KCS and Sjögren's syndrome the exposed parts of cornea and conjunctiva are graded. Such grading is inexpedient in cases of vitamin A deficiency (xerophthalmia) or climatological dry eye. The latter affects nonexposed regions. Vitamin A deficiency affects the epithelium below and above the cornea, and the climatological type particularly that below the cornea on the bulbar conjunctiva (cf. cauterization).

Rose-bengal staining is graded in KCS (according to Bijsterveld [20]) from 1 to 3 (slight, moderate, intense staining) on the exposed part of the cornea. Analogous scores are given to the exposed triangular areas of the medial bulbar conjunctiva and the corresponding lateral bulbar conjunctiva. These scores are added. Maximum staining at all the three sites thus yields a maximum score of 9 points for one eye. A score of 3.5 or higher is pathological. Specificity and sensitivity are reported as 95% and 96% [20]. Other workers have found 100% specificity and 58% sensitivity [77]. This grading is practical and universally accepted.

With a view to controlling changes of dryness and effect of local treatment I have employed a similar grading to a maximum score of 15 points [6].

In vitamin A deficiency, staining with rose bengal (or lissamine green) visible at a distance of 0.5–1 m is pathological (Fig. 16). Staining of the exposed part of the bulbar conjunctiva is given grade I, staining also below the cornea grade II, above and below the cornea grade III, and staining including the cornea grade IV [78]. Most likely only cases of fresh xeroph-thalmia (see Sect. 10.1) are positive [79].

The grading in climatological dry eye is based on estimation of jointly stained spots on the bulbar conjunctiva, nasally and temporally. Franck [63] has estimated the number of dots in the largest group and judged whether it was below 10, 10–50, or over 50 within this group, corresponding to grades I, II, and III, respectively.

In benign mucosal pemphigoid rose bengal staining is localized mainly in the tarsus (in one half of cases), more rarely on the exposed parts of cornea and conjunctiva [10]. The diagnosis is based on the deficiency of mucus (see Sect. 6).

8.3 Lissamine Green Staining

Lissamine green has been used for dyeing foodstuffs. It has color index number 44090 and the following synonyms: wool green S, BS, BSNA, pontacyl green, food green, calcoid green S extra, acid green S. Its formula is $C_{27} H_{25} N_2 Na O_7 S_2$; its molecular weight is 576.6. It is an acidic, synthetically produced organic dye containing two aminophenyl groups as tetrazolium salts. Neither carcinogenic nor toxic tendencies have ever been detected. Lissamine green was introduced as a vital stain for eyes in 1973 [80]. Strangely, its staining properties in a 1% solution equal those of 1% rose bengal, even though the two stains differ widely in chemical composition.

The advantage of lissamine green over rose bengal include its better color contrast to blood vessels and hemorrhage (green against red) and the fact that it causes practically no smarting. Lissamine green is therefore particularly suitable for screening in labor-hygienic investigations [63] and in field surveys of vitamin A deficiency [78,79]. As for the latter, some workers regard it as superior to the time-consuming night blindness test and blood retinol test (the liver depot is more important than the blood level). Bitôt's spots become stained by lipid-specific stain (Sudan III). Bitôt's spots are sequels of vitamin A deficiency or merely represent unspecific keratinization (Fig. 17). Draft in the eye while motoring has been found to reduce the BUT but to give no vital staining [54]. *Grading* of lissamine-green staining is identical to that of rose bengal (Fig. 18).

8.4 Fluorescein Staining

Staining with fluorescein is carried out with the sodium salt of resorcinol phthalein $C_{20}H_{10}N_2O_5$ a 1% aqueous solution, in a quantity of $10\,\mu l$ from a single-dose container (Smith and Nephew). Cobalt-filtered blue light (cor-responding to Wratten filter 47 B Kodak) is employed in the slit lamp in a dark room. The staining is observed as soon as is possible through the still

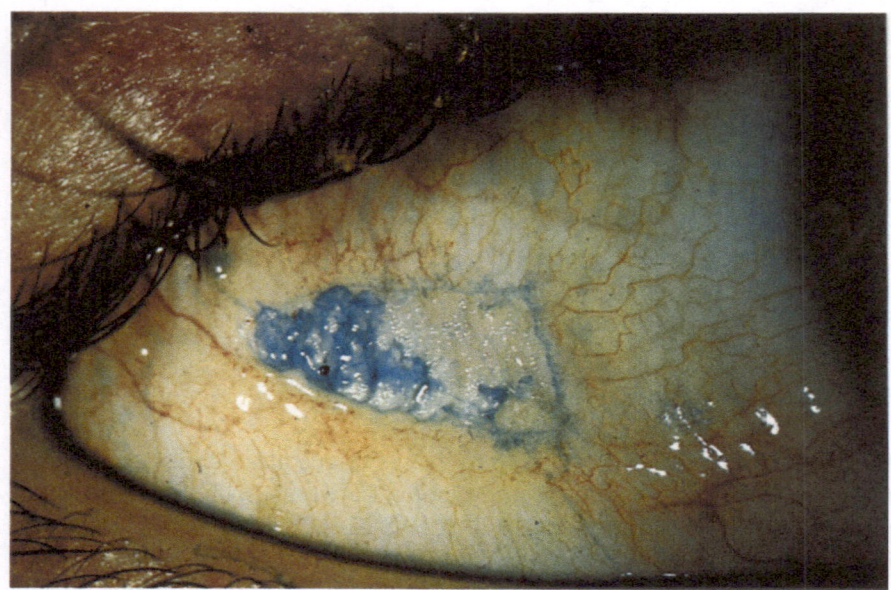

Fig. 17. Bitôt spot (keratinization) on the bulbar conjunctiva, surrounded by mucus. (Alcian blue)

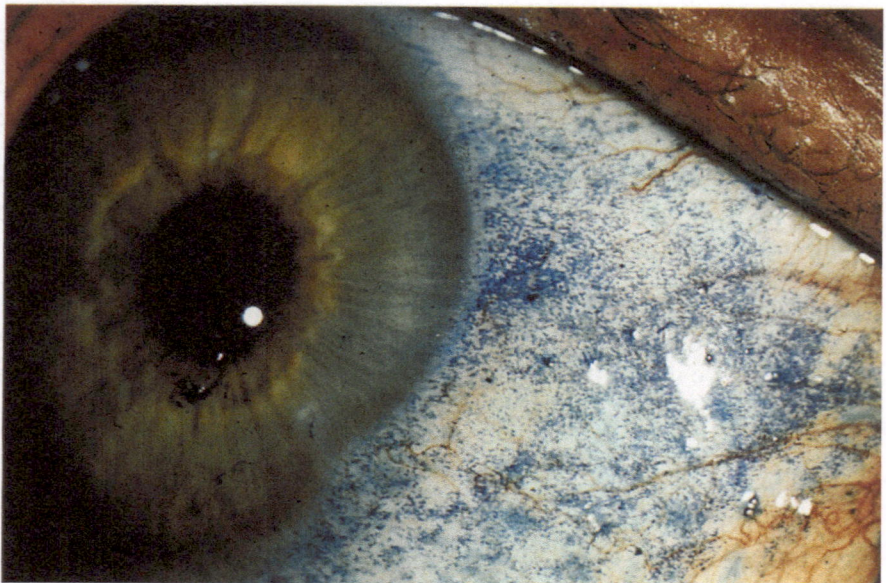

Fig. 18. A case of keratoconjunctivitis sicca. Grade 1 on cornea, grade 3 on bulbar conjunctiva (according to Bijsterveld). (Lissamine green)

fluorescein-stained lacrimal film. Repeated examinations within the first few minutes is recommended to be able to distinguish between genuine and false staining. The latter soon fades (uneven corneal surface, lacrimal fluid left in the dellen, corneal excavation, around filaments on the cornea). Genuine staining, on the other hand, means nonfading staining by fluorescein penetrating through defects extracellularly into the epithelium. Fluorescein does not stain dessicated epithelial cells but shows defects in the epithelial layer by penetrating into the intercellular space.

In normal eyes micropunctate staining is most often seen in the lower nasal regions of cornea and conjunctiva, increasing in intensity with increasing age. In subjects below the age of 60 years one rarely sees more than five to nine dots, but in older subjects there are a greater number scattered over the entire cornea [6]. In pathological cases an increased number is observed in the dry eye, also provoked by working conditions (rock wool fibers particularly on the nasal area of the bulbar conjunctiva [3]). Fluorescein staining is also noticed in many other states (contact lens wearers, keratitis, erosion, cauterization).

In video films one can estimate the proportion of stained to unstained corneas after instillation of 2% fluorescein [81].

8.5 Fluorexon Staining

Fluorexon is a fluorescein derivative with a larger molecule (molecular weight 710 against 376 for fluorescein). Fluorexon combines in one molecule the staining properties of fluorescein (fluorescing epithelial defects) and rose bengal (dark brown nonfluorescent staining of dead and degenerate cells). However, even in a 2% dilution it stains less intensely than the above stains. Hence rose bengal is still preferable in KCS.

8.6 Marx' Line on Lid Margin

Marx' line is stained by rose bengal or lissamine green. The line runs along the lid margin in relation to the base of the tear meniscus (lacrimal streak, lacrimal river) just behind the orifices of the meibomian glands. It forms an imprint, as it were, of the course of the streaming lacrimation. It may be irregular, especially in elderly persons. The line normally continues to and further down into the canaliculus. A wrong direction may disclose dry eye, as a result of ectropion where the line passes behind the lacrimal point [6,11]. Marx' line is rudimentary in pemphigoid with a concurrent reduced tear flow [10].

9   Other Methods

9.1   Blink Frequency, Height of Tear Meniscus, Foam in the External Part of the Eye

An increased blink frequency (greater than 12 per minute) is seen in primary Sjögren's syndrome. Increased blink frequency is correlated with reduced BUT [82].

The normal height of the tear fluid along the lower eye lid margin is not less than 0.2 mm (pathological value <0.2 mm or disrupted river). It can be measured on a magnified video film, by means of which this measure may become an important factor in the estimation of a dry eye (H.-W. Roth, personal communication).

Foam develops in the external part of the eye by blinking. It consists of lipids from the meibomian glands possibly combined with dermal fat. In normal subjects we find an average amount of $1.1 \, mm^2$, most of it laterally ($0.9 \, mm^2$), depending on age, with a maximum in those aged 30–50 years [73]. Foam is rare in patients with lagophthalmos, normal in KCS. It vanishes when silicone emulsion is applied [83], and is reduced in fat-soluble environment [2].

9.2   Specular Wide-Field Microscopy

Analysis of the rose bengal–fluorescein stained corneal epithelium was introduced by Lemp in 1984.

In KCS there is increased rose bengal staining. Lemp et al. [84] found a statistically significant shift to small cells, suggesting accelerated exfoliation.

9.3   Tear Evaporimetry

Goggles with defined moisture and temperature can be used for measuring evaporation from the eye surface. The normal value is $4.07 \pm 0.40 \times 10^{-7} \, g \, cm^{-2} \, s^{-1}$ ($n = 52$) and is independent of sex and age. Increased evaporation is seen in KCS, being perhaps the cause of hyperosmol a rity in such cases. Increased evaporation is also seen in conditions with defects in layers of lipid or mucus [85].

9.4   Corneal Sensitivity

The sensitivity is measured with Cochet and Bonnet's nylon thread esthesiometer. I have found normal sensitivity in KCS [18], others a reduced sensitivity in Sjögren's syndrome [86]. In pemphigoid the sensitivity is reduced diffusely over tarsal conjunctiva, fornix, bulbar conjunctiva, caruncle, and occasionally cornea, but never the lid margin [18].

9.5 pH Buffer Capacity

In KCS the conjunctival fluid has a normal pH [87]. An instilled buffer of pH 5.0 takes longer to become normalized in patients with KCS and pemphigoid [88].

9.6 Leukocyte Esterase Tear Stix

Tear stix is used on suspicion of bacterial infection of dry eye (see Sect. 1). A small tuft of cotton (2–3 mm wide and 20 mm long) is inserted laterally in the inferior fornix. After about 20 s the tear-moistened cotton is taken out, placed on the two distal test fields, and covered by the two proximal test fields on the turned-in urine test strip between the central fields (Nephur-test-leuco, Boehringer-Mannheim). The fields are pressed together for a few seconds, and the test pads are read exactly 60 s after contact with the cotton. The esterase field becomes red on positive response, indicating an increased amount of tear leukocyte esterase enzyme (sensitivity 89%, specificity 98%, overall agreement 96%; $n = 262$ normal subjects and 84 with infectious conjunctivitis [89]). The albumin field (blue reaction) serves as control of absorption of tear fluid in the cotton.

10 Laboratory Tests

10.1 Lactoferrin

Lactoferrin is produced mainly in acini of the lacrimal glands. Its tear concentration is therefore a suitable parameter of the diagnoses of KCS and Sjögren's syndrome [90]. Lactoferrin is tested by enzyme-linked immuno-adsorbent assay (coefficient of variation 5%). The method permits measurement of concentrations as low as 1 ng/ml [91]. Tear lactoferrin can in ophthalmological practice be measured by means of a commercially available Lactoplate, a radial immunodiffusion test. The diameter of the precipitation ring is read after 72 h.

10.2 Lysozyme

Lysozyme is an enzyme decomposing the wall of certain bacteria. The tear concentration can be measured by inserting a 5-mm Schirmer's paper in the conjunctival sac, withdrawing the tear-moistened paper, and transferring it to an agar plate containing a suspension of the bacterium *Micrococcus lysodeikticus*. The inhibition zone is measured after 24 h at 37°C. The immunoassay technique is now generally preferred. Aine employed the immunoturbidimetric method [92] and found age variations and normal values as follows: ages 10–60, 0.75–3.3 mg/ml; ages over 60, 0.65–2.9 mg/ml (average 1.68 ± 0.63). There is no difference in sex incidence. The lysozyme level is reduced in KCS and in nutritive xerosis.

10.3 Electrophoresis

Crossed immunoelectrophoresis and immunoblotting produce not only lactoferrin and lysozyme but also serum albumin, IgA, IgG, IgM, transferrin, etc. In normal subjects one finds 25 different compounds. During electrophoresis of ocular mucus it is possible to study glycoproteins – also in Sjögren's syndrome and Steven-Johnson syndrome [93].

10.4 Scintigraphy of Lacrimal Gland

After intravenous administration of 3 mCi ^{67}Ga citrate the accumulation of Ga in the lacrimal gland is measured. Ga is present in a reduced amount in Sjögren's syndrome [94].

10.5 Tear Fluid Osmolarity

The osmolarity of tear fluid is tested with a freezing-point osmometer on a tear sample of approximately 0.2 µl. The osmolarity is increased (>312 mosmol) in KCS [95], but the osmolarity varies according to the site of sampling: most often hypertonia in the inferior fornix compared with the center of the inferior tear meniscus. This may be due to a slower flow in the inferior fornix with accumulation of breakdown products [96].

10.6 Tear Cytology

A semiquantitative conjunctival cytological test (Figs. 19–22) gives normal values in KCS, but secondary bacterial infection is disclosed in patients with neutrophilia [6]. An increased number of nuclear squamous epithelial cells indicates the presence of pemphigoid (Fig. 21).

10.7 Impression Cytology, Biopsy

The imprint technique [37] is suitable for determining of the density of goblet cells. Marner in 1980 [97] found snakelike nuclear chromatin in

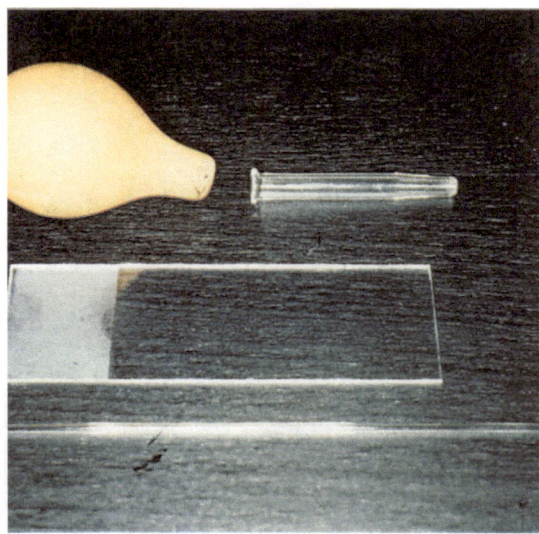

Fig. 19. Semiquantitative conjunctival cytological test (according to Norn). Instruments: standardized pipette, rubber bulb, glass slide and, glass capillary tube

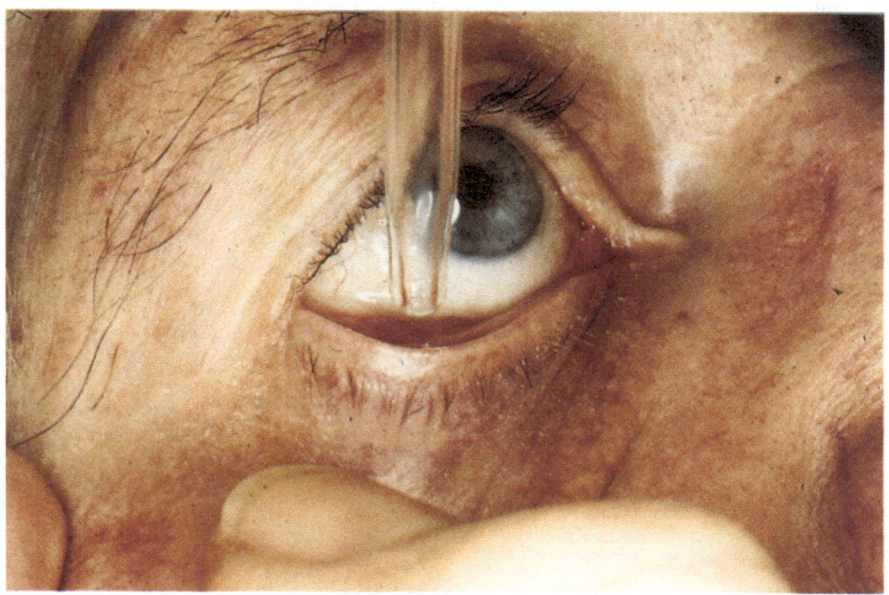

Fig. 20. Semiquantitative conjunctival cytological test, the bulb-mounted pipette sucks from the lateral part of the inferior conjunctival fornix

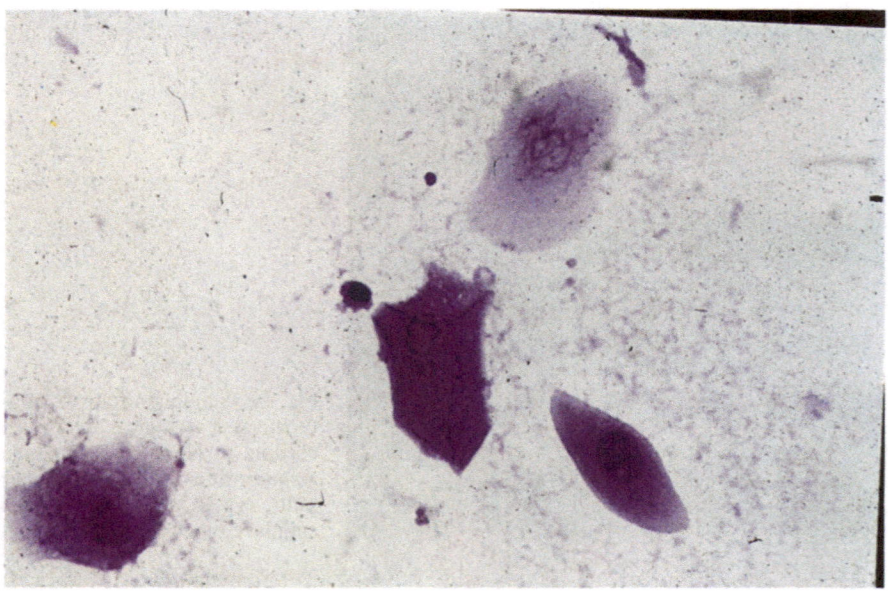

Fig. 21. Keratinized nucleated squamous cells from a case of benign mucous membrane pemphigoid (semiquantitative conjunctival cytological test)

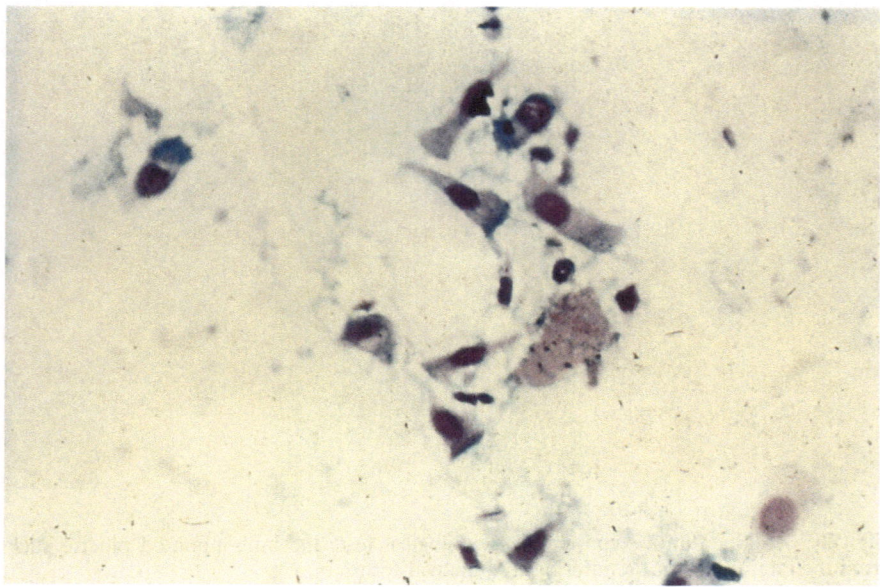

Fig. 22. Columnar epithelial cells (abnormal desquamation) from a case of environmentally induced dry eye (semiquantitative conjunctival cytological test). (×100)

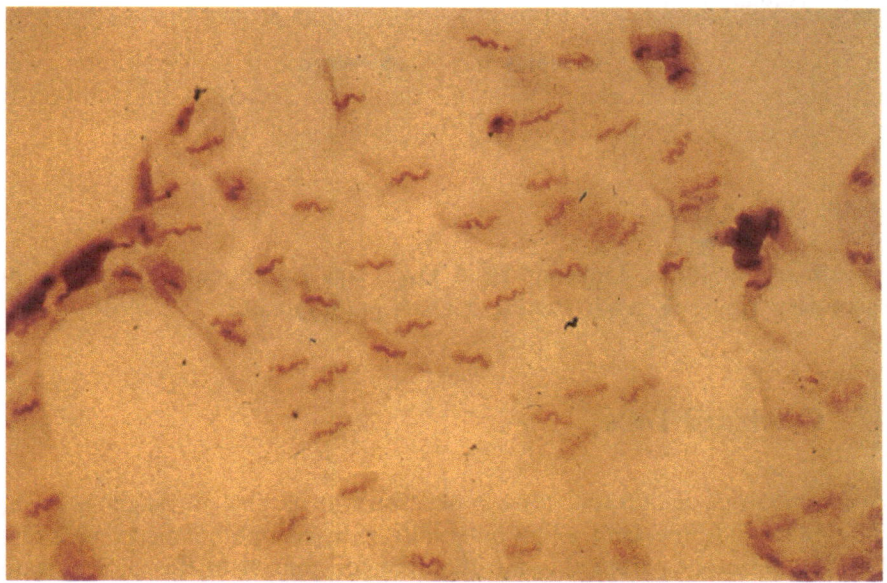

Fig. 23. Snakelike nuclear chromatin in conjunctival epithelial cells in a case of KCS (imprint technique according to Marner)

conjunctival epithelial cells to be characteristic of KCS. Such never occurs in normals (Fig. 23). Millipore MF type VS with pore size of 0.025 μm, presoaked in cold water and air-dried, is mounted on a tensiometer (Correx, Haag Streit) with tape adhesive on both sides. The filter is pressed against the superior bulbar conjunctiva for 2 s at a pressure of 25–30 mmHg. The S-shaped nuclei with condensed chromatin observed in KCS are present only in the conjunctival region above the cornea, not on the exposed part of the conjunctiva. The test was positive in 55 of 118 patients with primary Sjögren's syndrome and in 13 of 24 with secondary Sjögren's syndrome [98]. The cause of the phenomenon is obscure. A special vulnerability of the epithelial cells in this region is suspected. It is possible to transfer imprints from the primarily used Millipore filters to ordinary glass slides. This makes more specific histological investigation feasible. Proper biopsy is easily performed, for example, from the inferior fornix. In pemphigoid patients conjunctival shrinkage is aggravated after biopsy.

10.8   Lectin Analysis

Conjunctival mucus from goblet cells and from the second mucous system (subsurface vesicles) in normals present different sugar-linkage characters. The mucus in KCS links other sugar species. This can be studied in the electron microscope by lectin-gold cytochemistry [99] or in tear samples.

10.9 Autoantibody

In Sjögren's syndrome one finds increased erythrocyte sedimentation rate, antinuclear antibody, complement C3 antibody, anti-SS-A and anti-SS-B antibody (rabbit thymus), IgG, IgM-rheumatic factor, etc.

10.10 Tissue Types

In primary Sjögren's syndrome HLA Dw 2 and 3 predominate, whereas in secondary Sjögren's syndrome HLA Dw 4 predominates.

11 Combined Tests

A combination of different tests is necessary to be able to diagnose KCS, Sjögren's syndrome, and environmentally induced ophthalmic complaints. Further, different parameters are required for control of the clinical state and for assessment of therapy.

11.1 Criteria for Sjögren's Syndrome

Different criteria are employed for Sjögren's syndrome: the Californian, Greek, Japanese [102], and Copenhagen. As regards the Copenhagen criteria for Sjögren's primary syndrome, at least two of the three KCS criteria must be positive and at least two of the three xerostomy criteria. The Copenhagen criteria of KCS are the Schirmer's test I with closed eye showing <10 mm/5 min or below, BUT of 10 s or below, and rose bengal vital staining according to Bijsterveld score of at least 4 (in both eyes). The xerostomia criteria are based on sialometry, scintigraphy, and lip biopsy.

11.2 Criteria for Therapy

The value of KCS therapy can be assessed by Schirmer's test, BUT, and rose bengal score, supplemented by other tests, such as that for osmolarity.

11.3 Criteria for Environmentally Induced Dry Eye

Various investigations have produced results suggesting [2] that dry eye is due to reduction of the superficial lipid layer of the precorneal film (turpentine, n-butanol, sick building syndrome) [63]. In KCS, on the other hand, the lipid layer is not reduced. Hence, interference and possibly foam tests are recommended. BUT measurement and staining (rose bengal or lissamine green) are required. The grading of staining deviates from that of the Bijsterveld score because the staining is not diffuse over an exposed area but scattered in groups on the bulbar conjunctiva. The largest group of stained dots is assessed [63]. Quantitative cytological examination of the conjunctiva may disclose increased desquamation of cylindric epithelial cells (Fig. 22) and later neutrophilia [3,6].

12 Discussion

The result of a tear test depends on the type of tear, substances admixed, technique and site of sampling. Tear tests can rarely be carried out without interfering with the system. Instances of noninterfering tests include the nontouch BUT test and lipid analysis by the interference method. In the great majority of cases tear production is unfortunately reflex stimulated in an uncontrollable manner with resulting altered quality and quantity. Basal tears are rarely or never obtainable. Affectively provoked tears may have different characteristics. The levels of lysozyme and lactoferrin are considerably higher in reflex-stimulated tears than in more basal tears.

12.1 Technique of Sampling

The amount of lysozyme is smaller if absorbed by cell sponges than by filter paper (internal absorption in sponges) [100]. Capillary tube and filter paper yield parallel values for lysozyme and lactoferrin, but filter paper gives higher values for albumin, transferrin, and IgG, presumably because the paper causes mechanical stimulation of the conjunctiva [101].

12.2 Site of Sampling

The most reliable site for sampling tears must be the lacrimal gland duct, where tears can be collected from the main lacrimal gland by finely drawn glass capillary tubes. So far this has been done only in certain animal experiments, however. In human patients we must be content to collect tears from the tear meniscus, the inferior conjunctival fornix, etc., unfortunately with admixture of other elements.

Quantitative cytological samples from different conjunctival regions are not equal [6], and hyperosmolarity has been detected in the inferior fornix compared with the tear meniscus [97]. Both observations seem to indicate a slow flow in the inferior fornix compared with the fast (cleaner?) flood of tears in the tear meniscus (lacrimal river). This compartment theory shows how important it is to standardize and to choose the right site of sampling.

The samples contain ingredients originating exclusively from lacrimal glands (lactoferrin, lysozyme, secretory IgA), from the blood stream (albumin, IgG, emigrated cells), from goblet cells, from epithelium (secondary mucous system, among others), from meibomian glands, and possibly from cutaneous sebum (transferred by blinking via foam).

The composition of the tear sample depends on these admixtures, which again depend on the site and technique of sampling.

13   Diagnostic Methods in Practice

What to do in a busy practice in cases with suspicion of dry eye? Among the many diagnostic methods I recommend first the use of the BUT test and staining with rose bengal. In suspected KCS I also perform Schirmer's test later. In cases of suspected environmental keratoconjunctivitis, I also use the interference method in the slit lamp (lipid layer of the tear film).

References

1. L. Mc Monnies CW (1984) Detection and management of dry eye problems in contact lens wearers. 4th Scandinavian contact lens meeting, Sweden
2. Franck C (1991) Fatty layer of the precorneal film in office eye syndrome. Acta Ophthalmol (Copenh) (to be published)
3. Stokholm J, Norn M, Schneider T (1982) Ophthalmologic effects of man-made mineral fibres. [Scand] Work Environ Health 8:185–190
4. Edmund J (1951) Photoelectric measurement of the corneal gloss. Danish Science, Copenhagen, pp 136
5. Trobe JD, Laibson PR (1972) Dystrophic changes in the anterior cornea. Arch Ophthalmol 87:378–382
6. Norn M (1983) External eye, methods of examination, 2nd edn. Scriptor, Copenhagen, pp 212
7. Graves (1923) Trans Ophthalmol Soc UK 43:386
8. Duke-Elder S (1962) System of ophthalmology VII. Kimpton, London, pp 254–255
9. Boyd HH (1970) In: Sampson WG, Feldman GL (eds) Contact Lens medical seminar, vol I. Thomas, Springfield, p 138
10. Kristensen EB, Norn M (1974) Benign mucous membrane pemphigoid. I. Secretion of mucus and tears. Acta Ophthalmol (Copenh) 52:266–281
11. Norn M (1985) Meibomian orifices and Marx' line, studied by tripple vital staining. Acta Ophthalmol 63:698–700
12. Schirmer O (1903) Studium zur Physiologie und Pathologie der Tränenabsonderung und Tränenabfuhr. Arch Ophthalmol 56:197–291
13. Henderson JW, Prough WA (1950) Influenzia de la edad y el sexo en el flujo lacrimal. Arch Ophthalmol 43:224
14. Murube del Castillo J (1982) Dacriologia basica. Madrid
15. Prause JU, Frost-Larsen K, Isager H, Manthorpe R (1982) Tear absorption in the filter-paper strips and in the Schirmer-I-test. Acta Ophthalmol (Copenh) 60:70–78

16. Holly FJ, Beebe WE, Esquivel ED (1984) Lacrimation kinetics in humans as determined by a novel technique. In: Holly FJ (ed) The preocular tear film. Dry Eye Institute, Lubbock, pp 76–88
17. Hansen T, Kiehn O, Kristensen J et al. (1983) Schirmers tear test. (In Danish with an English summary.) Ugeskr Laeger 145:2573–2575
18. Norn M (1975) Conjunctival sensitivity in pathological cases. Acta Ophthalmol (Copenh) 53:450–451
19. Norn M (1977) Outflow of tears and its influence on tear secretion and break up time. Acta Ophthalmol (Copenh) 55:674–682
20. V Bijsterveld OP (1969) Diagnostic tests in the sicca syndrome. Arch Ophthalmol 82:10–14
21. Zappia RJ (1972) Fluorescein dye disappearance test. Am J Ophthalmol 74:160–162
22. Shiavi L, Lazzaroni F, Ghini M et al. (1986) Effect of oral contraceptives on tear secretion. IVth international symposium on the lacrimal system. Abstract Book, Pavia
23. Farris RL, Gilbard JP, Stuchell RN, Mandel ID (1983) Diagnostic tests in keratoconjunctivitis sicca. CLAO J 9:23–28
24. Shapiro A, Merin S (1979) Schirmer's test and break up time of tear film in normal subjects. Am J Ophthalmol 88:752–757
25. Rieger G (1986) Schirmer's test with topical anesthesia with opened or closed eyes? Fortschr Ophthalmol 83:179–180
26. Jones LJ (1966) The lacrimal system and its treatment. Am J Ophthalmol 62:47–60
27. Lamberts DW, Foster SC, Perry HD (1978) Schirmer's test after topical anesthesia and the tear meniscus height in normal eyes. Arch Ophthalmol 97:1082–1085
28. Jordan A, Baum J (1980) Basic tear flow, does it exist? Ophthalmology 87:920–930
29. Clinch TE, Benedetto DA, Felberg NT, Laibson PR (1983) Schirmer's test, a closer look. Arch Ophthalmol 101:1383–1386
30. Makie JA, Seal DV (1981) The questionable dry eye. Br J Ophthalmol 65:2–9
31. Jonasdottir E (1987) Schirmer-I test with and without modifications. Acta Ophthalmol (Copenh) 65:657–660
32. Holly FJ, Laukaitis SJ, Esquivel ED (1984) Kinetics of lacrimal secretion in normal human subjects. Curr Eye Res 3:897–910
33. Jones LT, Malcolm M, Vincent NJ (1972) Lacrimal function. Am J Ophthalmol 73:658–659
34. Kurihashi K (1984) Diagnostic tests of lacrimal function using cotton threads. Abstract 91 and 93. In: International tear film symposium program 1984. And in: Holly FJ (ed) The preocular tear film. Dry Eye Institute, Lubbock, pp 84–116
35. Norn M (1965) Tear secretion in normal eyes. Acta Ophthalmol (Copenh) 43:567–573
36. Norn M (1966) Tear secretion in diseased eyes. Acta Ophthalmol (Copenh) 44:25–32
37. Royer J (1985) Dry eye. Klinn Monatsbl Augenheilkd 186:436–441
38. Brandt HP, Fritsche G (1967) Klinische Erfahrungen mit dem Tränenstreifen-Verdünnungstest und Norn MS. Acta Ophthalmol (Copenh) 45:166–176
39. Port M (1980) The photographic assessment of tear flow. Contacto 24(6):10–20
40. Sørensen TB (1984) Studies on tear physiology, pathophysiology and contact lenses by means of dynamic gamma camera and technetium. Acta Ophthalmol [Suppl] (Copenh) 167:54
41. Mishima J, Gasset A, Klyce CD, Baum JL (1966) Determination of tear volume and tear flow. Invest Ophthalmol 5:264
42. Occhipint JR, Mosier MA, Motte J, Monji GT (1988) Fluorophotometric measurement of human tear turn over rate. Eye Res 7:995–1000
43. Puffer MJ, Neault RW, Brubaker RF (1980) Basal precorneal tear turn over in the human eye. Am J Ophthalmol 89:369–376
44. Norn M (1987) Ferning in conjunctival-cytologic preparations. Acta Ophthalmol (Copenh) 65:118–123

45. Sole A (1955) Die Stagoskopie der Tränen. Klin Monatsbl Augenheilk 126:446–451
46. Tabbara KF, Okumoto M (1982) Ocular ferning test, qualitative test for mucus defiency. Ophthalmology 89:712–714
47. Rolando M (1984) Tear mucus ferning test in normal and keratoconjunctivitis sicca eyes. Cibret. Int Ophthalmol 2:32–41
48. Rolando M, Baldi G, Calabria A (1984) Tear mucus ferning in KCS. International tear symposium abstract. Genova, p 35
49. Liotet J, Bijsterveld OP, Bletry O et al. (1987) L'oeil sec. Masson, Paris, pp 213–233
50. Norn M (1988) Quantitative tear ferning. Acta Ophthalmol (Copenh) 66:201–205
51. Calabria G, Rolando M (1984) Fisiopatologia del film lacrimale. Symp 64, Congres Soc Oftal Italiana, pp 240
52. Recupero SM, Castaniti G, Garufi C et al. (1986) Modifications of tear secretion during treatment with high doses of folinic acid and 5-fluorouracil in advanced colon cancer. IVth international symposium on lacrimal system. Abstract Book, Milano
53. Calabria GA, Rolando M (1986) Biochemistry of the tears. IVth international symposium on the lacrimal system. Abstract Book, Pavia
54. Wyon NM, Wyon DP (1987) Measurement of acute response to draught in the eye. Acta Ophthalmol (Copenh) 65:385–392
55. Norn M (1969) Desiccation of the precorneal film. I. Corneal wetting time. Acta Ophthalmol (Copenh) 47:865–880
56. Norn M (1969) Desiccation of the precorneal film. II. Permanent discontinuity and dellen. Acta Ophthalmol (Copenh) 47:881–889
57. Lemp MA, Holly FJ, Iwata S, Dohlman CH (1970) The precorneal tear film. Arch Ophthalmol 83:89–94
58. Fenton PJ (1965) Applanation tonometry using anaesthetic-fluorescein mixture. Br J Ophthalmol 49:504
59. Norn M, Opauszki A (1977) Effects of ophthalmic vehicles on the stability of the precorneal film. Acta Ophthalmol (Copenh) 55:23–34
60. Dilly PN, Makie IA (1981) Surface changes in the anaesthetic conjunctiva in man, with special reference to the production of mucus from the non-goblet cell source. Br J Ophthalmol 65:833–842
61. Marquardt R, Stodtmeister R, Christ T (1984) Unreliability of the tear film break up time. A modified BUT test. Inteational tear film sympornsium, abstract 3
62. Lemp MA, Hamill JR (1973) Tactors affecting tear film break up time in normal eyes. Arch Ophthalmol 89:103–105
63. Franck C (1986) Eye symptoms and signs in buildings with indoor climate problems. Acta Ophthalmol (Copenh) 64:306–311
64. Mengher LS, Bron AR, Tonge SR, Gilbert DJ (1985) Effect of fluorescein instillation on the precorneal tear film stability. Curr Eye Res 4:9–12
65. Norn M (1963) Mucus on conjunctiva and cornea. Acta Ophthalmol (Copenh) 41:13–23
66. Norn M (1972) Tetrazolium-alcianblue mixture. II. Acta Ophthalmol (Copenh) 50:285–294
67. Norn M (1969) Mucous flow in the conjunctiva. Acta Ophthalmol (Copenh) 47:129–146
68. Forst G (1986) Struktur des Tränenfilms beim Lidschlag. DOZ Kl 5:92–93
69. McDonald J (1969) Surface phenomean of the tear film. Am J Ophthalmol 67:56–64
70. Norn M (1979) Semiquantitative interference study of fatty layer of precorneal film. Acta Ophthalmol (Copenh) 57:766–774
71. Norn M (1987) Expressibility of meibomian secretion. Acta Opthalmol (Copenh) 65:137–142
72. Norn M (1986) Meibomian glands and lipids of the precorneal film in Eskimos. Arctil Med Res 44:53–55
73. Norn M (1987) Foam in the external part of the eye. Acta Ophthalmol (Copenh) 65:143–146

74. Josephson JE (1983) Appearance of the preocular tear film lipid layer. Am J Optom Physiol Opt 60:883–887
75. Olsen T (1985) Reflectometry of the precornal film. Acta Ophthalmol (Copenh) 63:432–438
76. Tiffany JM (1985) The role of meibomian secretion in the tears. Trans Ophthalmol Soc UK 104:396–401
77. Farris RL, Gilbart JP, Stuchell RN, Mandel ID (1983) Diagnostic tests in keratoconjunctivitis sicca. CLAO J 9:23–28
78. Sauter J (1976) Xerophthalmia and measies in Kenya. Denderen, Groeningen, pp 235
79. Kusin JA, Sinaga HSR, Marpaung AM (1977) Xeropthalmia in North Sumatra. Trop Geogr Med 29:41–46
80. Norn M (1973) Lissamine green. Vital staining of cornea and conjunctiva. Acta Ophthalmol (Copenh) 51:483–491
81. Iishi A (1985) Studies on staining test for keratoconjunctivitis sicca. I. Quantitation of fluorescein test by image analysis (Japanese). Acta Soc Ophthalmol Jpn 89:1359–1365
82. Prause JU, Norn M (1987) Relation between blink frequency and break up time? Acta Ophthalmol (Copenh) 65:19–22
83. Norn M (1963) Foam at outner palpebral canthus. Acta Ophthalmol (Copenh) 41:531–537
84. Lemp MA (1984) The ocular surface and keratoconjunctivitis sicca. Am J Ophthalmol 98:426–428
85. Refojo MF, Rolando M, Belldegrun R, Kenyon KR (1986) Tear evaporimeter for diagnoses and research. In: Holly FJ (ed) The preocular tear film. Dry Eye Institute, Lubbock, pp 117–126
86. Frost-Larsen K, Isager H, Manthorpe R, Prause JU (1980) Sjögrens syndrome. Ann Ophthalmol 12:836–846
87. Norn M (1988) Tear fluid pH in normals, contact lens wearers and pathological cases. Acta Ophthalmol (Copenh) 66:485–489
88. Norn M (1985) Tear pH after instillation of buffer in vivo. Acta Ophthalmol [Suppl] (Copenh) 173:32–34
89. Norn M (1989) Tear stix tests for leucocyte-esterase, nitrite, haemoglobin and albumin in normals and a clinical series. Acta Ophthalmol (Copenh) 67:192–198
90. Jansen PT, Bijsterveld OP (1983) The relations between tear fluid concentrations of lysozyme, tear specific prealbumin and lactoferrin. Exp Eye Res 36:773–779
91. Jensen OL, Gluud BS, Birgens HS (1985) The concentration of lactoferrin in tears. Acta Ophthalmol (Copenh) 63:341–345
92. Aine E, Môrsky P (1984) Lysozyme concentration in tear-assessment for reference values in normal subjects. Acta Ophthalmol (Copenh) 62:932–938
93. Wells PA, Ashur ML, Foster CS (1986) SDS gradient polyacrylamide gel electrophoresis of individual ocular mucus samples from patients with normal and diseased conjunctiva. Curr Eye Res 5:823–831
94. Tanabe M et al. (1984) Lacrimal gland accumulation of ^{67}Ga citrate in patients with Sjögren's syndrome. Eur J Nucl Med 9:233–236
95. Gilbart JP (1985) Topical therapy for dry eye. Trans Ophthalmol Soc UK 104:484–488
96. Benjamin WJ, Hill RM (1989) Tonicity of human tear fluid sampled from the cul-de-sac. Br J Ophthalmol 73:624–627
97. Marner K (1980) Snike-like appearance of nuclear chromatin in conjunctival epithelial cells from patients with keratoconjunctivitis sicca. Acta Ophthalmol (Copenh) 58:849–853
98. Prause JU, Manthorpe R, Marner K (1984) Snakelike nuclear chromatin in imprints of conjunctival cells from patients with Sjögren's syndrome. In: Tear symposium program, abstract 97

99. Versura P, Maltarello MC, Caramazzo R, Laschi R (1989) Mucus alteration and eye dryness. Acta Ophthalmol (Copenh) 67:455–464
100. Copeland JR, Lamberts DW, Holly FJ (1982) Investigations of the accuracy of tear lysozyme determination by the quantiplate method. Invest Ophthalmol Vis Sci 22:103–110
101. Stuchell RN, Feldman JJ, Farris RL, Mandell ID (1984) The effect of collection technique on tear composition. Invest Ophthalmol Vis Sci 25:374–377
102. Yamada K, Hayasaka S, Setogawa T (1990) Test results in patients with Sjögren's syndrome defined by the Japanese criteria. Acta Ophthalmol (Copenh) 68:80–86

Chapter 6

Therapy of Dry Eye

R. Marquardt

1 Introduction

Although important advances have been made in many branches of eye therapy over the past 100 years, we still have no fully satisfactory treatment method available to us today as regards keratoconjunctivitis sicca (KCS), generally known as dry eye. The words of the German surgeon August Gottlieb Richter in his *Fundamental Background of the Art of Surgery* (1790) still apply: "Chronic inflammations of the eye do not necessarily mean that there is a high risk of actually losing this organ, but rather that they are for the most part more difficult to heal than acute forms, as their causes are in most cases very involved, deeply rooted and difficult to discover."

KCS, or *Katarrhus siccus* as Peters termed it in 1891, is also to be classified among these chronic inflammations of the conjunctiva.

Since antiquity, physicians have occupied themselves with the phenomena produced by dryness of the eye. In classical Greece, egg white and goose fat were applied, in addition to irritants for inducing the lacrimal reflex such as wines or wine vinegar. These remedies changed little throughout the Middle Ages down to the nineteenth century. In 1790 Richter recommended eye baths made up of a decoction from palm leaves or the diluted mucilage of quinces. He had at that time already recognized that mucilaginous or similar substances improve the symptoms of dry eye.

In the nineteenth century, physiological saline solutions which had been thickened with gelatin were then applied for this purpose. However, eye ointments were still principally applied during this period. Although they permit the most intensive form of external ophthalmological application, they nevertheless have two crucial disadvantages in long-term therapy, particularly for dryness of the eyes: first, the ointments restrict vision, and second, they reduce the stability of the lacrimal film unless the patient keeps his eyes continuously closed. This is why such ointments are no longer used in the long-term therapy of the dry eye.

M.A. Lemp/R. Marquardt (Eds.) The Dry Eye
© Springer-Verlag Berlin Heidelberg 1992

Treatment with aqueous eye drops, on the other hand, also has a negative aspect; their short period of retention on the surface of the eye means that an approximately constant level of active substance can be obtained only with a high frequency of application. For this reason, as a viscosity-increasing factor in the therapy of dryness of the eye, aqueous solutions of methylcellulose were introduced by Swan [1] in 1945. In the following period, similar polymers such as hydroxyethylcellulose, hydroxy-propylmethylcellulose or hydroxypropylcellulose were used in eye drops as so-called artificial tears. All these aqueous solutions of polymers have a more or less pronounced viscosity, thus extending the retention period on the conjunctival and corneal surfaces.

In 1964 Krishna and Brown [2] first applied eye drops containing polyvinyl alcohol for treatment of dry eye. Up to the present day, both the methylcellulose derivates and macromolecular polyvinylalcohol are the most frequently used classes of substance in the treatment of disturbed and/or insufficient precorneal film.

In the search for substitutes with an increased eye surface retention capacity, and thus with the aim of reducing their application frequency, artifical tears of the gel type based on polyacryl were consequently intro-duced for dry eye treatment [3]. Treatment with solutions of viscoelastic substances were also quite successful. In 1977 the first trials with inserts were undertaken [4], in which soft solid polymers taking 6 h to dissolve were introduced into the conjunctival sac. Both the subjective and objective symptoms of KCS can be alleviated in this way. The long retention period of the inserts here provide a particular advantage due to the fact that stabiliz-ing agents are no longer necessary, since the inserts have previously been thoroughly sterilized via irradiation.

Substances capable of stimulating tear secretion are a further class of therapeutics in the treatment of KCS. However, these are capable of taking effect only if functional glandular/lacrimal tissue is still present. Promis-ing treatment results have also been found with vitamin A in the form of ointments or oils, provided that tear production has been retained and a squamous metaplasia of the conjunctival and corneal epithelium is present [5].

Preservatives in ophthalmological preparations present a special prob-lem. Over recent years, their toxic effect on both bacteria and tissue, as well as the extended retention period of various preservatives in the conjunctiva and cornea, have produced, at an ever-higher degree of frequency, intoler-ance in patients with KCS who depend on the long-term and continuous application of wetting agents, thus obliging them to discontinue an otherwise necesssary therapy. Wetting agents in disposable containers free of preserva-tives (which have been applied for and whose registration is presently subject to legal dispute in some countries) whould here be one possible solution.

2   General Aspects in the Treatment of KCS

This eye condition of KCS is more difficult to treat than any other in ophthalmological practice. This is due not least to the fact that disturbances in maintaining a moist surface (i.e., a thin film of liquid) over the eye result from a wide range of different causes of a both general and specifically ophthalmological nature. In addition to this, we are confronted here with a chronic condition for which no satisfactory therapy is yet available. Another difficulty is presented by the fact that substitutional therapy – and this applies in the majority of cases where dryness of the eye is presented – has been, up to the present, mostly of an empirical nature. For the patient's part, one may prefer a method of alleviating his or her condition which is by no means useful to the next. Here again, this is due to the most varied causes and manifestations of the complaint.

For therapy, it is particularly important to know which component of the precorneal tear film is disturbed and to what extent. First of all, careful elucidation of the patient's history and diagnosis is needed to determine the underlying causes before undertaking a therapy – which must always be on an individual basis. This is because both the selection of a possible therapy and the dosage involved must be related to the particular condition encountered. In the long run, we are still far from the desired aim of healing dry eye to the extent of reestablishing a stable film of moisture without restricting visual capacity, avoiding the frequent application of drops, and preventing epithelial damage to conjunctival and corneal surfaces. Reestablishment of lacrimal secretion and normalization in the composition of disturbed precorneal tear films are here the most worthwhile aims of therapy.

As we have seen, such disturbances in the ability to keep the eye surface covered with moisture have many causes and no uniform patient history. Accordingly, therapy must have many facets, being individually adapted in accordance with origin and manifestation. This is at present the only way of assessing the patient's condition and providing him with a treatment schedule fully suitable for his specific condition. Therefore, the following factors must be considered when treating dryness of the eye: (a) a careful search for the causes capable of producing a patient's specific form of dryness; (b) analysis of the disturbing factors with the aim of their exclusion; and (c) reestablishing an undisturbed visual capacity in the patient by using the most appropriate therapeutic measures.

2.1   Causes of Dry Eye

2.1.1   Subtypes of Dry Eye

First of all, the causes underlying the particular symptoms produced in dryness of the eye must be sought. Without this knowledge, no treatment specifically adapted to the form encountered is possible. The most important conditions capable of resulting in KCS are presented in Chap. 4. A knowledge of such causes constitutes the first step in the treatment of KCS. This

large number of possible factors causing dry eye shows how important it is to obtain a thorough, detailed, and specific description of the patient's history in this context. As dry eye generally requires long-term treatment, the therapist should take his time at the beginning of treatment and attempt to uncover those factors causing the conjuctivitis in question and, in the long run, capable of producing a disturbance of the precorneal tear film. As a rule, such an approach, together with a careful analysis of possible or prevailing disturbances, allow for a proper diagnostic classification and a therapy specifically adapted to the complaint.

2.1.2 Anaphylactic Reactions

If an allergy is the cause of KCS, it is sometimes possible by means of allergy tests to discover the allergen involved and to eliminate it or at least to bring about a decisive improvement in the patient's condition via specific hyposensitization. In particular, cosmetics, cleaning agents for contact lenses, and the contact lenses themselves if they are of the soft type, as well as ophthalmological preparations and those preservatives present in most commercially available forms of eye medication, may be considered as possible allergens in the eye condition.

2.1.3 Drugs

In cases of medicational side effects the irritative product in question must, after consultation with the prescribing physician, be replaced by another. First and foremost, beta-adrenoceptor blocking agents must be considered here. This is because they are administered systemically for hypertension and have found widespread topical use for glaucoma, resulting in a more or less pronounced, reversible reduction in tear fluid. This applies principally to earlier beta-adrenoceptors, particularly bupranolol, which is purported to reduce tear turnover by more than 50%. Apart from their ability to produce withdrawal symptoms, the unpleasant adverse effects produced by this group of substances in ocular conditions are also dose dependent.

A further group of systemically administered substances also capable of producing dry eye is that of psychopharmaceutical agents, primarily benzodiazepines, but also antidepressants and neuroleptics. In addition, long-term therapy with corticoids can also cause symptoms of insufficient tear supply, or dacryopenia.

Many women during menopause show dry eye symptoms which vary from moderate complaints to servere problems. In these cases mostly the wetting component of the precorneal tear film is found to be reduced.

Alterations in the different components of the tear film have also been observed in women receiving ovulation inhibitors. These observations suggest that hormones at least influence the structure and stability of the precorneal tear film. Clear-cut proof of this relationship has not yet been found, but some authors point out that therapy with estrogens shows a beneficial effect in patients suffering from dry eye disease.

Results also confirm that cigarette smokers show a reduced tear film stability compared to nonsmokers, i.e., a reduced tear film break-up time. Therefore it seems obvious that cigarette smoking also influences the precorneal tear film negatively.

2.1.4 Environmental Disturbances

Before using a medication, all possible environmental disturbances must be found and eliminated; these may be factors which are either connected with the causes of dry eye, or which aggravate its symptoms.

Generally, patients suffering from dry eye should as far as possible live in dust-free conditions; both dust and smoke, particularly where the aqueous component of the precorneal tear film is absent, change the surface pH value to such an extent that a patient's complaints can be aggravated to an intolerable degree. This also applies where the ambient air humidity drops below 50%, which frequently occurs in centrally overheated rooms during the winter months. When one considers the fact that within 10 s after opening the thickness of the precorneal tear film covering the eye of a healthy person is reduced from 10 μm to 4 μm, the degree to which a considerable reduction in air humidity is able to affect a patient suffering from dry eye becomes clear. This can be remedied by using air humidifiers, a wide range of which are commercially available. Fan-blower heating systems used in various types of vehicles also cause an increase in drying of the eyes' surface if their hot air is directed at the face.

The long-term effect of specific chemical agents prevalent in our environment is also able to produce or aggravate dry eye conditions. Traffic policemen at busy intersections, for example, often suffer chronic conjuctivitis with symptoms of dryness due to the high concentrations of noxious substances in the air around them. The same is true of persons occupied in various activities exposing them to chemical irritants or toxic substances.

One should also mention disturbed binocular cooperation and uncorrected errors of refraction. Both ametropia and phoria have a particularly unfavorable effect on dry eye. As a rule, apart from a sensation of pressure and heaviness, they produce headache and disturbed vision, with particularly the latter increasing during the course of the day. Patients suffering from dry eye find considerable relief as soon as such irritative factors are eliminated.

2.2   pH Value in the Treatment of KCS

In every form of therapy for KCS, it is important to know to what extent the pH value, the osmolarity, and the surface tension between the corneal surface and a disturbed and/or insufficient tear film have been pathologically changed by the condition encountered and whether, or in what way, therapy must be adapted as a result of such conditions [6].

The pH value of the normal precorneal tear film varies between 7.2 and 7.45, with both daily and individual variation. Patients suffering from KCS, however, have a hypertonic tear film. Such a pathologically increased pH value is one of the factors responsible for the objective and subjective symptoms of the disease. A logical consequence (i.e., possible alternative) would be to treat KCS with hypotonic tear substitutes. Studies also demonstrate that a slightly alkaline tear substitute (pH 8.45) is tolerated better than a neutral agent in the case of dry eye [7]. This has not remained uncontested, however. As a rule, slightly alkaline isotonic or almost isotonic moistening agents are preferred in its treatment. Accordingly, most commercially available tear substitutes are maintained at a pH value between 7.23 and 7.5.

2.3   Osmolarity in the Treatment of KCS

Another important factor is tear film osmolarity. Normally, this is between 303 and 305 mosm/l. In patients with dry eye, however, this is increased by up to 30–40 mosm/l. Studies involving tissue cultures have shown that such high osmolarity is toxic to the corneal epithelium. The conclusion was drawn that, in the context of KCS, this increase in osmolarity is responsible at least for changes in the cornea. Consequently the attempt was made to reduce this increased osmolarity by applying agents with half the value (150 mosm/l). Here too, however, the results have been contradictory. Therapy with reduced osmolarity agents of this type were in part preferred by patients with dry eye, although other tests showed no difference between the results of treatment with hypo-osmolar or normally osmolar substances. In the same way as the pH value, it is certain that osmolarity is merely an irritative factor. However, colloidosmotic pressure and viscosity do have a value which should not be underestimated [8–10].

2.4   Surface Tension in the Treatment of KCS

The primary function of the tear film is to maintain the optical transparency of the cornea by constantly wetting the epithelium, compensating for irregularities in the epithelial surface, and thus providing an optically intact surface. When the eye is affected by dryness, this constant moistening may no longer be sufficient if the mucin component is absent or reduced. To

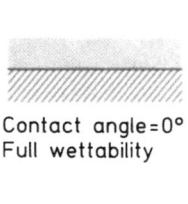

Contact angle=0°
Full wettability

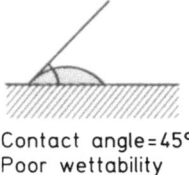

Contact angle=45°
Poor wettability

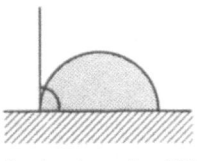

Contact angle=90°
Bad wettability

Contact angle=180°
No wettability

Fig. 1. Contact angle; parameter for wetting

restore this, substances must be sought which are able to spread themselves over the hydrophobic corneal surface. This is possible only if their surface tension is less than the adhesive force exerted by the surface of the cornea.

The contact angle or wetting angle is one of the physical parameters for the ability of solid surface to maintain a liquid layer. This is the angle formed by a liquid with a solid surface (Fig. 1). It is obtained by constructing, at the point where the drop and the solid surface meet, a tangent at the spherical surface represented by the drop and determining the angle. If this angle is greater than zero, the surface tension of the wetting liquid is greater than that of the corneal surface, so that the wetting function is either incomplete or absent. This means that wetting liquids must have a surface tension lower than that of the corneal surface. Under normal conditions, this is fulfilled by the physiological mucin of the conjunctiva alone; the hydrophobic surface becomes completely wettable only when this is present. As the surface tension of the aqueous tear film is thought to be only 3 dyne/cm below the critical adhesion force of the epithelial surface with its mucin layer, the wetting reserve is extremely slight. Such an unstable condition means that a whole series of different factors are able to disrupt its balance or even cause it to break down. This is therefore an extremely complex and instable biophysical system [11,12].

Since this was recognized, groups of substances have been sought whose aqueous solutions on the eye had approximately the surface tension of a normal aqueous tear film. Up to now, no applicable wetting agent has been found which meets this requirement. Purified animal buccal mucus has achieved the best results and is the only substance able satisfactorily to reduce the angle of contact and surface tension (Table 1). Thus, although it has not yet been made available for therapy, mucus would be optimal as a

Table 1. Viscosity, angle of contact, and surface tension of several tear substitutes. (From [11])

	pH value	Angle of contact	Surface tension (dyne/cm)
ATF	7.24	47 ± 2°	71.1
ATF + 0.67% protein	7.25	43 ± 3°	59.6
ATF + 0.5% purified bovine buccal mucus	7.24	26 ± 3°	43.2
ATF + protein + bovine buccal mucus	7.23	23 ± 3°	51.0

ATF, Artificial tear fluid

Table 2. Viscosity, angle of contact, and surface tension of several tear substitutes

	Viscosity	Angle of contact	Surface tension (dyne/cm)
Hydroxypropyl-methyl cellulose	200.00	67°	40
Povidone + hydroxyethyl cellulose (Adsorbotear)	58.90	68°	42
Polyvinylalcohol	3.65	67°	40
Adapt	8.25	84°	43

substance for artificial tear. Unfortunately, all our artificial tear agents constitute a more or less inadequate substitute. Information on the viscosity, angle of contact, and surface tension of some commercially available artificial tear agents are presented in Table 2 [13]; polyvinyl alcohol and hydroxypropylmethylcellulose have the most favourable characteristics.

The substitution or reconstitution of precorneal tear film as normal as possible in cases of KCS thus makes high demands on the pharmaceutical industry and on the therapist. Presently we are still far from having therapeutic agents satisfactory even regarding their effect.

3   Surgical Methods for the Treatment of KCS

A number of irritative factors can be relieved or eliminated by surgical measures. These include the following (the surgical techniques involved discussed at greater length below):

– Insufficient closing of the eyelids
– Positional anomalies of the eyelids

- Traumatic coloboma of the eyelids
- Wide palpebral fissure
- Tumors of the eyelids
- Conjunctival tumors
- Cicatrization of the conjunctiva
- Irregularities of the corneal surface

4   Autosuggestive Treatment of KCS

The ocular symptoms of some conditions producing incomplete or infrequent blinking rate of the eyelids can be influenced at least partly by the patient's own volition, for example by controlled blinking. This is principally so in the case of neuroparalytic keratitis, in which this protective reflex is largely absent due to a trophic disturbance of the cornea. This includes hyperthyroidism (Stellwag's sign), Parkinson's disease, senile dementia, damage to the brainstem, and to a certain degree exophthalmos. Care should be taken to maintain a frequency of no fewer than 12 blinks per minute.

Decisive steps toward relief or elimination of the conditions underlying dry eye can be taken when the above factors have been recognized and counter acted. Full use should always be made of these possibilities before considering a purely symptomatic therapy, for example, the application of wetting agents.

5   Pharmaceutical Treatmemt of KCS

If we are not successful in eliminating the causes and underlying irritative factors of dry eye, we must find a medication to eliminate or at least alleviate its troublesome subjective and objective symptoms. Even if it is not successful in stimulating tear secretion, the medication must aim at normalizing the disturbed physiological tear film over the corneal surface. This should be the case as far as possible in all conditions involving a quantitatively reduced or disturbed tear production, especially regarding the supply of so-called artificial tear substances. The main problem, which still remains unsolved, is to find a substance which has, apart from a good tolerance, high surface stability and thus as extended retention period on the cornea, but which is not too viscous, as this would have a negative influence on visual acuity [14,15].

5.1 Requirements for an Ideal Artificial Tear Product

An ideal tear substitute for the treatment of dry eye requires the following features:

- It must be well tolerated.
- It must not be toxic, even when applied frequently.
- It must be suitable for use as often as needed.
- To make the corneal surface hydrophilic, the substance must be adsorbable by it.
- It must have a long retention period, i.e., it should not be diluted too rapidly by the physiological tear fluid and thus eliminated, while not being too viscous.
- It should not influence the vision of the eye.
- It should not impede or inhibit tear secretion or mucus production and secretion from the palpebral glands.
- It should not disturb corneal nutrition and/or metabolism.
- It should not emulsify lipids (apart from the outmost tear layer).
- It must be neutral.
- As far as possible, it should contain no foreign substances, such as irritative preservatives.

Considering these requirements in the context of all topically applicable, artificial tears, we must acknowledge that we have, up to now, no form of medication capable of replacing a normal human tear layer, even approximately. Thus, at the present time, all artificial tears remain strictly artificial.

5.2 Tear Film Substitution by Polymers

Substances described as wetting agents (often termed eye or ocular lubricants or ophthalmic solutions) are the most frequently used for dry eye. By comparison with other ophthalmological preparations, they lead the list both as regards quantity and market turnover. These are aqueous solutions of polymers able to meet the requirements of wetting agents, i.e., hydrophilizing the corneal surface and extending adhesion and retention periods in the eye. These include the following substances:

- Semisynthetic cellulose derivates as additives increasing viscosity when in solution at 0.5%–1.0%
- Polyvinyl alcohol, polyvinylpyrrolidone (povidone) in a 1.4% concentration
- Polyacrylic acid derivates in the form of drop gels
- Dextran solutions (0.9%)
- Hyaluronic acid in concentrations of 0.1%–0.2%.

With these more or less viscous solutions, care must nevertheless be taken that their viscosity remains within limits, as visual acuity is influenced above a certain concentration. This also results in the further disadvantage that the prescribed viscosity limit also has a negative influence on the substance's retention in the eye. Up to now, all efforts to find adequate and tolerable wetting agents in the therapy of KCS with an extended retention period have failed due to these problems. Available preparations consisting of aqueous polymer solutions reduce the surface tension of the tear fluid, afford improved corneal moistening, thicken and stabilize the precorneal tear film, and consequently produce the best possible relief of the symptoms of dry eye. However, they all have only a limited period of ocular retention, which means that patients with severe or moderate eye moistening disturbances must make frequent use of such preparations.

5.2.1 Wetting Interval of Artificial Tears

The maximum capacity of the conjunctival cul-de-sac is $25-30\,\mu/l$ and the average liquid exchange per blink $7\,\mu/l$. Only a part of an applied wetting agent therefore remains in the eye, and most escapes over the edges of the eyelids. Its dilution is accelerated by both the blinking reflex and the tear stimulation reflex. Thus less than half the liquid in the cul-de-sac remains available after a few seconds (taking, for example, physiological saline solution as a substitute). Further studies on commercially available wetting agents using radioactively marked vehicles have shown only 3% of a physiological saline solution, approximately 5% of a polyvinylalcohol solution, and approximately 10% of a methylcellulose solution in the precorneal tear film could still be found in the cul-de-sac afer 90 s. Results in healthy persons on the retention interval and extension of the tear film breakup time of different commercially available tear substitutes are shown in Table 3. These data illustrate the importance of the retention period, or useful life,

Table 3. Wetting time and duration of effect of different tear substitutes. (From [11])

Medication	Original BUT/s (basis)	BUT after application (s)	Duration of effect (min)
Adapt	24	43	120
Adapette	26	48	90
Adsorbotear	24	50	90
Isoptotears	23	33	62
Isopto-naturale	24	33	100
Liquifilm	23	40	65
Lytears	23	35	50

BUT, Breakup time

of a substance used in eye treatment; however, they also illustrate that treatment results in terms of retention have by no means been encouraging. With the substances available to us up to now we are still far from the goal of building up a tear film that is as stable as possible over an extended period of time in patients with KCS without influencing optic functioning and without an overly frequent application of drops. We also know that the instillation of viscous eye drops causes considerable interactions in an insufficient or damaged tear film involving the mucous, viscous, and lipid phases, and we are able to complement both the aqueous and the mucin component only to an insufficient extent.

5.2.2 Methylcellulose

In the form of various commercially available eye drops as 0.5%–1.0% solutions, cellulose derivates (water-soluble polymers) have been in ophthalmological use for conjunctival and corneal lubrication since 1945 [1]. The positive properties of this synthetic polymer are that it is chemically inert and nontoxic, that it has a stable pH value, and that the refractive index at concentrations of less than 1% is similar to that of the natural tear film. In addition, these aqueous solutions of polymers have a good lubricant effect, thus relieving the friction between cornea and eyelid. This type of substitute supplies, over a short period, a tolerable precorneal tear film which, however, due to its short retention period, disintegrates after approximately 10–20 min. This means that wetting agents composed of water-soluble polymers have to be applied frequently by patients suffering from dry eye.

Studies have shown that at a concentration of 0.5% methylcellulose increases the tear film breakup time by a factor of 1.4. A further increase is possible by increasing the concentration to 1.5%; however, such levels of viscosity are not tolerated as they cause a blurring of vision. Furthermore, this produces an increased crust formation on the eyelids, which is uncomfortable and cosmetically undesirable, as well as stickiness and adhesion of the eyelid edges. A further disadvantage, which is perhaps somewhat less important, is that the healing of wounds is slowed by eye drops containing methylcellulose at such a high concentration. Thus, there are limits t the modical use of these solutions for treating KCS [16,17].

As the ocular retention time of preparations containing methylcellulose is somewhat longer than, for example, that of those based on polyvinyl alcohol, methylcellulose eye drops are best suited for the therapy of medium to severe cases of dry eye [18].

5.2.3 Hydroxypropylmethylcellulose

Hydroxypropylmethylcellulose is a viscous cellulose derivate which due to its very good surface properties is considered somewhat superior to other methylcellulose preparations. According to available studies, five applications ought to provide considerable relief in subjective complaints such as irritation from brightness, sensations of dryness or foreign bodies, and burning of the eyes, as well as providing healing in superficial punctate keratitis [12,16]. Unfortunately, however, this viscous lubrication agent does not improve tear film stability to the extent desired. In particular, it does not provide sufficient long-term coverage of the corneal surface. Although this form of lubricant eye drop is indeed able to relieve the symptoms of dryness, it is thus not able to eliminate them sufficiently and for a long enough time. Studies have also shown that these viscous substances slow the elimination of tear fluid as a result of their high molecular structure and the tendency of such molecules to form networks.

Hydroxyethylcellulose is another cellulose derivate that can be used in ocular lubricants. However, treatment results up to now have not been encouraging, especially as the surface tension is relatively high at 60 dyne/cm, which limits the surface activity of the substance [17].

5.2.4 Polyvinylalcohol

Polyvinylacohol is manufactured via hydrolyzation of polyvinylacetate and was applied in aqueous solution as a tear substitute for the first time in 1964 [2,18]. It is also a hydrophilic polymer with only moderate viscosity but good lubricating function. The most frequently used concentration is 1.4%. This can be increased to 3.0% if a higher lubricant effect is desired.

Regarding toxicity, animal experiments have shown that neutral eye drops at a concentration of 1.4% polyvinyl-alcohol and a molecular weight of 100000 cause no restriction or inhibition in wound healing. Even at concentrations of 10% it produced no irritations. Subconjunctival injections produce no tissue reactions worth mentioning. Intraocular instillation produced neither inflammatory reactions nor an increase in intraocular pressure.

The effectiveness of their lubricant and adhesive functions on the corneal surface have shown solutions of polyvinylalcohol to be of value in the treatment of KCS. The film-forming properties of polyvinylalcohol solutions reduce surface tension without restricting visual acuity. Studies have shown that in 1.4% solution the surface tension of polyvinylalcohol is only 46 dyne/cm. This surface tension corresponds approximately to that of human tear fluid, thus explaining the good wetting properties of the substance. Studies have also shown polyvinylalcohol capable of forming a thicker tear film on the corneal surface than cellulose-containing wetting agents. This is based on its ability to bind water to a high degree – higher than that of hydroxypropyl methylcellulose [12]. It is furthermore known to have certain properties similar to those of mucin, resulting in a comparable reduction in the interfacial air/tear and tear/epithelium surface tension of the eye.

According to some results, tolerance of this wetting agent is better when its pH value is somewhat higher.

A number of studies indicate that the ocular retention time of poly-vinylalcohol is longer (albeit by only a matter of minute) than that of cellulose derivates. Reports in the literature vary considerably, but a retention time of 3–10 min appears realistic. Tear substitutes based on poly-vinylalcohol are expecially preferred in milder cases of dry eye.

5.2.5 Tear Gels

In the search for artificial tear agents with longer retention period and thus lower frequency of application, gel type substances on a polyacrylic basis have found their way into the treatment of dry eye. The first positive test results with this agent were reported in 1984. In 1985 we tested a drippable artificial tear gel, an acrylic acid polymerisate which has now become firmly established as a therapeutic agent for dry eye in a number of European countries, especially in those patients suffering from pronounced and severe forms [3,19,20].

The advantage of this substance is its good distribution across the corneal and conjuntival surfaces without forming ocular striations. Compared with previously available tear substitutes, its relatively long retention period is particularly note worthy. Compared with substances based on poly-vinylalcohol, we found it to have an ocular retention time longer by a factor of 7. Our studies also showed it capable of exerting a positive influence on the tear film breakup time for up to 60 min. Consequently, for patients this considerably reduces the frequency of application, which is often found unpleasant. Even in severe forms of KCS, a mere three to four applications per 24 h is sufficient and still achieves a high degree of therapeutic effectiveness. Both objective and subjective conditions improved significantly in the patients treated. No forms of adverse effect were encountered, even when the substance was applied over an extended period.

Due to their favorable ocular retention period gel-based tear substitutes are thus particularly suitable for the long-term treatment of medium to severe forms of KCS.

5.2.6 Viscoelastic Agents

5.2.6.1 Hyaluronic Acid

Hyaluronic acid, a glycosaminoglycan, is an organic substance present in the tissues of practically all vertebrates. It has excellent viscoelasticity, a particular ability to bind water, and good adhesion to cell surfaces. Commercially, it is obtained from the comb structures of roosters.

Hyaluronic acid was first applied in the form of a 1% solution as a vitreous substitute. Thereafter its value in surgery was rapidly discovered, and its use has so increased that modern operating methods to implant artificial lenses for cataract are no longer conceivable without it. It is also chemically inert in solution and is nontoxic even in long-term use [21].

Its viscoelastic and wetting properties suggested its use in the treatment of KCS. The first instance of this was in 1982 [22]. Solutions of 0.1%–1% were tested, and lower concentrations showed the best treatment results and were best tolerated. Higher concentrations were found to be uncomfortable, particularly in patients with severe forms of the disease – who formed the major treatment group for this substance. Its high price, however, restricts the use of hyaluronic acid solutions to those cases in which other substances fail. A further difficulty is that only a 1% solution has been made commercially available up to now, and that this must be prepared on prescription, a process which is complicated.

With the exception of two studies showing no better results in comparison with preparations such as polyvinylalcohol or cellulose derivates, results have been positive. In particular, due to the good adhesion of this substance on the corneal surface together with its good water-binding properties, it has been possible to prevent premature breakup of the tear film between blinks. With this viscoelastic substance it has primarily been possible to treat severe forms of KCS successfully, both the subjective and the objective symptoms of the disease. In different cases its frequency of application is variously indicated: after applying drops only four times on a single day, the subjective and objective symptoms of KCS improved satisfactorily, although the necessity of applying drops hourly has been reported in other cases.

5.2.6.2 Chondroitin Sulfate

Solutions of chondroitin sulfate, another viscoelastic substance, have been used to treat KCS in various ways. Although up to now no preparation is available, and only few treatment results have been published, these results are very much worth discussing [23].

Solutions of chondroitin sulfate were well tolerated in all patients. They have a constant viscosity, and their good affinity to the corneal surface prevents premature breakup of the tear film on opening and closing of the eyes. This means, for example, that a 20% chondroitin sulfate solution (its therapeutically applicable concentration is 1%) has a lower viscosity than 1% methylcellulose but has a greater affinity to the corneal surface than other artifial tear substances. These advantages explain the value of chondroitin sulfate in dilute precorneal tear films, which are characteristic for KCS.

In a randomized prospective study, chondroitin sulfate showed better results in severe cases of KCS than solutions of hyaluronic acid or polyvinylalcohol, both in subjective and objective symptoms. Electron microscopy also showed its very good prospective property against dryness. No adverse effects have been found up to now.

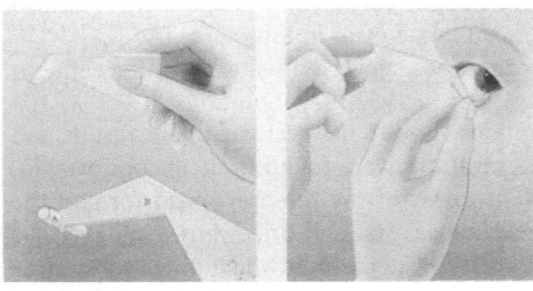

Fig. 2. Insert Application

5.2.7 Inserts

So-called inserts have been developed to obtain the longest posible retention time for tear substitutes and to avoid frequent drop applications by the patient with KCS. These are small, solid, yet soft polymers introduced into the cul-de-sac which, through continuous moistening by the natural tear fluid, take several hours to dissolve (Fig. 2). The first results were published in 1977 [4]. Solid insets measuring 6×12 mm made of water-soluble succinylated collagen with a dissolving time of 6 h were successful in patients with dry eye.

A few years later, inserts made of hydroxypropylcellulose [24] found their way into therapy. These relatively soft, rod-shaped plastic objects weigh 5 mg and are 1.27 mm thick and 3.5 mm long. They are introduced into the inferior conjunctival fornix, where they take approximately 6 h to dissolve, reaching maximum effect at 3 h. These inserts are previously sterilized via gamma-irradiation, are separately packed in sterile units, and contain no preserving agents. This means that patients need such medication only once or at the most twice per day, thus avoiding the frequent and inconvenient application of drops in patients suffering from more severe forms of dry eye. In addition, patients who have developed intolerance to preserving agents can use inserts without risk.

A considerable number of treatment results are available on the effects of these inserts. Although not yet available in the Federal Republic of Germany, they have gained a permanent place in therapy, particularly in the United States. Reports agree that inserts are especially preferred by by patients with severe forms of KCS, while patients with mild or moderate forms prefer drops for eye wetting. This reflects the fact that inserts are not without adverse effects. For example, transitory visual striation may occur during the dissolving phase. Inserts also transmit foreign body sensations to various degrees, and they are easily lost. These side effects, harmless in themselves, are still accepted by patients disappointed by conventional wetting agents. All studies also agree that inserts provide effective relief for both subjective and objective symptoms in most patients with dry eye, and that they may be applied without problem, even as a long-term form of medication. In addition, the inserts are fully inert and thus without toxicity.

Generally, these inserts have shown themselves to be an effective therapy for dry eye and constitute without doubt an important step forward and a genuine alternative in KCS therapy.

5.3 Tear Production Stimulants

5.3.1 Stimulation of the Secretory Tear System

Five different possibilities are recognized for stimulating the secretory tear system:

- Peripheral sensory stimulation: stimulation of the trigeminal (V cranial) nerve via the nasal nucosa or via the cornea; stimulation by cold or corrosive substances
- Reflectory stimulation: laughing, yawning, coughing, pain, heavily spiced foods
- Central nervous stimulation: crying
- Retinal stimulation: light stimuli
- Pharmaceutical stimulation (medication)

These forms of stimulation are directed principally at secretion of the orbital tear gland and less at that from accessory tear glands. In addition, stimuli must be relatively extensive to produce tear secretion and in dry eye are generally not sufficient. Apart from medication, of greatest therapeutic value has been cutting onions or taking snuff, both of which methods are, at the best, highly questionable and scarcely reasonable.

5.3.2 Pharmaceutical Stimulation

Bromhexine and eledoisin have been adopted into therapy. However, it must be emphasized that drugs for stimulating secretion are able to act only if a sufficient amount of functioning glandular tissue is still available. No medication is able to stimulate secretion from an atrophied gland.

5.3.2.1 Bromhexine

Bromhexine-HCl was originally used in internal medicine for the systemic treatment of bronchial disease. In 1971 an affinity of this substance to the tear gland was radioangiographically established. Two years later it was possible to produce an increase in tear secretion in the rabbit via topic application of 0.2% bromhexine-HCl drops. Consequently, the topic application of 0.2% bromhexine-HCl two to three times per day has been adopted for treatment of dry eye. Reports on the extent of treatment success in cases of pathologically reduced tear secretion are nevertheless contradictory. Examination of these studies shows that findings are principally from inhomogenous groups comprising patients with residually active lacrimal tissue either present or absent, or with pathological conditions of varying severity. Furthermore, the drug is expensive. Apart from the fact that the success of this kind of therapy is often questionable, another negative aspect to consider is that the patient experiences a burning sensation when the substance is applied. Therefore bromhexine has not up to now found wide application in KCS therapy [25,26].

5.3.2.2 Eledoisin

Chemically,. eledoisin belongs to a group of polypeptides (endecapeptides). More specifically, its physiological action resembles that of other tachykinins, and it is closely related to physalaemin. Eledoisin was discovered in the dorsal salivary glands of various species of Mediterranean octopus.

Studies on this substance involving animals initially concentrated on reducing blood pressure via peripheral vasodilation. An increase in tear secretion was at first seen as an undesirable side effect until eledoisin was first applied topically in 1973 to actually increase lacrimal secretion [27]. It was quickly recognized that this drug produced very favorable results particularly where severe forms of KCS had developed and particularly in patients with pronounced dryness of the eye in whom other tear substitutes no longer provided relief.

Eledoisin, which is very expensive, has now become fully synthesizable. The preparation available at present consists of a dry ampule with lyophilized eledoisin powder and an ampule with sterile solvent. The freshly prepared solution can be kept at room temperature for 30 days, just the time it takes to use the whole amount at one drop three times per day.

Reported treatment results in the literature are contradictory. Failures have been reported a number of times. We participated in a prospective randomized study in cooperation with the Ophthalmology departments at the Universities of Heidelberg and Cologne [28]. Particularly in severe forms of KCS, our rate of success was very good. The standard dose that we arrived at consisted of three drops per day. Patients who received permanent help with this substance were then unable to do without it. Even in the case of long-term application (now over 10 years) no form of adverse reaction has been found. The results of our study confirm that eledoisin is effective in severe and otherwise hopeless forms of KCS. Nevertheless, we recognize that the substance is not a universal elixir for the wide range of conditions subsumed under the heading of dry eye [29].

The mechanism of action of eledoisin is not yet known. The increase in tear secretion produced is doubtless connected with a hyperemia due to local vasodilation, although the quantitative increase in the aqueous phase of the tear film is certainly not the only effect involved. Eledoisin appears to have an additional stabilizing effect on the tear film.

The originally feared side effect of systemic hypotension is in any case ruled out, as the dose applied is so low.

5.4 Mucolytic Agents

In the areas of their indication, mucolytically active substances are restricted to those rare forms of KCS in which an excessive accumulation of mucus occurs in the precorneal tear film. These substances have an exclusively dissolvent action on thickened and tough mucus.

5.4.1 Acetylcysteine

Acetylcysteine has shown itself to be of value as a mucolytic. Its effect is based on its ability to split large glycoprotein polymers. It is used particularly for breaking down, i.e., dissolving, bronchial mucus. In eye therapy, acetylcysteine was first applied in the form of 20% N-acetylcysteine eye drops [30]. The ophthalmological effect of this substance, which only has a limited shelf life in aqueous solution, is difficult to quantify. It is generally used in the form of 10% eye drops. The application of drops twice a day is recommended as dosage. The fact that acetylcysteine eye drops, due to their fourfold ion concentration, cause a burning sensation is no inconsiderable disadvantage. On a general basis, this drug has not found wide application in the treatment of KCS [31].

5.5 Eye Ointments as Lubricants

In advanced and severe cases of KCS, especially where the cornea is also affected, consquently producing greater irritation and pain, it is often not possible to dispense with the application of an ophthalmic ointment with a good lubricant effect. Ointments, however, in the same way as drugs suspended or dissolved in oil, may damage the precorneal tear film and thus drastically reduce the breakup time. This means that this film breaks within a few seconds when the eye is open, thus producing an ophthalmic defect as deep as the corneal epithelium [14]. Furthermore, the flow of tear fluid is limited when the eye is opened and closed, as the ointment is not able to mix with the tear film. A blocking of the lacrimal ducts then also becomes unavoidable. For these reasons, ointments and oleaginous substances are, when properly considered, contraindicated in the case of KCS, at least during the waking period; ointment application during the daytime also produces a considerable visual restriction. Overnight, however, it is possible to use an ointment in cases where eye drops have an insufficient moistening action. As an ointment base, paraffin has shown itself here to be effective on corneal and conjunctival surfaces due to its good lubricant action and long adhesion period [32].

It is clear that any ointment base is more or less an inconvenience where the tear film has undergone primary damage and insufficiency as found in KCS.

5.6   Vitamin A

Over the last three decades, vitamin A acetate has been recommended for the treatment of KCS, either by itself or together with eye drops and either in the form of an ointment or that an oleaginous solution [5]. In the publications available at present, the therapeutic successes obtained are highly contradictory; this can be explained in terms of the mechanism of action of vitamin A and its indication.

In its pronounced form, a lack of vitamin A in the eye produces xerophthalmia, a keratinization and drying out of the conjunctiva and cornea, which may produce blindness and represents an extremely serious problem in underdeveloped areas. Normally, vitamin A is stored in the liver, and where nutrition is otherwise normal, this quantity is sufficient to cover one's entire requirement for a year; only in the case of chronic undernourishment do serious changes occur. The connection between undernourishment and xerophthalmia was first recognized in the seventh century by the Greek physician Paul of Aegina; in the past century, the Brazilian ophthalmologist Chilario de Gouvea was the first to treat the condition known as ophthalmia braziliana successfully with cod-liver oil. Later, researchers recognized the mode of action of vitamin A, of which a large amount is contained in the liver of the cod and other fish. Today it enjoys systemic and topical use for xerophthalmia and is a veritable blessing in developing countries. Xerophthalmia involves a metaplasia of the normally nonkeratinized epithelium of the cornea and conjunctiva. In its first stage this leads to a loss of goblet cells, in the second stage to an increased stratification and flattening of the epithelia, and finally in a third stage to keratinization or formation of a horny layer. In the literature, this process has been recorded as squamous metaplasia of the ocular surface. The three stages described may either occur simultaneously or overlap each other. The exact pathogenesis of squamous metaplasia has not yet been completely explained. It is certain that there is a loss in vascularization of the conjunctiva as well as secondary phenomena facilitating epithelial metaplasia [33].

Treatment with vitamin A thus suggested itself for specific eye diseases in which a similar process could be observed. The results of various studies have confirmed that success can be expected only in the absence of mucin, but not with a simultaneous loss of the aqueous phase. Vitamin A acid applied topically in oleaginous or ointment form can only have a local effect in squamous metaplasia of the conjunctiva producing mucus. This means that prior to initiating this therapy it must be determined whether KCS with an insufficiency of the lacrimal glands or a pathological picture involving extensive isolated atrophy of the conjunctiva is present. Treatment is also not successful in the case of lacrimal gland insufficiency with secondary loss of goblet cells as a result of the subsequently increased tear film osmolarity. Preparations containing vitamin A acid are therefore not generally effective in treating KCS. Its applicability is restricted to those patients with a loss of goblet cells but whose aqueous phase of the tear film has been retained to a considerable extent. Success may therefore be expected primarily in Stevens-Johnson syndrome, ocular pemphigus (benign mucosal pemphigoid), pseudopemphigoid, trachoma, and ocular changes following radiation.

The indication for therapy with vitamin A must consequently be established with great care and be limited to those conditions resulting in the symptoms described. If this rule is observed, vitamin A can be a highly effective therapy. Application in eye conditions is usually in the form of a 0.01% or, less commonly, 0.1% ophthalmic ointment. Local overdose of vitamin A is less dangerous than is systemic overdose. One should also, for the sake of completeness, recall that vitamin A plays an important part in the regeneration of visual purple.

5.7 Corticosteroids

Drugs containing cortisone do not provide a therapeutic possibility for dry eye. At best, they are applied to treat systemic aspects, such as Sjögren's syndrome and sarcoidosis. It is the hope of the therapist here to stimulate tear secretion via systemic application. The results of some studies support this, and others do not [34]. It is the opinion of Sjögren himself that the doses of corticosteroids required in chronically progressive Sjögren's syndrome and their resultant side effects are sufficient argument against their use on a long-term basis. This also applies in cases of benign pemphigoid and erythyma multiforme exudativum [35].

6 Preservatives in Topical Ophthalmological Agents

6.1 General Aspects

Preservatives are substances which protect pharmaceutical preparations, particularly those in multiple-dose containers, against bacterial contamination and the growth of pathogenic micro-organisms. The necessity of such preserving agents in ophthalmic preparations is subject to controversy. A number of points speak in favor of their use, but a number of others against it. It is in any case certain that the risks and the sequelae of infection via contaminated eye drops without preservatives are far greater and more serious than those of the possible side effects actually produced by preservatives [36].

6.1.1 Preservatives and Their Necessity

The precorneal tear film and the hydrodynamics of the tear removal system allow aqueous pharmaceuticals only a short retention period on eye surfaces. To obtain a continuous and adequate active spectrum in the eye from the pharmaceutical substance used, repeated application is necessary. For this, ophthalmic preparations in multiple-dose containers are necessary. Continuous applications from such containers, however, are subject to contamination by their very nature. While industrial preparation under sterile conditions is no longer a problem, improper handling by the patient or even inadequate sealing devices may result in secondary contamination by pathogenic micro-organisms. From the literature we know that the sequelae of contaminated ophthalmic preparations are potentially serious and may even result in the loss of an eye. A study carried out in 1973 showed that in 60 freshly prepared dispensers obtained from 54 public pharmacies, 33 contained bacterially contaminated eye drops [37].

Iatrogenic superinfections with *Pseudomonas aeruginosa* are the most problematic. This pathogen is resistant to most antibiotics and to most preserving agents, and even to heat. Due to its ability to produce collagenase, it is capable of causing corneal ulcerations. In addition, its wide effective range between pH 3.0 and 11.0 in aqueous solutions enables it to multiply practically unchecked. The same applies to fungoid organisms which also have a wide pH tolerance range. For all these reasons, legal administrators in most countries have made the use of preserving agents obligatory in multiple-dose containers for eye drops.

Since all preservatives have toxic properties to a greater or lesser extent, they too constitute a not inconsiderable stress on ocular functioning. It is unlikely that a preserving agent will ever be developed which provides a sufficient protection for ophthalmic preparations while having no form of influence on the precorneal tear film or conjunctival and corneal surfaces.

6.1.2 Requirements for Preserving Agents

An optimal preservative must meet the following requirements:

- Efficacy even at low concentrations and within a wide pH range.
- A wide spectrum of activity due to bacteriostatic and fungistatic or, better, bactericidal, sporicidal, and fungicidal effects, even against problem pathogens such as *P. aeruginosa*.
- Stability even under long-term storage.
- Sterilizability in autoclaves.
- Good solubility in water.
- Effects not inhibited by the pH of the medication it protects nor by its active substance, auxiliary substance, or the container.
- It does not restrict the chemical tolerance of the active ingredient(s).
- It has no toxic side effects and causes no allergy even when used frequently and over an extended period.

6.1.3 Mode of Action of Preservatives

With the exception of organic mercury compounds, the preserving agents used today act primarily against the cell membrane, damaging or destroying it. However, the exposed membrane of bacteria is the actual site of their metabolism, this being the opposite in tissues. In other words, the ability of a bacterial cell to live depends on the safety of its outside wall and cell membrane. Any disturbance of the functioning of the bacterial outer membrane thus has far-reaching consequences for its metabolism, normally producing cellular breakdown (lysis). According to its structure and function, a tissue cell is, by contrast, much more resistant. As a result, any effect of a preservative in attacking cell walls or membranes makes it is bactericidal. Organic mercury-conserving agents are an exception here as they inhibit protein synthesis or other metabolic processes, although this is basically the same as regards their bacteriostatic properties [38,39].

6.1.4 Side Effects of Preservatives

There are no preserving agents of any type which possess sufficient efficacy against pathogens but which lack toxic side effects in the eye and produce no allergies when the patient has a corresponding disposition. This affects primarily those aptients who must apply ophthalmic preparations regularly and over long periods, in the same way as wearers of contact lenses must immerse their lenses in commercially available storage or cleaning liquids. Although severe and irreparable ocular impairments resulting from preserving agents are rare, their toxic or allergic side effects often force their users to discontinue use of otherwise necessary substances in multiple-dose containers. We are thus faced with the problem, on the one hand, that severe eye conditions may arise through the contamination of medication free of preservatives, but, on the other hand, that the presence of such preservatives may force a discontinuation of the required pharmaceutical agent due to adverse reactions of a toxic and/or allergic nature [40,41].

How can this be explained? The high storage capacity of the cornea and conjunctiva make them practically predestined for toxic reactions from preserving agents, such as redness, burning, foreign body sensation, a sensation of dryness, avoidance of brightness, frequent blinking, and superficial punctate keratitis. Studies have shown, for example, benzalkonium chloride and chlorhexidine are stored in the cornea of the rabbit for longer than 24 h [42]. Even if the storage ability of the human cornea and conjunctiva is different from that of the rabbit, and even if only due to the fact that the animal blinks less frequently than a human, we must nevertheless assume that, when applied a number of times per day, a considerable concentration of such a preservative in the eye can be reached. We also know that even at low concentrations these substances reduce ion transport to a minor degree but epithelial resistance of the cornea quite considerably. According to electron microscopic studies, even at a low concentration of preservative substances, there is a loss of microvilli and a detachment of intercellular substance on the corneal surface, through which the corneal diffusion barrier and the intake of oxygen is changed [41,43]. It is also known that the healing of epithelial lesions can be prolonged as a result of the corneotoxic effect of preservatives. It has been shown that benzalkonium chloride attacks the lipid barrier of the precorneal tear film, which especially in the case of dry eye results in additional drying.

The results of further studies show that the preservative substances in eye preparations may produce genuine allergic reactions. Thimerosal is here the principal culprit.

6.1.5 Classification of Preservatives

According to their molecular structure, we can differentiate between: alcohols, phenols, cationic substances, and organic mercury substances. In alcohols, the antimicrobial effect lies in their ability to dissolve lipids. This changes the lipid structure of cell membranes and, consequently, their permeability. Phenols are linked to the cell membrane and are thus also able to change membrane permeability. Cationic substances have a pronounced effect on cell surfaces. Organic mercury compounds react with sulfhydryl groups and enzymes, destroying in this way the cell's metabolism. Compared with the other types of preservative, the point of attack is here principally the intracellular metabolism.

6.2 The Most Commonly Used Preservatives

6.2.1 Benzalkonium Chloride

Benzalkonium chloride, a quaternary ammonium base from the cationic group of substances, is applied at a dilution of 0.01% and is the most used preservative in eye medication (Fig. 3). Compared with other substances, it has a high surface activity, is absorbed by bacterial cell membranes, and increases permeability. This is due to the fact that, as the result of electrostatic interaction, its positively charged head associates with the phosphate group of the phosphorus lipids in basal membranes, whereas the uncharged part of the molecule penetrates into the hydrophobic interior of the cell membrane, which finally results in the lysis of the bacteria. As a result of this active mechanism, benzalkonium chloride exerts a very rapid and sure bactericidal action with a wide effective spectrum, even including, although not in the same optimal way, the problem pathogen *P. aeruginosa*.

However, because of its surface activity, benzalkonium chloride is also toxic for the eye at higher concentrations. Scanning electron microscopic studies have shown damage to the microvilli of the corneal surface and detachment of intercellular bridges in the corneal epithelium. Nevertheless,

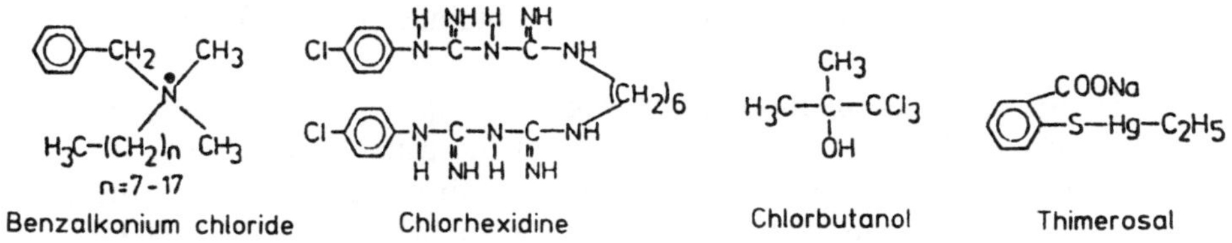

Benzalkonium chloride   Chlorhexidine   Chlorbutanol   Thimerosal

Fig. 3. The most commonly used preservatives

there is general agreement that at a concentration of 0.01% this preservative only very rarely produces side effects even when applied over an extended period and is generally well tolerated. In addition, however, benzalkonium chloride also has a negative influence on the stability of the precorneal tear film [44].

One difficulty is the high storage capacity of the cornea and conjunctiva for benzalkonium chloride in patients dependent on a long-term and frequent application of eye drops containing this substance as a preservative, as this can result in toxic phenomena. Furthermore, benzalkonium chloride can trigger an allergy if the patient's disposition is susceptible.

To summarize, benzalkonium chloride has the following properties:

- It is a bactericidal which starts acting rapidly.
- Even at a low concentration it has a wide range of action against gram-positive and gram-negative pathogens, yeasts, and fungi (molds).
- It is chemically stable and storeable between pH 6 and 8 and is effective between pH 3 and 8.
- In the eye, benzalkonium chloride at higher concentrations (above 0.01%) results in a loss of microvilli on the corneal surface, damage to the intercellular bridges, epithelial loss, breakup of the precorneal tear film and allergization; in addition, benzalkonium chloride can be stored by the cornea and conjunctiva over extended periods.

6.2.2 Chlorhexidine

Chlorhexidine digluconate, a strongly alkaline compound, is a cationic substance with a surface activity similar to that of benzalkonium chloride, although this activity is much less pronounced than with the latter. It also has an aggressive action on bacterial cytoplasmic membranes, destroying their semipermeable character. It is water-soluble and thus suitable as a preservative of aqueous solutions. Its active range is wide, both in the gram-positive and gram-negative sectors, and its action against the otherwise highly resistant *P. aeruginosa* is optimal. Chlorhexidine digluconate also has a good inhibitory action against the growth of fungi, although it has no effect on spores and viruses. As with benzalkonium chloride, the concentration necessary to keep a liquid preparation free of pathogens is between

0.005% and 0.01%. Its optimum effect is obtained in the alkaline range at pH 8.

Its toxic effects on the eye are slight; histopathological studies on the rabbit cornea showed no sign of damage at the usual dose. Due to its wide spectrum of activity against pathogens this substance is ideal for the preservation of eye drops. This is especially valuable due to the fact that, at therapeutically effective concentrations, it produces no disturbances in corneal permeability. Chlorhexidine digluconate also only rarely has an allergizing effect. When its tolerance is compared with that of other preserving agents, chlorhexidine shows very good results.

6.2.3 Chlorobutanol

Chlorobutanol belongs to the group of alcohols. In comparison to nonhalogenic substances, the chorine atom in its molecule increases the lipid solubility of the alcohol used and its surface activity. The antimicrobial effect of this well-tested preservative is thus based on its ability to draw lipids out through the bacterial membrane. This makes it primarily a bacteriostatic and, at higher concentrations (0.5%), a bactericide. Its range of action comprises both gram-positive and gram-negative bacteria, with inhibiting properties on fungal growth. This means an irreversible though slow-acting destruction of the problem pathogens *P. aeruginosa* and *Staphylococcus aureus*.

A 0.5% solution has been found to be both effective and tolerable. Chlorobutanol acquires an additional importance due to its effectiveness and stability only in the acid pH range (6.0 or below).

On the other hand, chlorobutanol has toxic effects on the cornea, even at lower concentrations than usually applied. It reduces the adhesability of the epithelia and inhibits the oxygen-processing capacity of the cornea. A local anesthetic effect of this preservative should also be mentioned. This explains its popularity as a preservative of local anesthetics.

The question as to which substance, chlorobutanol or benzalkonium chloride, has the greater toxic effect on the cornea, is still the subject of discussions.

In any case there appears to be no negative influence of chlorobutanol on the healing of epithelial lesions, which makes it an ideal preservative in a number of different fields. A possible disadvantage is a cumulative storage effect when used frequently.

6.2.4 Thimerosal

Whereas the preservatives discussed above have a primary action on the (bacterial) cell membrane, the effects of thimerosal (USP; thiomersal, BP), the most important of the organic mercury compounds, are based on an interaction with enzyme sulfhydryl groups. Here, the organic mercury cations produced by dissociation are an important active agent inhibiting those enzymes necessary for the metabolism of the microbial cell.

Thimerosal has a good bactericidal effect. To kill *P. aeruginosa* – for which, nevertheless, 6 h is necessary – a concentration of 0.0125% is sufficient, this still being within the tolerance limits. Concentrations of up to 0.01% are generally described as being well tolerated. Its optimum active range is between neutral and slightly alkaline limits.

In the eye, cytotoxic damage does not occur until a concentration higher than 0.02% is reached. At therapeutic dosages, impairments to permeability are minimal, although a storage of mercury salts by the cornea may become a negative factor when thimerosal is applied frequently. According to cytological studies, this preservative may be considered, at a concentration of 0.01%, as toxicologically safe. Through combination with chlorobutanol this concentration, otherwise necessary, may be reduced.

When one compares the different spectra of activity of the most frequently used preservatives, the cationic compounds benzalkonium chloride and chlorhexidine show the best results, although benzalkonium chloride is not optimally effective against *P. aeruginosa*. On the other hand, thimerosal, although it has a wide active spectrum, has a principally bacteriostatic effect. It should also be mentioned that considerably more favorable effect are obtained by combining individual preservatives.

Concerning toxicity, after all that we know about preservatives for ophthalmic preparations in multi-dose containers, there is still no ideal substance for this purpose and probably will not be in the future. This can be particularly unfortunate for patients having to apply ophthalmic preparations frequently and for extended periods due to the more or less pronounced cytotoxicity and allergizing properties. Practice has taught us that the number of these patients has increased over recent years. Single-dose containers without preservatives or inserts are becoming available as a necessary alternative; some of these have already been registered, and some are still awaiting registration by the authorities concerned. We are concerned here principally with treatment for dry eye and glaucoma. Table 4 provides information on the preservatives in various commercially available tear substitutes.

7 Surgical Treatment of Dry Eye

7.1 Tarsorrhaphy

Although tarsorrhaphy – the suturing together a portion of or the entire upper and lower eyelids – is quite simple, it is cosmetically disfiguring. Its aim is to shorten or entirely close the palpebral fissure to reduce or avoid a

Table 4. Preservatives in different tear substitutes

Isopto-Fluid AT	Hydroxypropylmethylcellulose	Benzalkonium chloride
Isopto-Naturale AT	Dextrose, hydroxypropylmethylcellulose	Benzalkonium chloride
Lytears	Hydroxymethylcellulose	Benzalkonium chloride
Oculotect AT	Hydroxypropylmethylcellulose	Benzalkonium chloride
Protagent AT	Polyvinylpyrrolidone	Benzalkonium chloride
Siccaprotect AT	Dexpanthenol, polyvinylalcohol	Benzalkonium chloride
Uligin AT	Dexpanthenol, polyvinylalcohol	Benzalkonium chloride
Vidisept AT	Polyvinylpyrrolidone	Benzalkonium chloride
Vistofilm	Polyvinylalcohol	Benzalkonium chloride
Vidisec Gel	Polyacrilic acid	Cetrimide (cetrimonium bromide)
Liquifilm AT	Polyvinylalcohol	Chlorobutanol
Adsorbotear	Hydroxymethylcellulose	Thimerosal (Thiomersal)
Thilo-Tears Gel	Carbomer	Thimerosal (Thiomersal)
Protagent SE	Polyvinylpyrrolidone	Without preservative in single pack
Coliquilm AS	Paraffins, vaseline, sterols, and alcohols from pure wax in vaseline	
Contafilm AT	Polyvinylalcohol	Ethylmercurithiobenzoci acid

drying out of the precorneal tear film between individual blinks. This should be undertaken only where damage to the cornea is progressive in spite of medicational therapy and an occlusion of the outgoing lacrimal canaliculi has brought no relief.

7.2 Ectropionization of the Lower Lacrimal Point

As an alternative to occlusion of the lacrimal points, it is possible by means of a simple surgical method to reposition the lower lacrimal point at the outer edge of the eyelid so that tears from the lacrimal lake are no longer able to enter it, and contact with the conjunctiva is avoided [45]. This process has the advantage of being reversible if required. Up to now, surgery of this type has been carried out on eight patients suffering from keratoconjunctivitis; of these, seven operations were successful (Fig. 4).

7.3 Transposition of the Parotid Duct

In desperate cases of KCS, the rechanneling of fluids to substitute tears from other exocrine glands into the conjunctival sac offers an alternative [46]. The parotid salivary gland is here an obvious choice, and its outward duct is transplanted into the lower conjunctival fornix. The disadvantages of such an operation are, first, that the parotid gland secretes approximately 1 l of saliva per day in comparison with about one teaspoonful of natural tear

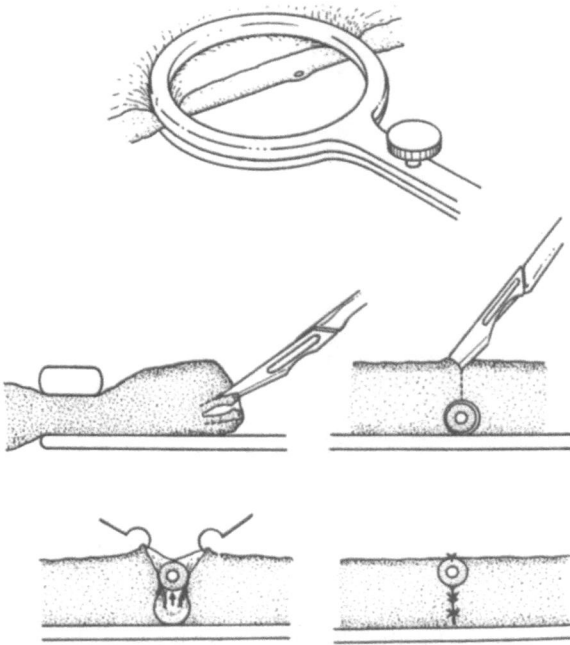

Fig. 4. Ectropionization of the lacrimal point (Murube del Castillo [45])

secretion over the same time. Secondly, the diverted fluid has a different composition. Thirdly, atrophy often occurs sooner or later, with a subsequent occlusion of the artificial duct. This is not a usual procedure and should be restricted to genuinely desperate cases.

8 Temporary or Permanent Occlusion of the Lacrimal Point

In advanced cases of KCS, occlusion of the lacrimal points is able to provide a permanent improvement of both objective and subjective complaints [6]. The fact should nevertheless be considered that, in patients with widespread insufficiency of the precorneal tear film, such a measure is often not sufficient in itself but must be accompanied by other forms of therapy such as medicational substitution. Another factor to be considered is that, once the lacrimal ducts have been closed permanently, the patient suffers considerable limitations due to permanent epiphora (illacrimation) when tear secretion recommences. Consequently, great restraint must be exercised in treating acute forms of dry eye or symptoms of a fairly recent nature. Prior to undertaking a permanent occlusion of the natural lacrimal drainage system, the following three criteria should be present: (a) the precorneal

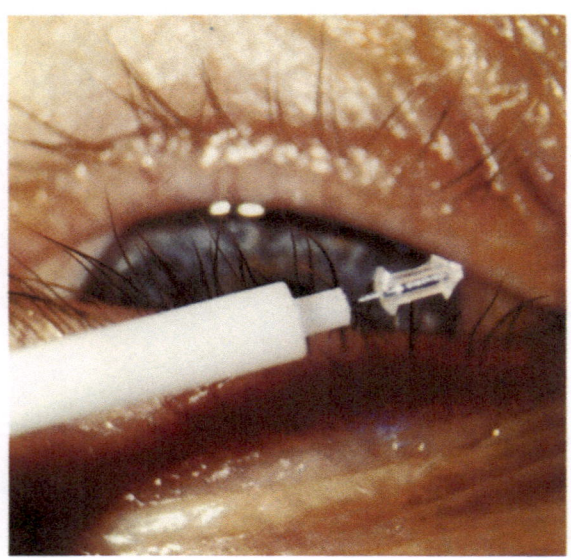

Fig. 5. Temporary occlusion of the lacrimal point

tear film must have been impaired or insufficient over an extended observation period; (b) long-term results obtained with Schirmer's test should be below 5mm; (c) damage to the corneal epthelia must have reached an extensive stage.

First of all, temporary occlusion of the lacrimal points or canaliculi should be aimed at. Formerly, this was carried out using a silk thread passed via a puncture on the nasal side of the lacrimal point through the lower eyelid and knotted. This compressed the duct involved, and it was possible to observe whether improvement occurred or not. Nowadays, temporary occlusion of the lacrimal point is performed more favorably using gelatin rods or, especially quite recently, with plastic stoppers, of which a number of various types are commercially available (Fig. 5). These are simply inserted. If such a temporary measure is successful, permanent sclerosing or dessication of the lacrimal canaliculi can be performed, or else the plastic stopper simply removed without affecting the patient in any way [47,48].

When a permanent occlusion of the lacrimal canaliculi is the objective, both the canaliculus and the lacrimal point of the upper *and* the lower eyelids must be sclerosed. If occlusion in the lower eyelid only has brought little success, the patient will hardly agree to a further occlusion in the upper eyelid. The sclerotization of both canaliculi (upper and lower) in one eye and during one session is therefore recommended, with a repetition shortly after in the other eye. If, after initial success, aggravation occurs, a careful search should be undertaken to determine whether one or the other occlusion has reopened or not.

The following possibilities are given as regards operative sclerotization of lacrimal canaliculi:

- Electrocoagulation via diathermy; this is the most frequently applied method and has the greatest rate of success.
- Argon laser occlusion: not enough experience has been gained with this method as yet.
- Occlusion with histoacrylic tissue adhesive: we urgently counsel against this method due to the fact that persistent inflammation – abscess formation has also been described – can occur, thus resulting in complaints of a considerable nature as well as cosmetic disfigurement.

9 Additional Methods

In severe cases of dry eye, stimulation and the substitution of absent or reduced tear secretion are not always sufficient to improve objective and subjective complaints satisfactorily. This applies particularly to patients with Stevens-Johnson syndrome, ocular pemphigus, or following severe chemical corrosion in which the goblet cells have been destroyed via atrophy or cicatrization of the conjunctiva, and the resulting permanent lack of mucin constitutes the major disturbing factor of the pathological process involved. In such patients, evaporation of the residual tear volume occurring when the eye is open must be reduced as far as possible or prevented through additional measures.

9.1 Tight-Fitting Goggles

Whereas a normal pair of spectacles with large glasses provides a certain degree of protection against loss of humidity from the tear film, a pair of more or less tightly fitting protective goggles can improve this factor considerably (Fig. 6). In place of such goggles, normal spectacles can be modified by the optician relatively economically by fitting protective side panels reaching up to the eyebrows. In addition, it is possible to buy a specially designed set of protective glasses. In this context, swimming goggles should also be mentioned as they are worn by men and women with sensitive eyes or chronic allergic inflammations such as conjunctivitis as protective devices when swimming in chlorinated water. When properly fitted, these goggles are approximately equivalent to a moist chamber (watchglass compress). They provide a damp chamber without additional aeration, accumulate condensation as a result of the damp microclimate inside, but are scarcely suitable as a long-term therapy procedure.

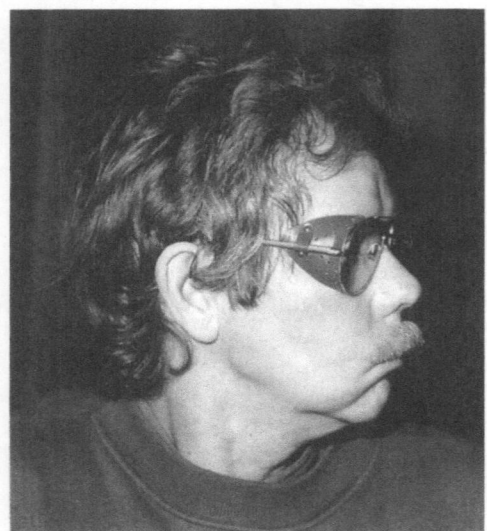

Fig. 6. Tight-fitting goggles

9.2 Moist Chambers

The remarks on goggles also apply to moist chambers (watchglass compresses), which are generally applicable in ophthalmic therapy: these are not suitable on a long-term basis.

9.3 Hot Eye Patches

Hyperemizing agents such as hot compresses (eye patches) may also be considered. A towel or flannel cloth is immersed in hot water, wrung out, and applied over the eyelids for a few minutes. As a result, the rate of secretion from the meibomian glands is increased to thicken the outer layer of the precorneal tear film, thus producing a slight drying out of the tear fluid over an extended period.

9.4 Infusion Pumps

In extreme cases, spectacles have been constructed with an infusion pump located in the side arm. A continuous flow of liquid is ensured by a tiny pump operated by an electric motor installed in the side arm. This liquid is passed via a small plastic tube with a T-shaped end into the lower conjunctival fornix. This T-shaped end practically does not come into contact with the inner canthus, which means that a continuous supply of liquid can be passed into the eye throughout the day without great inconvenience. Thus, at a low flow rate of $1-3\,mm^3$ over a 12-h day, individual patients can find relief in the quite considerable complaints such as extreme dryness or where other therapeutic measures have failed [49]. Nonetheless, this and similar infusion devices are individually constructed systems which are only to be applied with many reservations, and which, due to the high price involved as well as the risk of infection, must remain restricted to very extreme cases.

10   Strategies of Therapy

A whole range of different ophthalmic and systemic conditions, all of which have resulted in an insufficiency either of the aqueous or the mucous components of the tear film or in a mixed form involving both, are subsumed under the diagnostic term of dry eye as a symptomatic complaint. This makes therapy more difficult. It also means that there can be no universal therapy for such a general condition; what helps one patient may not bring even slight relief in another. In spite of this, we should still try to design possible therapies for those affected, although there is certainly no advantage in doing so on rigid lines and without being able to adapt from case to case. I recommend the following procedure as useful in therapy:

1. A detailed and comprehensive patient history should be taken, including factors such as environment, professional and social surroundings, etc.
2. Diagnostic procedures:
   - Determination of visual acuity
   - Testing of binocularity
   - Examination of the anterior eye segments
   - Testing of eyelid closure
   - Measurement of the blinking frequency
   - Minimal tests to assess the precorneal tear film: Schirmer's test, tear film breakup time, staining with rose bengal solution
3. Therapeutic measures:
   - Treatment of any specific underlying condition or disease, if present
   - Elimination of risks or aggravating factors, including professional exposure, air humidity, refractory errors, disturbed binocularity, etc.
   - Medication

We are concerned here primarily with the substitution of absent or pathological components of the precorneal tear film. As the therapeutic agents available are different as regards their pH value, osmolarity, and viscosity, we should be sure to use, as far as possible, that form of medication which is most convenient to the patient (optimum tolerance). As practically all topically applicable substitutes contain preservatives, the individually determined drop frequency should be limited to ten applications per day at most to avoid undesireable side effects from the preservative. If intolerance to preservatives in the eye drops occurs, therapy must be shifted either to a preparation containing a different preservative or to a one without preservatives in single-dose containers. The patient must be instructed on how to administer the drops. It is here of special importance to build up a permanent compliance, as therapy of the dry eye is a long-term procedure which cannot be carried out without a good relationship of trust between patient and physician. The patient must know that the physician is able to bring healing to his or her condition only in the rarest of cases, as one is dealing with a chronic condition which can only be brought under control when treatment is regular and continuous.

Where conditions of dry eye are mild, i.e., without corneal involvement (repeatedly measured Schirmer values of 6–10 mm in 5 min), we first recommended trying a tear substitute with low viscosity. For this purpose, a wetting agent based on polyvinylalcohol and applied as far as possible no more often than four times per day has been found the most useful solution.

In the case of more pronounced cases of dry eye (repeatedly measured Schirmer values of 3–5 mm in 5 min), the frequency of eye drop application must be increased to ten times per day where necessary. For this purpose, a tear substitute with greater viscosity is found to be of value. Preparations on a cellulose basis here come into consideration or, to avoid an excessive eye drop frequency, gel drops which generally need not be applied more frequently than four times per day. If the cornea is involved, the application of a neutral eye ointment (such as Bepanthen AS) brings relief overnight.

In cases of highly pronounced dryness of the eye (repeatedly measured Schirmer values below 3 mm in 5 min), the application of commercially available tear substitutes is frequently in sufficient. A too frequent use of these preparations may result in toxic or allergic reactions due to a cumulative effect of the preservatives, a reason sufficient by itself to prohibit their use, as the wetting function of the actual preparations would no longer suffice. At this stage of the disease, the following recommendations can be made:

Early Morning. Hot wet compresses on the eyelids, followed by eye drops or eye gel.

During the Day. Application of gel drops or inserts. The latter have the advantage that they contain no preservatives and must only be used twice a day as a rule, but the disadvantage that an insert located in the lower conjunctival fornix produces the sensation of a foreign body being present in the eye, or they may occasionally cause mild striated vision while being dissolved. Nonetheless, the advantages outweigh the disadvantages, especially in professionally active patients with pronounced forms of dry eye. In cases of intolerance to preservatives in eye drops, we recommend single-dose preparations and/or inserts free of such additives. In cases of extreme dryness, therapy with eledoisin drops may be effective. As a rule, patients responding to this substance need to apply the drops only about four times per day.

Overnight. The use of a neutral eye ointment (such as Bepanthen AS) is generally of advantage. In desperate cases, temporary occlusion of the relevant lacrimal ducts should be performed. When results are positive, all ducts should be then be closed permanently. Protective spectacles or goggles are further able to improve symptoms. Tarsorrhaphy may be recommended in cases where the palpebral fissure is too wide.

With the forms of medication and additional measures available to us up to now, we are able to improve the inconvenient and often irritating symptoms of this condition in a great majority of cases, thus enabling the patient to go about his or her daily business without hindrance – provided that patient-physician compliance is completely intact.

To conclude, it should not go unmentioned that, in view of the wide range and diversity of causes and symptoms involved in dry eye, any recommendations as to therapy can only be guidelines at the best. The optimum therapy must always always be reached through trial in each individual case. In this context, it is not possible to ignore one major handicap. i.e., that all therapeutic measures available to us up till now are for the most part symptomatic and are causal only in exceptional cases as regards their effect on the dry eye. This will most probably remain so in the future.

11   Perspectives

Over the past 20 years, important knowledge and insight have been gained on the physiology, pathophysiology, and diagnosis of dry eye. In spite of this, much remains to be done as regards the therapy of this condition. All forms of artificial tear – most forms of therapy – that we have been able to make use of are more or less artificial. If, in 1790, Richter, as quoted at the beginning, recommended "jelly of quince" and a decoction of palm leaves to treat chronic conjunctivitis, we have not advanced much further over the intervening 200 years. This is why it should be demanded of research and the pharmaceutical industry to develop substances possessing good surface-active properties and thus a longer retention period, which are as close as possible to the natural precorneal tear film. We must still continue all our efforts on behalf of our patients, and, not least, because the number of persons suffering from dry eye is increasing from year to year.

References

1. Swan KC (1945) Use of methylcellulose in ophthalmology. Arch Ophthalmol 33:378–380
2. Krishna N Brown F (1964) Polyvinyl alcohol as an ophthalmic vehicle. Am J Ophthalmol 55:99–106
3. Marquardt R (1986) Die Behandlung des trockenen Auges mit einem neuen tropffähigen Gel. Klin Monatsbl Augenheilkd 189:51–54
4. Bloomfield SE et al. (1977) Soluble arteficial tear inserts. Arch Ophthalmol 95:247–250
5. Tseng SCG et al. (1980) Topical retinoid treatment for various dry-eye diseases. Ophthalmology 92:717–727
6. Jones BR Coop HV (1965) The management of keratoconjunctivitis sicca. Trans Ophthalmol Soc UK 85:379–389
7. Lemp MA (1973) Artificial tear solutions. Int Ophthalmol Clin 13(1):221–238
8. Wright P et al. (1987) Effect of osmolarity of arteficial tear drops on relief of dry eye symptoms. Br J Ophthalmol 71:161–164
9. Gilbard JP et al. (1978) Osmolarity of tear microvolumes in keratoconjunctivitis sicca. Arch Ophthalmol 96:677–681
10. Gilbard JP Farris RL (1979) Tear osmolarity and ocular surface disease in keratoconjunctivitis sicca. Arch Ophthalmol 97:1642–1646
11. Lemp MA et al. (1970) The precorneal tear film. I. Factors in spreading and maintaining a continuous tear film over the corneal surface. Arch Ophthalmol 83:89–94
12. Benedetto OA et al. (1974) The instilled fluid dynamics and surface chemistry of polymers in precorneal tear film. Invest Ophthalmol 14:887–902
13. Lemp MA et al. (1975) The effect of tear substitutes on tear film break-up-time. Invest Ophthalmol 14:255–258
14. Norn MS Opauski A (1977) Effects of ophthalmic vehicles on the stability of the precorneal film. Arch Ophthalmol 55:23–34
15. Lemp MA (1973) Artificial tear solutions. Int Ophthalmol Clin 13:221–229
16. Lemp MA (1973) Tear substitutes in the treatment of dry eye. Int Ophthalmol Clin 13(4):145–153
17. Lemp MA, Holly FJ (1972) Ophthalmic polymers as ocular wetting agents. Ann Ophthalmol 4:15–20
18. Krishna N, Mitshell B (1965) Polyvinylalcohol as an ophthalmic vehicle. Am J Ophthalmol 59:840–864
19. Leibowitz HM et al. (1984) Gel tears: a new medication for treatment of dry eyes. Ophthalmology 91:1199–1204
20. Marquardt R et al. (1987) Gelartige Tränenersatzmittel und unspezifische Augensalben auf Intensivstationen und in der perioperativen Anwendung. Anästh Intensivther Notfallmed 22:235–238
21. Balazs EA (1983) Sodium hyalurate and viscosurgery. In: Miller D et al. (ed) Healon: a guide to its use in ophthalmic surgery. Wiley, New York, pp 5–20
22. Polack FM, Niece MT (1982) The treatment of dry eyes with Na-hyalurate (Healon). Cornea 1:133–136
23. Limberg MB et al. (1987) Topic application of Hyaluronic Acid and Chondroitin Sulfate in the treatment of dry eye. Am J Ophthalmol 103:104–107
24. Leibowitz HM et al. (1984) A new medication for the treatment of dry eyes. Ophthalmology 91:1199–1204
25. Van Bijsterveld OP, Westers JCE (1980) Therapie bei Keratokonjunktivitis sicca. Klin Monatsbl Augenheilkd 177:2–57
26. Prause JU et al. (1984) Lacrimal and salivar secretion in Sjögren's syndrome: the effect of systemic treatment with bromhexidine. Acta Ophthalmol (Copenh) 62:489–497

27. Bietti GB et al. (1973) Zur Anwendung eines neuen Medikamentes, des Eledoisins zur Behandlung der Keratokonjunctivitis sicca. Ber Dtsch Ophthalmol Ges 73:399–407
28. Jaeger W (1988) Die Behandlung schwerer Verlaufsformen der Keratoconjunctivitis sicca mit Eledoisin. Klin Monatsbl Augenheilkd 192:163–166
29. Jaeger W et al. (1985) Eledoisin – a successive therapeutic concept for filamtary keratitis. Trans Ophthalmol Soc UK 104:496 (abstract)
30. Messner K, Leibowitz HM (1971) Acetylcysteine treatment of keratitis sicca. Arch Ophthalmol 86:357–359
31. Wright P (1971) Diagnosis and management of dry eyes. Trans Ophthalmol Soc UK 91:119–128
32. Graham WP et al. (1976) Keratoconjunctivitis sicca symptoms appearing after blepharoplasty. Plast Reconstr Surg 57(1):57–61
33. Soong HK et al. (1988) Topical retinoid therapy for squamous metaplasia of various ocular surface disorders. A multicenter, placebo-controlled double-masked study. Ophthalmology 95:1442–1446
34. Cook JR et al. (1972) Lacrimal sarcoidosis treated with corticosteroids. Arch Ophthalmol 88:513–517
35. Sjögren H, Bloch KJ (1971) Keratoconjunctivitis sicca and the Sjögren syndrome. Surv Ophthalmol 16(3):145–159
36. Krieglstein GK (1981) Konservierungsstoffe in ophthalmologischen Arzneimitteln. Z Prakt Augenheilkd 2:59–70
37. Ertel E et al. (1973) Über die Qualität rezepturmäßig hergestellter Augentropfen. Klin Monatsbl Augenheilkd 163:462–467
38. Kreiner CF (1980) Die Biochemie von Konservierungsstoffen, welche zur Anwendung am Auge bestimmt sind. Contactologia 2D:130–137
39. Leopold JN (1945) Local toxic effect of detergents on ocular structures. Arch Ophthalmol 34:90–105
40. Gasset AR et al. (1974) Cytotoxicity of ophthalmic preservatives. Am J Ophthalmol 78:98–106
41. Burstein NL (1985) The effects of topical drugs and preservatives on the tears and corneal epithelium in dry eye. Trans Ophthalmol Soc UK 104:402–409
42. Champeau EJ, Edelhauser HF (1986) Effect of ophthalmic preservatives on the ocular surface. In: Holly FJ (ed) The precorneal tear film in health, disease and contact lens wear. Dry Eye Institute, Lubbock, Texas
43. Brewitt H et al. (1981) Zytotoxizität von Konservierungsstoffen in Augenmedikamenten – eine rasterelektronenmikroskopische Untersuchung an der Kaninchencornea. Beitr Elektronenmikrosk Direktabb 14:543–548
44. Tønjum AM (1985) Effects of Benzalkonium chloride upon the corneal epithelium studied with scanning electron microscopy. Acta Ophthalmol 53:358–368
45. Murube del Castillo J (1986) Ectropionisation of the lacrimal punctum in Sjögren's syndrome. Scand J Rheumatol [Suppl] 61:268–269
46. Bennett JE (1969) The management of total xerophthalmia. Arch Ophthalmol 81:667–682
47. Freeman JM (1975) The punctum plug: evaluation of a new treatment for the dry eye. Trans Am Acad Ophthalmol Otolaryngol 79(6):OP 874–OP 878
48. Dohlmann CH (1978) Punctual occlusion in keratoconjunctivitis sicca. Trans Am Acad Ophthalmol Otolaryngol 85:1277–1281
49. Dohlmann CH et al. (1971) Mobile infusion pumps for continuous delivery of fluid and therapeutic agents to the eye. Ann Ophthalmol 3:126–128

Chapter 7

Dry Eye in Wearers of Contact Lenses

H.W. Roth

1 Outlining the Problem

An impairment of tear secrection and its therapy are always a special
problem for wearers of contact lenses, as the integrity of the tear film is of
utmost importance for comfortable wearing of a contact lens. Hard contact lenses need a cushion of tears to swim on upon the cornea, and soft
lens materials need a certain quantity of water to keep them elastic and
transparent.

A deficit of lacrimal fluid or a disturbance of its qualitative composition
in a patient without contact lenses leads only to irritations of the outer
segments of the eye when a certain degree of severity is reached. In the
contact lens wearer, these irritations are observed much earlier as the steady
stimulus caused by his contact lens significantly disturbs the physiology of
the outer segment of the eye. Disturbances of the physiological environment
of the anterior segments of the eye by wearing contact lenses include the
following:

Formation of deposits
Decrease in corneal sensibility
Alteration in osmotic pressure
Variation in pH value
Alteration in anterior eye temperature
Alteration in surface tension
Shift in electrolytes
Electrostatic shifts
Decrease in O_2 offered to the cornea
Increase in CO_2 in the lacrimal fluid
Decrease in glucose content in the cornea
Variations in the refractive index

Therefore more lacrimal fluid is needed than would be necessary without a
contact lens. Pathophysiological reactions of the conjunctiva and cornea are
by no means rare. Numerous examinations [1] showed that more than 60%
of all contact lens intolerance phenomena that were not caused by handling

M.A. Lemp/R. Marquardt (Eds.) The Dry Eye
© Springer-Verlag Berlin Heidelberg 1992

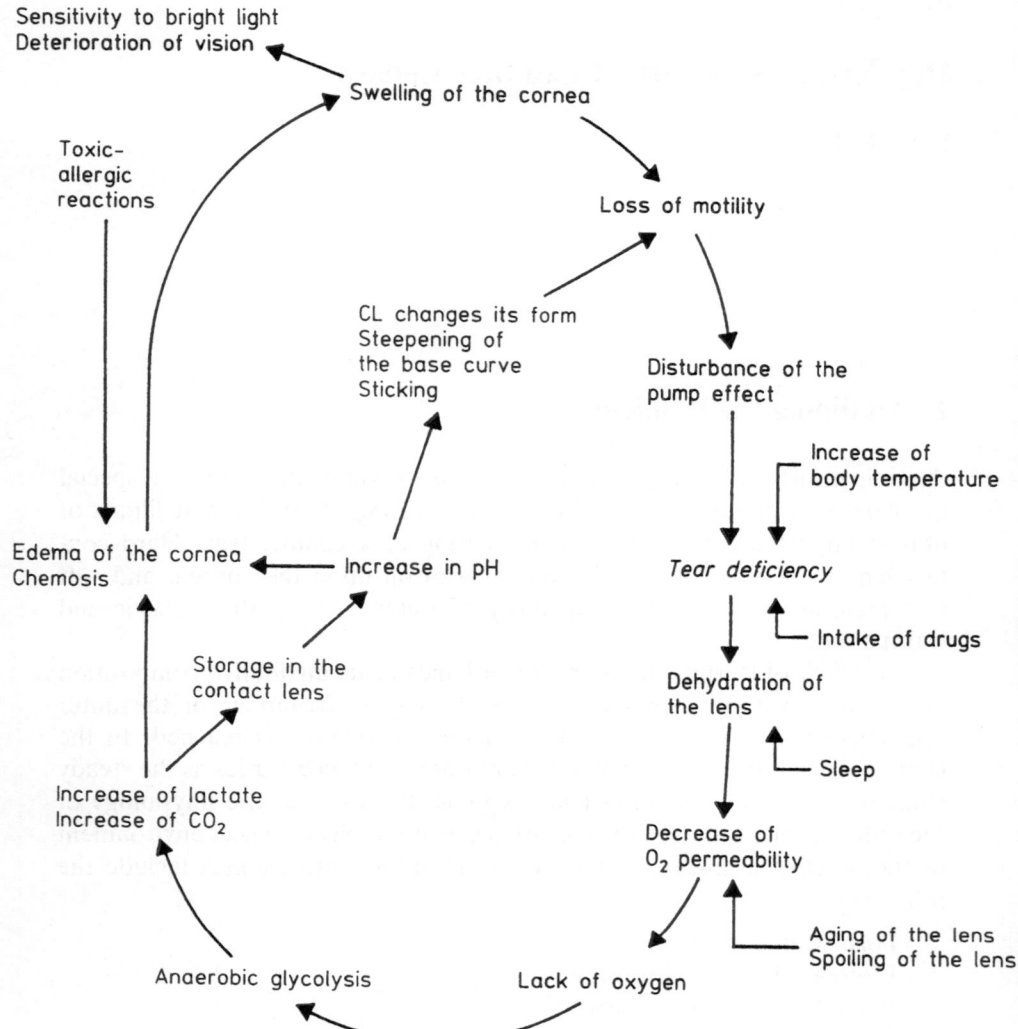

Fig. 1. Disturbance of the corneal physiology of the eye in contact lens wearers (schematic diagram)

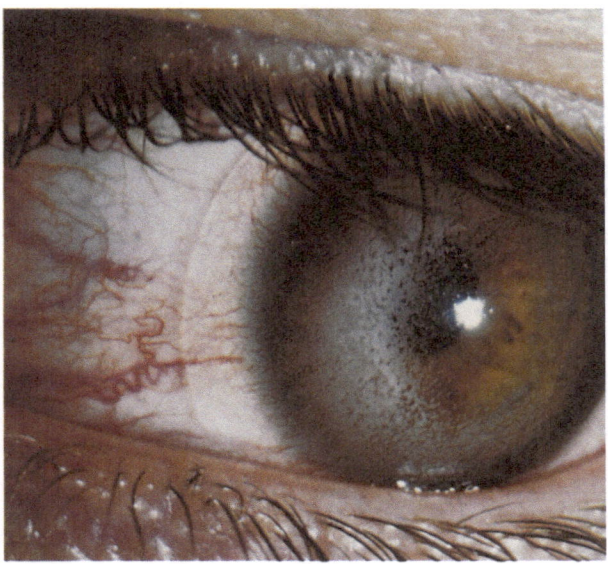

Fig. 2. Protein deposits on a soft, hydrophilic contact lens (extended-wear lens). Especially in extended wear of lenses, a lack of tear secretion (Schirmer's test 2 mm; wettening time 7 s) leads to dehydration and increased crystalline deposits. Normally these are difficult to remove, and the lens must be exchanged

mistakes or wrong care were caused by tear deficiency or desiccation of the lens in the eye (Fig. 1). As a rule, a person who wears glasses lives without complaints in an intact environment if a daily quantity of 1.0 ml lacrimal fluid is produced. This is different in the contact lens wearer. According to the type of lens, fitting technique, and individual factors, he needs several times this quantity (Fig. 2).

Typical symptoms of the dry eye in the contact lens wearer are the following:

Objective symptoms
Increased deposits
Jelly bumps
Three- and nine-o'clock injection on the conjunctiva
Changing of the lens parameters
Stainability with rose bengal
Increased thickness of cornea
Cell detritus in the tear lens
Giant papillary conjunctivitis
Induced contact lens torus
Air bubbles in the lacrimal fluid
Frequent loss of lenses

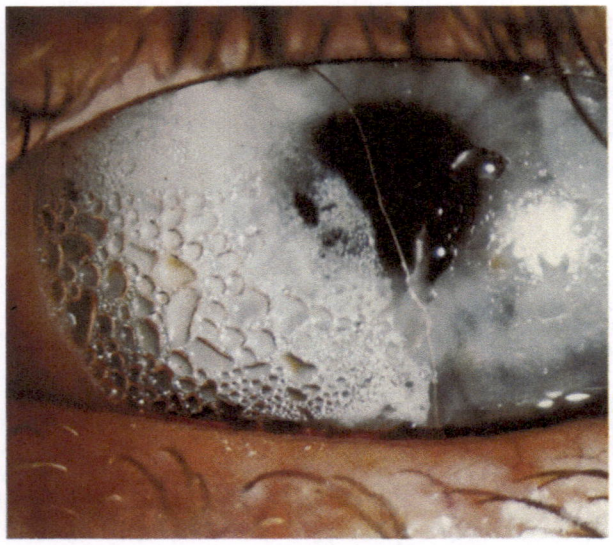

Fig. 3. Soft, hydrophilic lens after several hours of wearing time. The lens is desiccated, disturbed vision and increased sensitivity to light is reported

Subjective symptoms
Variation in visus
Increased sensitivity to bright light
Visual acuity improved by blinking
Blurring vision
Halo vision
Increased sensation of foreign body

Figure 3 shows the typical course of pathological reactions.

1.1 The Influence of Lacrimal Fluid on the Optical Effect of the Contact Lens

Not only does the tolerance of the contact lens depend on a sufficient supply of lacrimal fluid but also the acuity of vision that can be achieved with this lens. Desiccated dry lenses look dull and no longer have an optical effect. When the light comes directly from the front, scatter effects occur, and the sensitivity to bright light increases. The wearer of soft lenses does not only look through the lens material – the optical effect system is formed by the liquid stored in the lens' molecular structure together with the structure of the lens-shaped plastic material.

For the wearer of hard lenses, the water reservoir between the corneal anterior surface and the reverse side of the contact lens is a part of the optical compensation. According to the fitting technique and topography of the corneal anterior surface, an optical lens is formed by the lacrimal fluid, which may be bent to a convex, plane, parallel, concave, or astigmatic form (Fig. 1) and thus compensate a part of the error of refraction. The power of refraction of the tear cushion, which shows a central strength of 100–200 µm, is calculated by the following formula:

$$D_{TLC} = \frac{n_C - n_T}{r_C}$$

$$D_T = \frac{d_T}{n_T} \cdot \frac{(n_T - 1)^2}{r^2}$$

D_T = refractive power of the tear lens
D_{TLC} = refractive power of the reverse side of the tear lens
n = refractive index
D = refractive power
r = inner radius of the contact lens
T = lacrimal fluid, tear lens
C = contact lens

In corneal astigmatism, irregular cicatricial astigmatism, and keratoconus this form of optical compensation (contact lens and lacrimal fluid) is of special importance. Furthermore, the wearer of hard or semihard, gaspermeable contact lenses needs a tear film on which the lens may glide over the cornea during lid movements, and when the line of sight is changed. If there were no tear film, the plastic material would come into direct contact with the corneal surface. This would result in an electrostatic charging of the contact lens, disturbance of the corneal physiology, and increased irritation by foreign body.

A certain tear lens is also formed in wearers of soft lenses, but this is of only limited optical effect because the lens to a large degree clings to the cornea. A deformation of soft lenses on a toric corneal surface is observed so that even with a sufficient supply of lacrimal fluid, an optical compensation of the corneal torus is often not satisfying. The wearers of soft lenses need additional lacrimal fluid to keep the plastic material transparent and soft (Fig. 3). Corresponding to the type of lens, size, weight, and especially water content, different minimum quantities of lacrimal fluid are necessary. The total quantity of these – apart from the chemical configuration of the lens material – depends on numerous other factors, such as the environment and individual patient data. The quantity of necessary lacrimal fluid is especially critical with highly hydrophilic permanent-wear lenses (extended-wear lenses) having an H_2O content above 60%. These may stay in the eyes

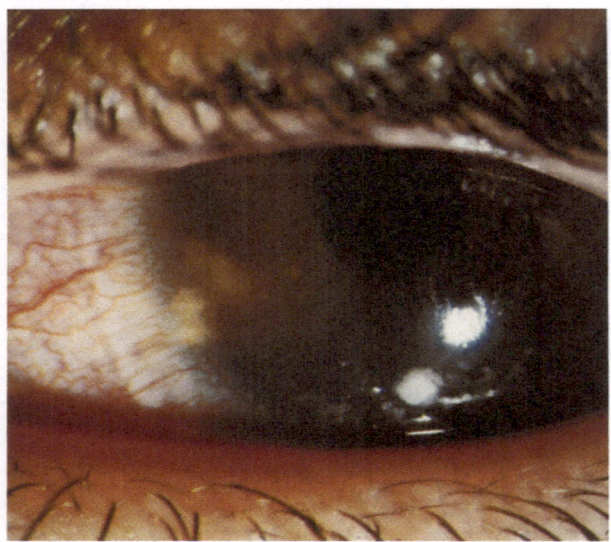

Fig. 4. Tight-lens syndrome. Due to lack of tears (Schirmer's tests I and II 1 mm; breakup time 5 s), a highly hydrophilic lens desiccated and stuck to the cornea during extended wear

overnight, when the tear secretion subsides almost completely. A decreased flow of tears may lead to changes in the lens parameters, and the plastic material may thus dry (tight-lens syndrome) [2]. Dangerous complications in the eye may result from this (Fig. 4).

1.2 Importance of Temperature Stabilization

Although it is often possible to fit a patient with reduced tear secretion of less than 8 mm in Schirmer's test II with contact lenses, the intolerance to the lenses becomes critical when other, mainly external disturbing factors occur which require an additional supply of lacrimal fluid. During a long automobile drive with the fan on, in air-conditioned or overheated and dry rooms, or during activities which lead to a decrease in blinking (e.g., when working at a computer screen), the contact lens may become dry and cause a sensation of foreign body. At the same time, the temperature of the anterior surface of the eye rises by 1°–2°C due to the increasing dehydration and loss of evaporation. This means that the pathophysiological situation caused originally by the wearing of contact lenses deteriorates further. Such a rise in temperature influences the reaction speed of the corneal metabolism, but most of the enzymatic reactions in the corneal metabolism can take their course only in a very narrow temperature range.

It is recommended to test the patient after fitting of lenses in a climatic stress situation to avoid complications [3]. Patients with a relative deficiency of lacrimal fluid report an increased sensation of foreign body after exposure to the warm air stream of an electric hair dryer for a few seconds. Within a few minutes, conjunctival injection is found during a slit lamp examination.

1.3 Special Diseases of the Eye Associated with Lacrimal Fluid Deficiency

Numerous diseases of the eye which require a contact lens for medical and optical reasons are associated with disturbed tear secretion. This is the case, for example, in a patient who must wear a contact lens to correct one-sided aphakia. Because of his age, there was not enough lacrimal fluid produced to keep the lens moist. Although this problem has lost importance in recent years due to the increasing number of implantations, there are still patients who must wear a contact lens after surgery has failed, and wearing a lens is indicated from an optical and medical point of view.

Disturbed tear secretion has been observed mainly in keratoconus. In 64% of all cases, this is connected to a deficiency of lacrimal fluid [4]. It could not be clarified whether this is a reason for the development of a keratoconus, or whether it is only an accompanying syndrome. Some authors [4] are of the opinion that tear deficiency and the resulting chronic conjunctivitis indicate the risk of developing a keratoconus. For this reason especially keratoconus patients should be examined carefully for disturbances of tear secretion, particularly since patients with this disease show the highest infection rate of all contact lens wearers, and in connection with a contact lens a faster progress of the disease is observed. If the patient suffers from moistening disorders, stabilization of the lens in front of the swollen cornea is difficult. This may lead to damages of the epithelium in many cases if the mechanical irritation by the lens is not buffered by an intact tear cushion. It is recommended to keratoconus patients to wear their lenses only when a sufficient quantity of tears is available. If this is not the case, keratoplastic surgery should be carried out to avoid further complications (e.g., corneal ulcus) on the already predamaged cornea which is further damaged by wearing contact lenses.

1.4 Deposits on Contact Lenses

Hard contact lenses must also be surrounded by lacrimal fluid for other reasons. During the daily wearing, dust and particles of foreign bodies or exfoliated epithelial cells of the cornea and conjunctiva get onto or under the lens, where they can stick more easily than on the uncovered cornea. Microscopic examination of worn lenses even after a few hours show protein deposits, lipids, and particles of foreign bodies from the environment (Fig. 5). Because of a deficiency of lacrimal fluid, these mechanically dis-

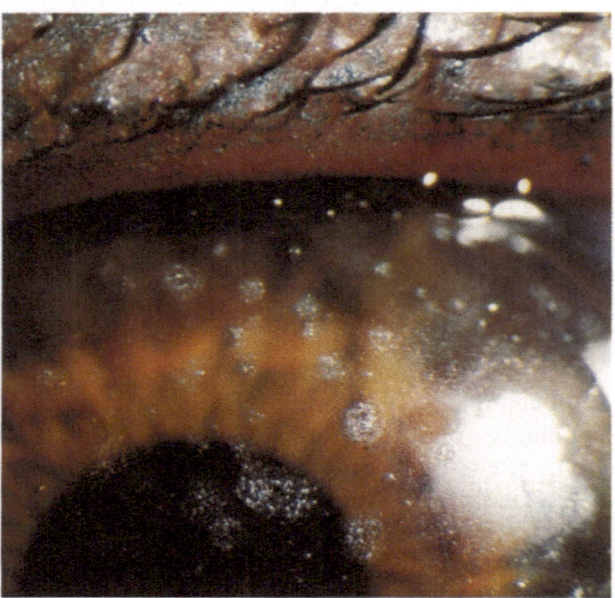

Fig. 5. Deposits of lipids, proteins, and pigments on a soft, hydrophilic contact lens. Due to insufficient care and decreased flow of tears, deposits developed on the surface of the lens. After switching to a hard lens together with application of an artificial lacrimal fluid, the patient was symptom-free

turbing deposits are not solved or rinsed off; they accumulate and destroy the integrity of the tear film, which further intensifies the vicious circle of the dry eye. This is especially the case when these deposits consist of hydrophobic particles disturbing the homogeneity of the tear film. It is even more complicated when foreign bodies get under the lens and cannot be washed out due to insufficient exchange of lacrimal fluid. Then they may cause a long-term irritation of the eye. Since contact lens wearers show decreased sensibility of the cornea, a corneal ulcus may develop more rapidly than in patients with a sufficient quality and quantity of tears.

Disorders of the aqueous layer of the tear film cause an increased deposition of proteins, lipids, and environmental substances (foreign bodies) on the surface of contact lenses. The form, structure, and extent depend primarily on the composition of the lacrimal fluid. Further important factors are material composition and physical condition of the lens surface, which may be impaired by aging of the material and handling mistakes. Regular deposition always points to qualitative or quantitative disturbances of the lacrimal fluid. It is known that components of the lacrimal fluid sticking to the lens surface may also indicate general diseases, for instance, disorders of lipometabolism or water equilibrium. A diabetic wearer of soft lenses whose lacrimal fluid shows an increased content of glucose, may be more susceptible to fungus infections of the eye [5].

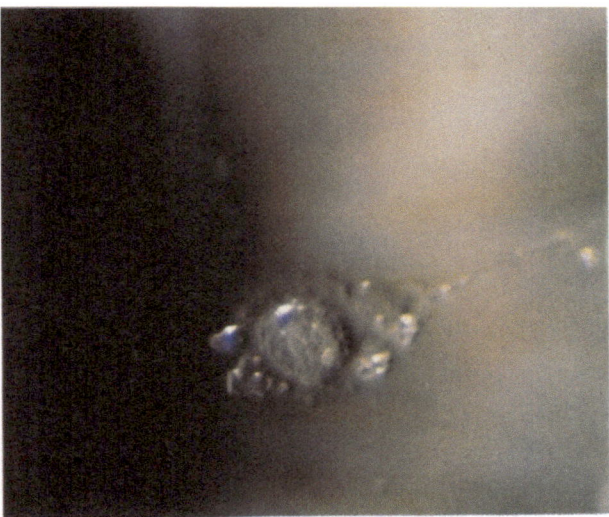

Fig. 6. Jelly bumps, early stage. These calcium-protein compositions are observed particularly in wearers of highly hydrophilic soft lenses in combination with disturbances of tear secretion. It is discussed whether the phenomenon may be caused by disorders in the calcium equilibrium of the lacrimal fluid

If jelly bumps – water-insoluble protein-calcium compounds which occur mainly on highly hydrophilic lenses (Fig. 6) – are found, disorders of the lacrimal fluid also should be considered. They are frequently observed in patients with an increased calcium level or osmotic pressure of the lacrimal fluid. This may, for example, be fostered by intake of certain drugs, especially hormones. Jelly bumps, may occur even after a few days of wearing, and they grow continuously until in the end they mechanically irritate the eye. Lenses once affected by jelly bumps may no longer be worn, because after removal of the jelly bumps new ones very soon form on the same site of the lens surface, which in most cases is damaged. In these cases it is recommended to use a type of lens that requires less water. Regular administration of artificial tears cannot stop the formation of jelly bumps but the process may be slowed down in connection with less water-storing lens material.

1.5 Immunological Disturbing Factors

Each tear deficiency in the contact lens wearer may be dangerous if the immunological defensces of the eye are impaired. Examples are the corneal ulcus [6] and the giant papillary conjunctivitis (Fig. 7) [7]. The latter is a typical immunological overreaction of the eye which is frequently observed in disorders of tear secretion together with the wearing of hard, but mainly

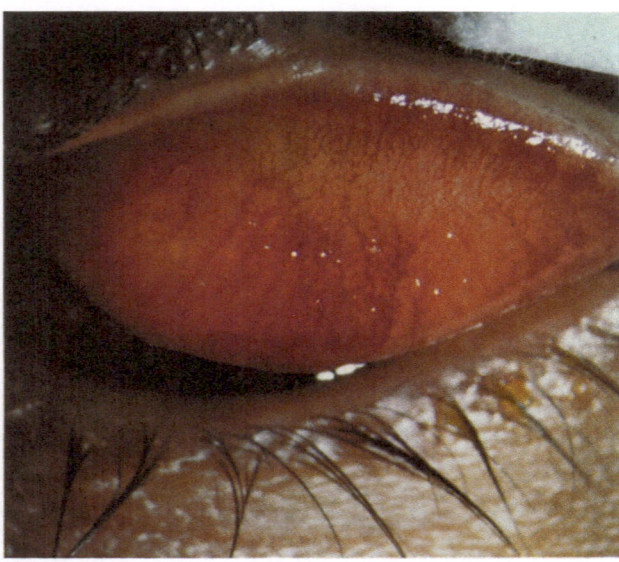

Fig. 7. Giant papillary conjunctivitis; lack of tears in combination with protein deposits on the lens surface led to a swelling of the papillae in the area of the conjunctiva tarsi. This disease is an immunoreaction of the anterior segments of the eye against denatured proteins, which deposit on the lens surface due to lack of tears

in soft, contact lenses. After several months of wearing the lenses, the patient complains of a slowly increasing burning, chafing, and sensation of foreign body. Sometimes the sensitivity to bright light is increased and the visual acuity with the lens diminished. In the area of the conjunctiva tarsi, a papillary hypertrophy is found, which resembles to vernal conjunctivitis in form and extension (Fig. 3). Immunological false reactions are discussed [8] as a reason. Proteins which stick to the lens surface due to insufficient lacrimal fluid are denatured by preserved cleaners and conditioning solutions. Therefore they are recognized as exogenous substances and develop antigenic character. They trigger a strong antigen-antibody reaction, which is diagnosed from a massive increase of IgE in the lacrimal fluid. Even the regular application of artificial tears is ineffective against this phenomenon. In the long run, only the change to a different lens material, such as polymethylmethacrylate, is possible, which tends less to protein deposits than hydrophilic lens material but is practically not permeable to oxygen. Therefore giant papillary conjunctivitis is of special importance, as it is observed in 8%–10% of all contact lens wearers and ultimately prohibits the wearing of contact lenses. In some cases it is possible to help the patient with a short-term lens combined with artificial tears, but the lens must be exchanged against a fresh one as soon as the first deposits occur. This may happen at intervals of only a few days [9].

1.6 Causes of Tear Deficiency in Contact Lens Wearers

The deficiency of tears in contact lens wearers has mainly the same causes as in patients who do not have a sight defect. A person wearing glasses who suffers from a relative lack of tears may find it difficult to switch to contact lenses for the reason that the necessary water is not available. Therefore it is important to examine all potential contact lens wearers before fitting the lenses for factors pointing to dry eye. The question whether drugs (especially hormones, psychopharmaceuticals etc.) are taken in is equally important as the question of thyroid dysfunction, diabetes mellitus, or rheumatic diseases.

Some symptoms of the dry eye in the contact lens wearer are found in Sect. 1. Fitting errors also may result in a relative lack of tears. If a lens is fitted too flat, the increased sensation of foreign body leads to an increased flow of tears and more fluid is needed which will be lost by tearing. If the water content of the lens is too high, the lens may store or bind the residual water in the case of a lack of tears, and thus the corneal metabolism breaks down.

2 Diagnosis

One should make sure before fitting a contact lens that the quality and quantity of tear film are sufficient to guarantee a symptom-free wearing of the lens.

The following tests are well established for preexamination and for controls: Schirmer's test I, Schirmer's test II, tear film breakup time, Rose bengal test, and, tear meniscus test. Schirmer's tests I and II are only to a limited extent suitable to answer the question whether contact lenses will be tolerated. This is particularly the case when the patient has been wearing lenses for quite some time. The reason is that, due to the stimulus exerted by each contact lens, the secretion at rest and upon stimulation are measured erroneously higher than they actually are, and seemingly optimal values result. There are also reports of a change in the composition of tears after several years of wearing contact lenses, for example, in the content of salt, proteins, and lipids [10].

If the impression arises that the tear film is not sufficient for wearing a lens, the tests should be repeated with the lens inserted in the eye. For Schirmer's tests I and II, only colorless paper should be used to avoid a staining of the lens. If Schirmer's test II values of less than 4 mm are then measured in a wearer of hard lenses or less than 6 mm in a wearer of soft lenses, long-term complications and intolerance phenomena can be predicted (Fig. 8). Table 1 shows the different materials and the quantity of lacrimal fluid that they require.

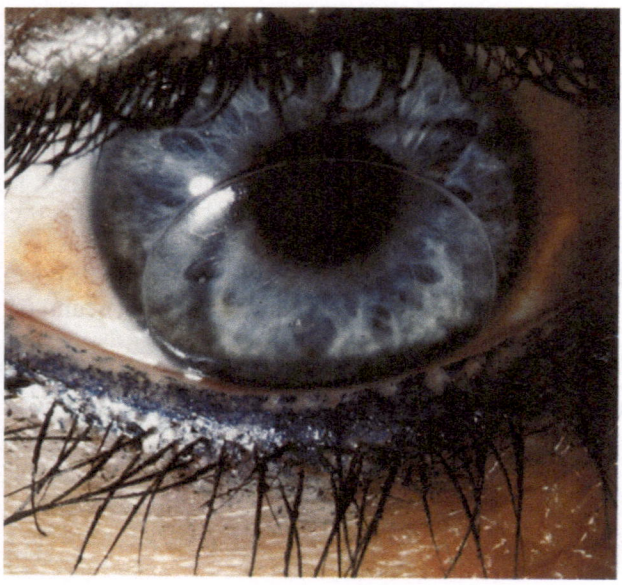

Fig. 8. Dry eye in contact lens wearer due to lack of lacrimal fluid (Schirmer's test I 3 mm; II, 1 mm). The lens desiccated; typical vasodilatation on the limbus occurred at 3 and 9 o'clock

Even more important than Schirmer's test is the test of tear film break-up time on the surface of the contact lens. This may not be shorter than 10 s (just as on the uncovered cornea). As experience shows, it is always slightly lower when measured on the lens surface than on the cornea itself. This is due to the fact that most contact lens surfaces, because of the properties of their material, do not possess the same hydrophilicity or the same contact angle as the corneal epithelium (Table 1).

The rose bengal test is also useful for evaluating dry eye in contact lens wearers. A staining of all areas where the lens has caused mechanically irritated or dry spots is observed (Fig. 9). Typically these are chafe traces and vasodilatations on the limbus at three-and nine-o'clock position in the wearer of hard lenses, if the lenses are not sufficiently moistened. The rose bengal test should always be carried out at the end of the daily wearing time, for evaluation then is optimal. Stainable defects are found where the lens has rubbed on the eye due to drying or fitting mistakes. An additional combination of the colorant with fluorescein at the same time makes it possible to see fine erosions of the cornea. Soft lenses always should be removed from the eye before this test to avoid staining of the lenses. The high molecular weight fluorexon is the only colorant which is not stored in soft contact lenses, but because of its low color intensity it is not suitable for this test.

Table 1. Contact angle for different contact lens materials (physiological saline)

Material	Contact angle
Polymethylmethylacrylate	58°
Cellulose acetobutyrate	37°
Fluorosilicone acrylate	25°
Silicone	82°
Paraperm	41°
Etafilcon	20°
Polycon	35°
Polymacon	25°
Anduran	39°

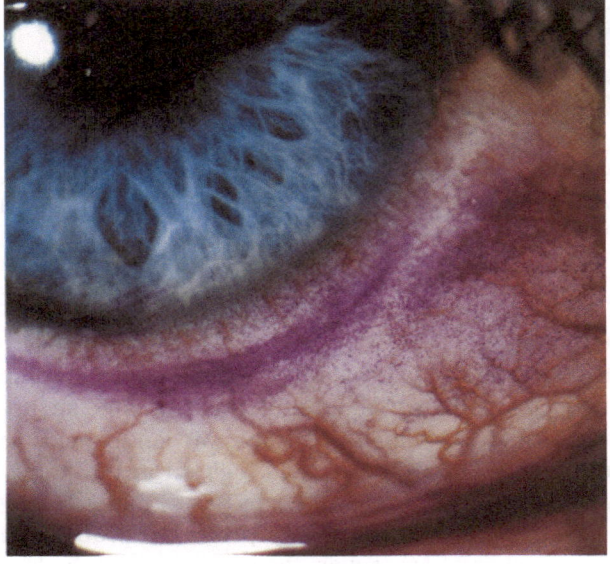

Fig. 9. Rose bengal test. Although the tear meniscus was measured to be 0.2 mm, the patient's lens dehydrated when he was working, and an increased sensation of foreign body was the result. Parallel to the limbus, chafing traces were found between 4 and 7 o'clock

Disturbed wettening can often be recognized from a patient's case history. Often the patient suffers from sight defects which point to a lack of mucin. Some patients report that they can see well for a few seconds after opening the lids (corresponding to the reduced breakup time), but then suddenly the picture blurs until the next blink. This problem of moistening, which can easily be detected by slit lamp examination, is not always caused by a lack of mucin. Sometimes deposits on the lens surface such as lipids or

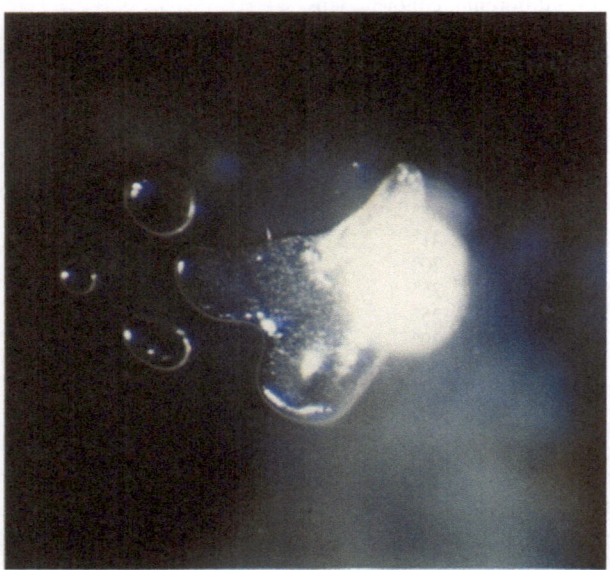

Fig. 10. Dry areas on a soft, highly hydrophilic contact lens in lack of tears (Schirmer's test 2 mm); aphakia lens; water content 60%. By regular administration of an artificial lacrimal fluid, the patient could continue to wear his lens without complaints. (×200)

denaturated proteins prevent a deposition of mucine as interim carrier for the improvement of lens wettability.

If the disorder is caused primarily by a lack of water, the lenses become dry (Fig. 10). The patient complains of rubbing of the lens and an unpleasant sensitivity to bright light. Repeated drying of soft lenses leads to early aging of the material, deformation, cracks, and higher rates of breakage. Periodic alterations in the water content of the lens plastic material may cause variations in the refractive power. This may present a problem in severe myopia, hyperopia, or aphakia. Moreover, the inner curve of the lens deforms in most plastic materials after drying, which also causes sight defects and a decrease in the motility of the lens. If at the same time the lid closure is insufficient, the lenses become dry in the area of the palpebral gap, and a toric effect in a 180° position develops. These symptoms may easily be examined by overrefraction or control of the lens parameters.

3   Therapy of Dry Eye in the Contact Lens Wearer

Therapy of dry eye in the contact lens wearer is the same as for a patient who does not wear lenses. It is important to differentiate whether a disturbance of water or mucine or both exists. The most simple way is experi-

Table 2. Artificial lacrimal fluid suitable for use by contact lens wearers

Name	Hard lens	Soft lens
Adapettes	×	×
Adapt	×	
Amilis	×	
Comfort Drops	×	
Contafilm	×	×
Contactol	×	
Contactolosol	×	
Hy Flow	×	
Lens Fresh	×	×
Lensine	×	
Liquifilm	×	
Mirasoft	×	×
Proculens	×	
Protagent S.E.	×	×
Transol	×	
Vidisept	×	
Vidisept N	×	
Vistofilm	×	

mentally to apply artificial tears and observe whether the patient's symptoms can be treated. If this is the case, sporadic or regular application of wetting eye drops is recommended. The dosage should be determined by individual requirements, lens material and lens type, and environmental factors. Just as in the patient without contact lenses, the preservative is of utmost importance in the choice of the artificial lacrimal fluid. For example, benzalkonium chloride is contraindicated for soft lenses, as it accumulates in the lens material.

Due to the low water content of hard lenses, the risk of preservatives accumulating in the material is lower, but most of the newly developed, highly gas-permeable plastic materials show a certain storage capacity for preservatives. Until further test results are available, the use of preservatives in artificial tears should generally be avoided in contact lens wearers. Table 2 lists artificial tears which are presently used by contact lens wearers. Their contact angle on the different lens surfaces must be observed.

Most commercial preparations may be applied several times a day. It is recommended to instruct the patient to apply one or two drops into the eye as soon as feeling the disturbance, an increased sensation of foreign body, or an increased sensitivity of light. It must be considered that exaggerated application of an artificial lacrimal fluid inhibits the endogenous tear stimulation, and thus that the physiological control system of tear secretion is further disturbed. Quality and quantity of the endogenous lacrimal fluid reduce quickly. The long-term administration of artificial tears to a person wearing contact lenses should be carefully considered. If the regular admin-

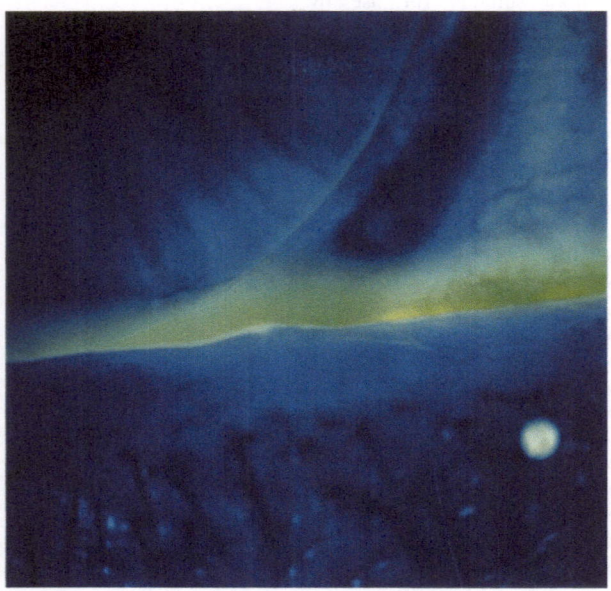

Fig. 11. Tear meniscus in a patient with dry eye after inserting a punctum plug after Freeman [11]. Due to the increased tear meniscus on the lower lid margin, the lens could be worn without complaints again

istration of artificial lacrimal fluid is inevitable for symptom-free wearing of the lens, the patient should not wear a lens, unless it is medically indicated. In cases of transient treatment with hormones, antibiotics, or other drugs influencing the tear secretion, a substitution should be attempted. The same applies to pregnancy and lactation period, during which contact lenses are often not well tolerated because the precorneal tear film dries faster. If it is not possible to diminish the complaints with an artificial lacrimal fluid, the lenses should – at least temporarily – not be worn.

Another method [11] is treating contact lens wears having dry eye with the punctum plug of Freeman or the flow controller. While the punctum plug (Fig. 11) temporarily completely closes the lower and – if necessary – upper lacrimal points, the flow controller (Fig. 12) reduces the rapid outflow of lacrimal fluid. In both cases the therapeutic effect may easily be controlled by measuring the tear meniscus on the lower eyelid with the lens inserted. Less than 1 mm is insufficient for a symptom-free wearing of contact lenses. The punctum plug as well as the flow controller should only be used in patients in whom the lens is medically indicated, and who show intolerance due to a disturbance of tear secretion. Regular ophthalmological controls must be guaranteed.

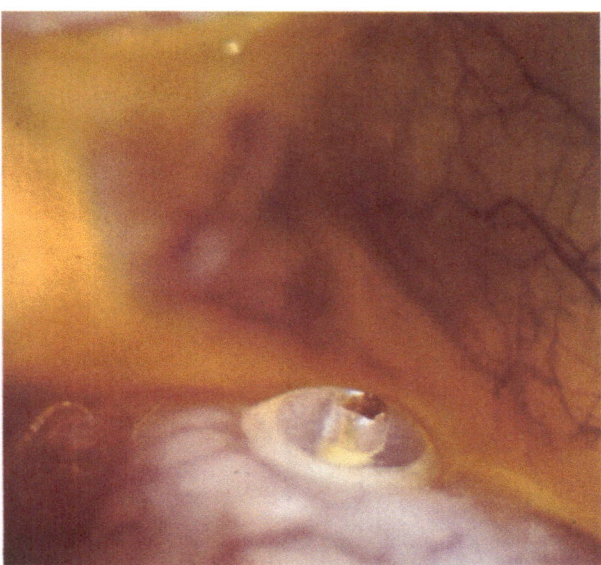

Fig. 12. Flow controller after MacKeen and Roth. By inserting a small silicone stopper (available with different diameters) into the lower lacrimal point, tear flow may sometimes be reduced, and the patient who must wear contact lenses may be treated successfully despite a lack of lacrimal fluid

3.1 Therapy of Dry Eye by Means of Contact Lenses

Contact lenses not only improve visual acuity but may also be used in the treatment of chronic or recurrent eye diseases. Extreme or absolute tear deficiency belongs to the range of indications which can be treated insufficiently only with conservative methods, and in most cases after infections and metabolic disorders of the cornea in the end lead to the loss of the eye.

The therapeutic system is to fit a soft, hydrophilic lens or a collagen lens [12] with a total diameter of more than 13 mm as a transparent bandage and water store. With these lenses, the anterior segments of the eye can be protected from dehydration if artificial lacrimal fluid is applied regularly. As a rule, soft contact lenses with a water content of 40%–80% are chosen for this treatment. The material in most cases is polyhydroxymethacrylate or a copolymer. Fluorosilicone carbonates have recently been recommended.

Hydrophilic lenses act as a water store (Fig. 13) which, together with an artificial lacrimal fluid, moistens the eye. This artificial lacrimal fluid should not consist only of water and mucins but rather should be a nutrient solution. The dropping frequency must be observed in any case because the

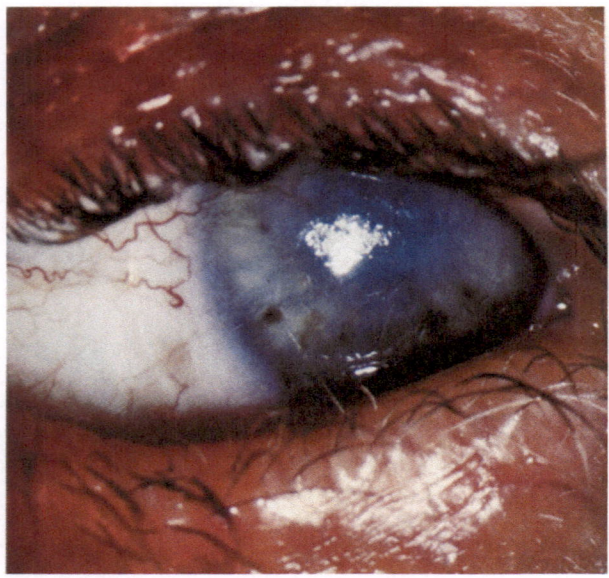

Fig. 13. Therapy of dry eye with hydrophilic bandage lenses. Due to destruction of the lacrimal gland, the eye desiccated. There were repeated keratides with subsequent scars on the cornea and vascularization. After fitting of a hydrophilic soft contact lens with a water content of 56% and application of Lens Fresh every 2h, progress of the disease could be stopped

dehydrated lens may stick to the cornea, which can lead to the tight-lens syndrome or corneal ulcus. If this should happen, the lens may not be removed from the eye before it has been thoroughly moistened with artificial lacrimal fluid or, better, with a buffer solution (5 × 5 drops in intervals of 5 min). Each attempt to remove the lens before this causes extended lesions in the corneal epithelium, which then sticks to the inner side of the lens. This means that contact lenses in the dry eye can be considered as a therapeutic measure only in rare cases. All questions concerning this therapy should be thoroughly clarified, and treatment should be performed only by a specialist.

3.1.1 Therapeutic Procedure

If the value on Schirmer's test II is above 2 mm, or the moistening time is more than 4 s, the attempt may be worthwile to treat dry eye with a soft contact lens. This therapy is very promising, especially in cases in which disorders of lid function such as ectropium or entropium, scarlike changes of the lid margins, or a lagophthalmus additionally complicate the situation. Successful treatment of dry eye with soft hydrophilic contact lenses mainly depends on the choice of the lens material, particularly on its water content, the fitting technique, and the composition of the added artificial tears.

Possible contraindications are to be excluded before fitting of the lenses; these include:

- Acute and chronical infections
- Technical fitting problems (microcornea, macrocornea, keratoconus, etc.)
- Schirmer's test I and II values under 2 mm
- Wetting time under 2 s
- Insufficient compliance by the patient

Foremost among these are acute and chronic infections. Since in 85% of all cases therapy is discontinued because of an infection, it is recommended to prepare a swab culture and wait with the fitting until the result is achieved. If pathogens are found, 2 weeks of treatment with antibiotics and a subsequent control examination are necessary. The relative contraindications also correspond to those of a soft lens: abnormalities of the anterior segments of the eye or other alterations which may impair stabilization of the lens in front of the cornea. If doubts arise, these may easily be diagnosed or excluded with a test fitting. Furthermore, it must be guaranteed that the patient shows the required understanding for this therapy and will regular attend the necessary control examinations.

3.1.2 Fitting Technique

The choice of lens parameters depends on the directions for the fitting of any other soft hydrophilic contact lens. The diameter should not be less than 13.5 mm to prevent the paralimbal sulcus vessels being compressed by the edge of the lens and tear circulation in front of the cornea being impaired or the metabolic situation of the cornea in dry eye being further deteriorated. The base curve (R_2O) should be chosen in a way that the lens motility during blinking (or eyelid closure) does not show values below 0.8 mm or above 1.2 mm. This is to guarantee that the tear film under the lens can be exchanged regularly. If the lenses are fitted too tight, the tight-lens syndrome normally develops, and the danger of an irreversible metabolic corneal disorder arises. If they are fitted too flat, or the lens motility is too high during blinking or eye movements, mechanical lesions of the corneal epithelium are caused in the long run. Moreover, the lens may drop from the eye more easily if the motility is too high. As experience shows, the best fitting results are achieved with lens diameter of 14.0–15.0 mm and basis curve of 8.8–9.2 mm. It is a well-established method to determine the central corneal anterior surface radius (K value) and take a value which is 1–1.2 mm higher for the base curve R_2O. If an exact keratometry of the anterior surface is not possible due to an irregular astigmatism or corneal scars, or if only one eye is affected, it is a good alternative to use the values of the other eye, which correlate with the values of the second eye up to about 80%. If doubts arise, a test fitting is necessary [13].

The refractive power of the lens is chosen according to individual requirements. Only a few soft contact lenses which are suitable for therapeutic use are available at values other than "plane." Particularly all the disposable-lens systems with refractive values between +4.0 and −8.0 may be fitted to compensate a sight defect at the same time. In aphakia patients this is a problem, although particularly in elderly patients dry eye is observed more frequently after cataract surgery. If the lenses are to be worn day and night, and no disposable lens is available, it is recommended to chose a material with a water content of 60%−80%. Otherwise the risk of an overwear or a tight-lens syndrome exists [14].

3.1.3 Fitting Procedure

If possible, a soft hydrophilic lens should be fitted early in the morning to control the motility and wettability after 20 min, 2 h, and 8 h. This is necessary because the motility of the lens decreases with increasing wearing time in dry eye. It can only be determined after several hours or days whether the system may be worn without presenting a danger to the eye. If no sticking of the lens is found after 8−12 h of wearing time and during follow-up controls, the lens may also remain in the eye overnight if this is medically indicated or the lens is an extended-wear lens. However, it is necessary in this case to control its motility, transparency, and moistening at short intervals.

3.1.4 Wearing Times

The wearing times of all therapeutic lenses are limited. As a rule, they should not be worn longer than 14−18 h daily. Only the extended-wear lenses may remain in the eye overnight, but according to present opinion [15] no lens should remain in the eye for more than 7 days without interruption. At least once per week the lens should be removed, cleaned, and disinfected in a suitable solution without preservatives. An overnight break in wearing should be observed, unless medical reasons speak against it (e.g., risk of epithelial damages). If a disposable-lens system is used, the lenses should not be cleaned and reinserted but replaced by new ones after 7 days. This system has become established for economic reasons.

3.1.5 Use of Drugs

Only in exceptional cases is a soft hydrophilic lens without further medication suitable to treat a lack of tears or to protect the cornea from dehydration. Normally, artificial lacrimal fluid must be added. It must be kept in mind that all preservatives either deposit on soft lenses or accumulate in them, which may lead to toxic keratopathy [16] after long-term application.

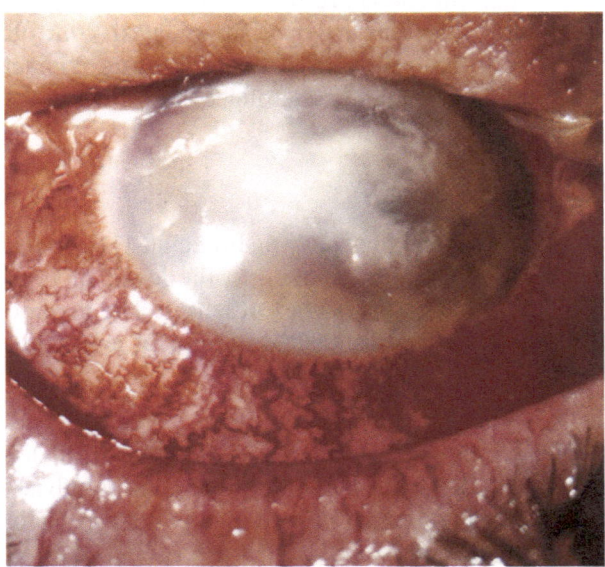

Fig. 14. Corneal ulcus caused by wearing a soft contact lens

Therefore, substitution with a fluid without preservatives is recommended. The dropping frequence should be chosen according to the initial situation. According to my own investigations [17], it is hardly ever necessary to insert more than one drop per hour. An average application of 5× daily has become established. According to the complaints, individual situation, and the kind of added lacrimal fluid, more or fewer applications are possible.

Oily, highly viscous tear substitutes or eye ointments are generally contraindicated in combination with soft lenses for the therapy of dry eye. These reduce the motility of the lens and may cause a sticking to the corneal epithelium and the tight-lens syndrome.

3.1.6 Complications

The most common complications from wearing of a therapeutic soft lens for the treatment of dry eye are infections, mainly those with the problematic bacteria *Pseudomonas*, *Haemophilus influenzae*, *Staphylococcus*, and *Pneumococcus* (Fig. 14) [18]. Often these are due to mistakes in handling and wearing, as the risk of an infection increases with increasing continuous wearing times. Sometimes the prophylactic application of antibiotic eye drops is recommended. This should be rejected particularly for longer wearing because of the risk of toxic reactions caused by an accumulation and potentiation of the substance in the lens material.

It is striking that the number of infections depends on the quantity of lacrimal fluid. The worse the values in Schirmer's test II and moistening test are, the more bacterial and fungal infections are observed on the conjunctiva and cornea. Particularly for this reason, ophthalmological controls should be carried out much more frequently in patients wearing contact lenses for therapy of dry eye than in patients wearing contact lenses for optical reasons.

3.1.7 Flow Controller, Punctum Plug

Apart from artificial lacrimal fluid a punctum plug of Freeman [11] or the flow controller of MacKeen and Roth can be applied to the lower or both lacrimal points without problems in connection with soft lenses. The method has become established in a too rapid or uncontrolled outflow of tears.

3.1.8 Collagen Shields

Instead of soft, hydrophilic lenses an increasing number of collagen shields have been fitted recently to treat dry eye. Their easy handling is advantageous. Generally they are used only once. Of proven quality are especially the shields Bio-Kor-24 H 3 (Bausch and Lomb). They are produced from sclera tissue of the pig which is a collagen type I with a few admixtures of type III. The diameter is 14.5 mm, and the base curve is 9 mm; thickness lies between 12 and 71 μm. They are inserted into the eye as is a contact lens; as the lenses dissolve in the eye, the stability normally lasts for only 24 h. The use of these shields is worthwile only for short-term treatment. Although this method up to now does not belong to the routine methods, it may be expected that with falling production costs, it will become a real alternative to the soft lens therapy in years to come.

References

1. Roth HW, Roth-Wittig (1980) Contact lenses. Harper and Row, Hagerstone
2. Roth HW (1986) The Tight-Lens-Syndrom: weitere Untersuchungen zur Ätiologie und Pathogenese. Contactologia 8:49.52
3. Holly FJ (1978) On the wetting and drying of epithelial surfaces. Academic, San Francisco, pp 439–450
4. Thomas CI (1955) The cornea. Thomas, Springfield
5. Neuhann T, Blassmann K, Roth HW (1978) Pilzwachstum auf weichen Linsen. Klin Monatsbl Augenheilkd 173:648–653
6. Roth HW (1990) Zur Ätiologie und Pathogenese des Hornhautulkus beim Kontaktlinsenträger. Contactologia 12:110–114
7. Allansmith MR, Korb DR, Greiner JV (1977) Giant papillary conjunctivitis in contact lens wearers. Am J Ophthalmol 83:697–708
8. Meisler, Krachmer JH, Goeken JA (1981) An immunopathologic study of giant papillary conjunctivitis associated with an ocular prothesis. Am J Ophthalmol 92:368–371
9. Wechsler S (1989) Disposable contact lenses. In: Weinstock FJ (ed) Contact lenses. Lippincott, Philadelphia

10. Farris RL (1986) Tear osmolarity in contact lens wearers. In: Holly F (ed) The preocular tear film. Dry Eye Institute, Lubbock, Texas
11. Freeman JM (1975) The punctum plug: evaluation of a new treatment for the dry eye. Trans Am Acad Ophthmol Otolaryngol 79:874–876
12. Pillunat LE, Marquardt R (1989) Klinische Erfahrungen mit einer therapeutischen Kollagenkontaktschale. Fortschr Ophthalmol 86:192–194
13. Marquardt R, Roth HW (1975) Weiche Kontaktlinsen, Indikation, Verträglichkeit. Bücherei Augenarzt 66:95–105
14. Roth HW (1991) Complications wearing contact lenses, and overview. CLAO J (in press)
15. Roth HW (1990) Kontaktlinsen für Einmalgebrauch, Indikation, Verträglichkeit. Contactologia 12:173–177
16. Krieglstein GK (1981) Konservierungsstoffe in ophthalmologischen Arzneimitteln. Z Prakt Augenheilkd 2:59–70
17. Roth HW (1990) Zur Therapie des trockenen Auges mit einer künstlichen Tränenflüssigkeit. Augenspiegel 11(90):44–51
18. Wilson LA, Schlitzer L, Ahearn G (1981) *Pseudomonas* corneal ulcers associated with soft contact lens wear. Am J Ophthalmol 92:546–554

Subject Index